NEGOTIATING REALITIES

Dedicated

to my mother

Helen Conkling Tilley

1918-1962

and

my father

Harvey Awyer Tilley

1915-1986

who loved

talk and voices.

Negotiating Realities

Making sense of interaction between patients diagnosed as neurotic and nurses

STEPHEN TILLEY

Avebury

Aldershot · Brookfield USA · Hong Kong · Singapore · Sydney

Published by
Avebury
Ashgate Publishing Limited
Gower House
Croft Road
Aldershot
Hants GU11 3HR
England

Ashgate Publishing Company
Old Post Road
Brookfield
Vermont 05036
USA

British Library Cataloguing in Publication Data

Tilley, Stephen
Negotiating Realities: Making Sense of Interaction Between Patients Diagnosed as Neurotic and Nurses
I. Title
610.7368
ISBN 1-85628-939-7

Library of Congress Catalog Card Number: 94-73716

Printed in Great Britain by Antony Rowe Ltd, Chippenham, Wiltshire

Contents

Why upon your first voyage as a passenger, did you yourself feel such a mystical vibration, when first told that you and your ship were now out of sight of land?...Surely all this is not without meaning. And still deeper the meaning of that story of Narcissus, who because he could not grasp the tormenting, mild image that he saw in the fountain, plunged into it and was drowned. But that same image, we ourselves see in all rivers and oceans. It is the image of the ungraspable phantom of life; and this is the key to it all...(p. 9)

But wherefore it was that after having repeatedly smelt the sea as a merchant sailor, I should now take it into my head to go on a whaling voyage; this the invisible police officer of the Fates, who has the constant surveillance of me, and secretly dogs me, and influences me in some unaccountable way - he can better answer that than anyone else...(Yet), now that I recall all the circumstances, I think I can see a little into the springs and motives which being cunningly presented to me under various disguises, induced me to set about performing the part I did, besides cajoling me into the delusion that it was a choice resulting from my own unbiassed freewill and discriminating judgment.

Chief among these motives was the overwhelming idea of the great whale himself...(pp. 10-11)

Herman Melville - *Moby Dick*

Foreword

In this book Steve Tilley explores the discursive production of social reality in psychiatric inpatient wards. He has collected a variety of empirical data concerning the 'positions' (Harré & Van Langenhove 1991) of nurses and patients in relationships with each other. His field notes derive from his own position as a participant in the society of the wards he observes. As well as the main interview material that he uses for analysis he has various notes which form the basis of his construction of nurses' systems for conceptualizing their work. The bulk of his data derive from his transcriptions of audiotape recordings of psychiatric nurses' and patients' accounts of their interaction with each other.

Each participant's account of the nurse-patient relationship provides a window not on reality, but on a set of shifting realities. Language and participants' use of language form narratives which define the selves of the narrators at the same time as they define the relationships between the narrators and their interlocutors.

Steve Tilley focuses therefore not on the individual participant but on the group, defined as two or more participants. His application in the field of the work of Harré and Secord (1972), Shotter (1984) and Vygotsky (1978) leads him to a conclusion similar to that reached later by Shotter (1993) who writes, 'the developmental relation between thought and speech has a variable, socially negotiated quality to it. Indeed, it develops within a rhetorical context of criticism and justification...' (p. 62). As a group converses, each person adopts a number of positions in which he or she expresses a sense of self, attempts to exert control over others, attempts to construct meaning. (This moral dimension of the nurses' accounts of their work may be amenable to further empirical evaluation. Wykes and colleagues at the Institute of Psychiatry are using the Stroop test to differentiate between mental health nurses' responses to apparently value-laden words and to apparently value-neutral words, examples of which occur repeatedly in the accounts recorded in this book: 'observation', 'chat, 'support', 'clinical', 'assessment', 'illness', 'problem'.)

A 'sender-receiver' model of communication is often used to teach novice nurses, implying that senders and receivers are self-enclosed individuals who initiate and respond to 'messages'. Shotter (1993) describes this as a causal model of social relationship. An ethical model of social relationships supposes that they are based on assumptions of propriety. Each individual's notion of what is 'proper' is based on his or her history and present context as much as on any cognitive process. A sense of propriety is developed socially, at first in the family of origin, then in preferred social groups. By looking at nurses' accounts it is possible to arrive at a view of the moral basis of their work. Such a view has three possibilities. It is likely to be different from the kind of ethical account given, say, in the UKCC Code of Conduct. It is likely to be a more accurate representation of nurses' moral feelings about their work than if they were asked to describe it in ethical terms. And it offers the beginnings of an explanation of often-observed phenomena: for example, that student nurses' behaviour reflects more closely the influences of the wards in which they are placed than the influences of the colleges of nursing in which they study; that loyalty to colleagues is more highly valued than loyalty to service users. Moreover, every casual as well as trained observer has noticed the multiple realities that a traditional psychiatric ward contains — most obviously the differences between shifts. So Steve Tilley arrives at the point where he watches a social construction of realities rather than of reality.

The management of self and others through discourse brings to mind firstly the Platonic dialogues to which Steve Tilley alludes early in this book, secondly Pirsig's *Zen and the Art of Motorcycle Maintenance*. Pirsig's (1974) epigraph sounds like but is not a quotation from Phaedrus (Hamilton & Cairns 1963) — 'And what is good, Phaedrus?' Later, Pirsig's narrator draws out the threads of ambiguity in a related but different question. 'What is the Good?' (p. 385) reminds us of Socrates' death as the narrator/Phaedrus realizes how dialogic discourse can be abused. Meanwhile he descends into the maelstrom from which he emerges with his memory ravaged by electroconvulsive therapy.

The 'good', according to Steve Tilley, is 'the development of understandings' (p. 357 in the text). Understanding and the communication of meaning occur through social interaction. 'Quality' or 'good' care might then be defined as interaction between a nurse and a patient and between members of the nursing team.

But Steve Tilley's observations confirm that nurses and patients do not necessarily communicate in order to share understandings but in order to 'reproduce...locally valued discourse' (p. 358 in the text). He directs our attention to the construction of moral orders and ideologies which may be repugnant to non-members of a group but which the members of the group value and which are used to confirm membership of the group (p. 183 in the text). Accordingly individual nurses rarely construct their accounts of patients' behaviour in isolation from other nurses. Collective discourse as well as collective observation strengthen collective and sometimes catch-all interpretations. 'Being responsible for oneself' defines an expectation of a patient and implies a sanction if the expectation is disappointed. 'Asking for help' may be understood as an expression of agency or as an expression of 'unhealthy' dependence. A description of a dream might simultaneously be taken as evidence of a 'normal' component of mental illness, and as evidence of the mental illness itself.

Steve Tilley has demonstrated empirical support for Shotter's (1993) critique of causal models of social relationships. Moreover, since the language of nurses mediates their relationships with patients a cause-and- effect model of good or 'quality' nursing care cannot work either. The quest by nurses for meaning in their work is summarized by Steve Tilley (pp. 2 and 360 in the text) in the question: 'What am I doing with this patient?' The answer takes the form of an explanation, conditional on the self of the participant as a person who shares or does not share the group's values and on his or her ability to share understanding on multiple levels. But nurses rarely conceptualize these multiple layers of meaning and inference. Steve Tilley suggests that only when nurses are able to analyse their own part in the social production of reality through critiquing their own and colleagues' shared language will they be able to desist from reifying the processes of relating to patients.

Sue Ritter
Lecturer in Psychiatric Nursing
Institute of Psychiatry
(University of London)

References

Hamilton E & Cairns H eds 1963 *The Collected Dialogues of Plato*, Princeton University Press Princeton, New Jersey

Harré R and Van Langenhove L 1991 Varieties of Positioning *Journal for the Theory of Social Behaviour, 21* pp. 393-407

Harré R and Secord PF 1972 *The Explanation of Social Behaviour*, Basil Blackwell, Oxford

Pirsig R 1974 *Zen and the Art of Motorcycle Maintenance*, Bodley Head, London

Shotter J 1984 *Social Accountability and Selfhood*, Basil Blackwell, Oxford

Shotter J 1993 Vygotsky: the Social Negotiation of Semiotic Mediation, *New Ideas in Psychology 11*, (1), pp. 61-75

Vygotsky LS 1978 *Mind in Society: the Development of Higher Psychological Processes*, Harvard University Press, London

Acknowledgements

This monograph is based substantially on my University of Edinburgh PhD thesis (Tilley, 1990). I was supported in carrying out the research for the thesis by a Scottish Home and Health Department Nursing Research Training Fellowship (1985-1988).

I acknowledge Penny Prophit's encouragement to pursue this work. I owe a great debt to my supervisors, Susan Sladden and Stewart Asquith, who provided support, counsel and good argument, without which I could not have understood some meanings of the work reported here, let alone completed it.

Professor Emeritus Annie Altschul and Dr. Kath Melia of the Department of Nursing Studies, University of Edinburgh gave listening time. In the Nursing Research Unit, Dr. Alison Tierney, members of the research staff, and secretaries Lynne Dyer and Margaret Semple provided a good environment for work. My thanks are also due to Tom McGlew and Rolland Munro for support and discussion.

Of the friends and fellow students in the Department of Nursing Studies whose companionship I valued during the course of this work I thank in particular Martha MacLeod, fruitful talks with whom fuelled me on the way; Fiona Shaw and Yvonne Ashley. Dr. Linda Pollock's comments on early material helped me steer a course. Dr. Miller Mair and his colleagues in the Department of Psychological Services, Crichton Royal Hospital, Dumfries, let me share with them the pleasures and challenges of dialogue. Staff in the Department of Health and Nursing, Queen Margaret College, Edinburgh, encouraged me; as did my 'manager', Tom MacLeod. Staff in the local hospital's Data Office helped unstintingly.

I owe a great debt to the nurses and patients in the two sites of this study, who in letting me share their lives and talk taught me more than I have been able to tell.

My sister, Sharon, and Monica Rushforth supported me. Eileen helped me see what it matters to see and did stand behind me when the game got rough.

Toby and Linda Morris have helped immensely with preparing the text for production.

The limitations of this work are my own. They would have been greater but for the help of those mentioned above and many others.

1 Introduction: Questions and argument

This monograph is a form of response to questions in psychiatric nursing practice and questions about psychiatric nursing practice. The study on which it is based was in the interpretive tradition. It was a descriptive, exploratory study of interaction between psychiatric nurses and patients diagnosed as neurotic in two psychiatric admission wards, as seen from the perspectives of the nurses and patients and as interpreted by myself on the basis of qualitative analysis of data comprising accounts of conversations, interviews, and participant observation fieldnotes.

The study sprang from three sources. In this chapter I introduce the main source, questions in practice. In Chapter 2 I describe the second source, the body of nursing literature to which this monograph contributes. In Chapter 3 I discuss the third source, theoretical work in the interpretive and ethogenic traditions, in particular the work of Berger and Luckmann (1967) and Harré and Secord (1972). In Chapter 4 I outline the methods of data collection and analysis and present views of the sites of the study. The main analysis and discussion of the data are presented in Chapters 5, 6 and 7. In Chapter 8 I draw conclusions and present recommendations based on the study.

I have chosen to recount the narrative of this research in the first person, partly in order to convey that the process of research was a process in which I was often self-consciously involved, in ways to be elaborated below, and partly because I can convey more easily in this voice that the research was based on dialogues, interchanges of personal and social being in interaction.

Accounting in practice: what am I doing with this patient?

This study stemmed from questions about psychiatric nursing practice. The claim of the monograph is not that I have answered the questions, but that I have advanced understanding of them. The original question that arose within my practice was 'What am I doing with this patient?'. I will present the background to this question and the further questions that flowed from it and informed the study.

Having trained and worked in Scotland as a psychiatric nurse I did further training as a nurse therapist specialising in behavioural treatment of 'adult neurotic outpatients' (Marks, 1977). During that course I conducted behaviour therapy with a man and wrote an article describing the treatment process and outcome (Tilley, 1985). The more I developed an account of the therapy which fitted the format for presentation in a behaviour therapy journal, the less I felt I was describing what really happened. I sent drafts of the paper to the man to ask whether he thought it reflected the work we had done together. His comments led me to conclude that another account could be given, and that though mine would be published as 'the' account, it had no privileged status. It was no more 'true' than his, and no less. His account, in his voice, competed with mine but would not be heard publicly. I realised that we could have negotiated new accounts. However, I could not form these alternative accounts without entering into a new dialogue with him, for the purpose of understanding what we had done. I felt unable to do this within the confines of the intellectual framework of practice, based on behavioural description and understanding, then available to me.

In later work I used clinical review sessions[1] to try out alternative accounts of the work I did with patients. I experimented with ways of accounting that made more sense to me, and 'read' the ways others heard and responded to my accounts. Listening to other practitioners intensified my interest in how they accounted for what they did in their work.

Personal knowledge and professional knowledge

Through the process of trying to give accounts of what the patient and I were doing I inevitably told about myself. What I said to psychologists in clinical review sessions was heard not only as my account, but as a nurse's account, or a behaviour therapist's account.

Through accounts I entered the micropolitical world of the institution. In telling what I did I participated in the definition of nursing for myself and for others. In order to further understanding of what I was doing in practice, I started dialogues with peers, asking nurse therapist colleagues to tell me more about what they did (Tilley and Weighill,1986). I was trying to develop a shared understanding of what we did in practice (Weighill et al, 1986).

From these dialogues in practice, with patients and with colleagues, stemmed the dialogic study reported here. The problem I found in practice became the problem of the study and this monograph: finding ways to understand, tell about, and feed understandings back into practice. I realised through the course of this research that what I wanted and needed were better ways to understand what I and the patient were doing in our work together. With hindsight I construe the questions that motivated the study as questions related to interpretation of action and definition of what was going on. What I lacked was some sense I could share with others, some common sense, of psychiatric nursing.

Common sense and argument

In this monograph I argue that the definition of psychiatric nursing with neurotic patients in two psychiatric admission wards depended on understanding the common sense the nurses and patients made or failed to make as they negotiated reality in their interaction. The background to understanding the meaning of this claim in the context of nursing knowledge is found in Chapter 2, where I set the questions from my own and colleagues' practice in the context of other works by and about nurses, especially psychiatric nurses in their interaction with patients diagnosed as neurotic. In Chapter 3 I discuss the concept 'common sense', as it is relevant to the argument of this monograph, in the work of Schuetz (1943) [Note: this is the spelling of 'Schutz' in the article], Schutz and Luckmann (1974), Garfinkel (1967), Harré and Secord (1972) and Shotter (1984). Here I will orientate the reader to the direction of the argument by reviewing a work (Billig et al, 1988) which addresses some of the concerns and clarifies some of the concepts central to this monograph.

Billig et al (1988) discuss common sense and its relationship to 'ideological dilemmas'. They construe common sense as a set of contradictory maxims and contrary themes available to members of a society, which are used as 'the *seeds*, not *flowers* of arguments'

(Bacon, cited in Billig et al, 1988; emphasis noted as in original).[2] The contradictoriness of common sense is held (Billig et al, 1988, p 17) to be the basis of rhetorical argument and social thought:

> In a real sense social argumentation can be seen as providing the model for social thinking...These are the arguments which arise *within* a particular sense, as people debate about the common sense they share. Moreover, these are the sort of arguments which people must have with themselves if they are to deliberate about matters. (Billig, 1987) (Italics in original.)

The term 'deliberate' will be seen as a crucial one in the nursing literature. There, however, 'deliberate' and 'purposeful' talk and action were opposed to common sense and lay reasoning as terms in the discourse on nursing action. I will argue that the notion of 'deliberate' talk in the main discourse in nursing literature was linked with an analytically and methodologically individualistic conception of nursing. The research methods adopted by previous nursing researchers did not permit adequate investigation of nurses' actual 'deliberations' in interaction with patients, other nurses and themselves.

To understand psychiatric nursing, a new methodology was needed, based on strategies for locating and occasioning dialogue and deliberation, the making of common sense. In Chapter 2 I suggest that the 'seeds' of such a methodology were implicit in Altschul's (1972) recommendation of accounting as a basis for understanding and developing psychiatric nursing. However, I argue in Chapter 3 that the methodology also depends on an adequate grasp of distinctions between accounts and theories, and between practical and theoretical knowledge. The aim of accounting as used in the method of this study is neither increased observability of the individual nurse's thought and action, nor examination of the response to the patient's 'stimulus' (Altschul, 1972, p. 137). Rather, this study can be seen in relation to a comment by Altschul (personal communication) that the problem with nurses' actions and explanations was that the nurses thought that what they did was the only thing that could have been done or said. One strand of the argument of this monograph is, therefore, that the central issue related to knowledge in and of psychiatric nursing is not the opposition between theoretical knowledge and common-sense knowledge. Rather, the central issue is the definition of the common-sense knowledge of psychiatric nursing: what is it, who will define it, and where will the definition take place?

In this monograph I will use the term 'ideologies' to refer to aspects of psychiatric nurses' discourse. The term has different meanings in different contexts. The term as I use it is intended to convey a relatively coherent and stable set of ideas which make sense in and of situations. This usage is related to Geertz's (cited in Adler and Asquith, 1981): 'systems of interacting symbols and patterns of interwoven meanings'. Billig et al (1988, p. 27) explore the relationship between common sense and ideology, regarding common sense as the 'lived ideology' of the culture:

> ('Lived ideology')...refers to ideology as a society's way of life. This sort of ideology includes what passes for common sense within a society. On the other hand there is 'intellectual ideology', which is a system of political, religious or philosophical thinking and, as such, is very much the product of intellectuals or professional thinkers.

Two points from this passage are relevant to the argument of this monograph. I will explore tensions and contradictions in the view of common sense in the nursing literature. These arise in relation to the question of what 'passes'[3] for common sense in psychiatric nursing, from the point of view of nursing researchers, and the demarcation between common sense and theoretical knowledge. My review of the nursing literature indicates that nursing researchers and theorists 'police' the 'lived ideologies' of nurses' practice and critique them from the perspective of 'intellectual ideologies'. Two main shortcomings of previous research are identified. Previous researchers have not considered, as I do in this study, nurses' roles in negotiating 'lived ideologies'. Moreover, I will argue that nursing researchers' critiques of nurses' common sense depend on common-sense reasoning; but that the researchers are privileged in having the last word in claims about what counts as common sense.

Billig et al (1988, p. 98) discuss the dilemmatic character of both 'illness' and 'health' and the work healthy people do to 'stay healthy by constantly patrolling the borders with illness'. In the description and exploration of the interaction of nurses and neurotic patients, I will refer to features which suggest that in it the nurses 'patrolled' illness and health, common sense and talk that indicated problems or illness. Through talk and accounting they participated in the accomplishment of the work of the sites[4]:

assessment and treatment of mental illness and problems. The empirical data of this study shed light on how 'what passes for common sense in a society' was negotiated between psychiatric nurses and patients. Their interaction will be interpreted as a set of practices through which distinctions were made between (judgements were made on 'what passes' for) common or social sense, on the one hand, and 'illness sense' on the other. The tensions in interaction with these patients will be discussed by locating it in the contexts in which nurses practised discretion in their work on the basis of distinctions between 'illness' and the residual category 'problems'.

Billig et al (1988) recommend hermeneutic interpretation 'to explore the dialectic of discourse meanings' (p. 24), and argue that the dialectic 'exist(s) in practice as well as in discourse' (p. 144). They claim (pp. 149-150) that:

> ...much of what is presented as 'interactional' or 'dialectical' social psychology and sociology, said to be inspired by a project in which the negotiations between social groups and classes is meant to be the central focus of interest and explanatory principle, has failed to fulfil the objective of examining social 'interaction' as expressing social dilemma....(Even) the main forms of 'post-structuralist' theory have...only produced new theoretical monologues, not displaced them with a perspective in which the truly dialogic principle and its necessary conditions are of prime concern. In short, argument is downgraded in modern sociology and philosophy. There is...a consistent avoidance of examining social life as dilemmatic... .

This monograph is the product of a process of handling the dilemmas and contradictions of discourse as I have interpreted them in the nursing literature; in disputes in interaction between nurses and patients, nurses and nurses, nurses and doctors about 'what happened'; and in 'disputes' produced through analysis of nurses' and patients' accounts of the 'same' conversations. The metaphor I have used to shape the production of the monograph is that of 'conversation'. This monograph is intended to be a contribution to the 'conversation' about nurse-neurotic patient interaction. An important part of the contribution is a claim that the 'conversation' is a potential argument.

Billig et al (1988, p. 163) conclude:

> If we have begun to examine dilemmas as ideological, as social situations in which people are pushed and pulled in opposing

> directions, it is because they are also seen to impose an assessment of conflicting values...(The) characteristics of dilemmas are revealed as fundamentally born out of a culture which produces more than one possible ideal world, more than one hierarchical arrangement of power, value and interest.

The theme of alternative and conflicting 'possible worlds' runs through this monograph. I use Berger and Luckmann's (1967) understandings of the social construction of reality to portray nurse-neurotic patient interaction as a form of 'therapy' intended to return patients to common sense through rhetorical persuasion. The subjectivities of nurse and patient and the objectivity of the world they share are at stake in that process.

The dilemmas include depending on common sense while having to know better (than another); knowing that the nurses can help but you have to do so much for yourself; having obligations to help patients who claim to need help when they appear to want it, in a context where others are seen as more clearly in need; being interdependent with patients who are seen as not wanting to 'work', being like the patient but unlike. I discuss in Chapter 5 how the nurses used working ideologies, based on an ideology of 'work', to manage these dilemmas. Competence in use of ideologies enabled them to give accounts of work on 'the main thing'. In Chapter 6 I explore the practices, based on the working ideologies: the practices of power in 'the working relationship'. The legitimation of the ideologies is discussed in Chapter 7: taking 'the right attitude' based on 'the kind of person' the nurse and patient were. I argue in this monograph that interaction between nurses and patients - interpreted as knowledge, power and moral order - was based on understanding achieved through participation in the dilemmatic discourses. In Chapter 8 I will advance the claim that the interaction is based on practical, not theoretical knowledge; and that within the practice is potential for development, through argument, of shared understandings of what in practice is best. Billig et al's (1988) notion of 'pushes and pulls' recalls Peplau's (1952) conception of nurse-patient interaction. In Chapter 8 I relate conclusions regarding knowledge, power and moral order in the nurses' and patients' interaction, to Peplau's (1952, 1978) and Henderson's (1966) conceptions of nursing.

Claims about knowledge and practice in nursing will be interpreted in professional and political contexts. This monograph centres on practical, day to day matters of accounting and accountability. All discussion of accountability in nursing is interpretable in terms of 'top down' codes (UKCC, 1984).[5] Moreover, decisions about who will command resources in the National Health Service (Secretaries of State, 1989; Scottish Health Service Planning Council, 1988) are increasingly linked to arguments about accountability, with implications for the valuing of professional judgement. More than ever, nurses' practices are scrutinised by those who command the resources for delivery of care (Wooff and Goldberg, 1988). These considerations can be used to justify investigations of nurses' accountability (ability to give accounts, as well as the enforceable obligation to give accounts: see Thompson et al, 1983). However, this study was not motivated by these considerations and it was conducted in such a way that it would be wrong to use it to answer questions posed from the above perspectives. This study explores the nature of nurses' and patients' interaction as interpreted through their accounts. It was not intended to answer questions of, and should not be interpreted in terms of effectiveness, efficiency, or resource planning. Nor was it intended to enable comparison of interaction between nurses and neurotic patients in psychiatric admission wards, with interaction between other (specialist or non-specialist) nurses and neurotic patients in other admission wards or other settings. Nonetheless, one conclusion that will be drawn from this study is that nurses would benefit from practice in accounting for their practice in ways that they can command, to answer the practical questions posed by their work. The context in which the study is intended to be interpreted is, therefore, one in which nurses and patients should be empowered to develop the resources for participating in systems of accountability.

Notes

1 The facility to do this was afforded by Miller Mair and others in the Department of Psychological Services, Crichton Royal Hospital, Dumfries. Various members of that Department are exploring themes related to those which run through this monograph.

2 In Chapter 6 the 'seed of argument' is seen as an apt metaphor for nurse-patient interaction.

3 See Berger and Luckmann (1967) on 'knowledge that passes'.

4 By 'sites' I mean throughout this monograph the wards in which the study was conducted.

5 For example, Clark (1988) refers to the UKCC Code of Professional Conduct in arguing that nurses' accountability rests on practice based on the best available knowledge.

2 A review of relevant literature on nursing

Introduction: the nursing literature as 'conversation' and discourse

In Chapter 1 I said that the primary source for this study was questioning in practice. I wanted means of understanding and telling about what I and others did as nurses. In order to plan a study to find out more about what psychiatric nurses and neurotic patients do in their interaction, and to interpret the knowledge I produced in relation to other nursing knowledge, I reviewed relevant nursing literature.

In this section I summarise the literature as it relates to the concerns of this monograph. Research-based knowledge about nursing with these patients is mainly found in larger studies on nurse-patient interaction, legitimation or developments in role. I will review in fuller detail the previous British study (MacIlwaine, 1980) specifically addressed to nursing care of neurotic patients in admission wards. I suggest that the literature on nurses and neurotic patients reflects in microcosm the concerns in the broader literature on psychiatric nursing. I critique the literature on theoretical and methodological grounds, and will argue on the basis of this review that theoretical and methodological issues are closely related in attempts to describe and explain psychiatric nursing. In the second part of the chapter I review literature that addresses some of the issues raised in this critique, and conclude the chapter with a note on the development of the present study in relation to the literature.

Adopting the metaphor of this monograph as a contribution to a 'conversation' about nursing, I review the common topics in the conversation and discuss issues related to who gets heard and whose voice - that of patient, nurse, nurse researcher - is 'privileged'. I use the term 'privileged' in this context to mean that which is regarded as the grounds for claims of truth and the good, the greater 'presence' of which is valued (Selden, 1989, seminar discussion). Voices and terms are privileged in discourse. By 'discourse' I mean both talk and text, specifically the overt and 'covert rules and prohibitions which constitute the knowledge of a "native speaker" of a language - the rules outside the rule book for ordering concepts, the materials which are acceptable, and the valid formulations for those who are inside the group' (Arens, 1989, p. 35). I am not arguing that there is a single psychiatric nursing discourse. Nonetheless, interpreting the literature as a discourse enables me to identify themes that run through the literature, and to identify some of the ways in which knowledge in psychiatric nursing is constituted.

The main themes in the nursing literature: defining psychiatric nursing

One of the main concerns of the body of work on British psychiatric nursing is the definition of psychiatric nursing. Each work in British psychiatric nursing has had to address this issue because there is no agreed paradigm of psychiatric nursing practice (Kuhn, 1970; see also Cormack, 1983; Altschul, 1980, 1984a and 1984b). Each contribution can be regarded as reflexively defining psychiatric nursing through the process of research. I have structured this review of the literature around a central work, Altschul (1972), because in that work are defined or discussed issues addressed by subsequent British psychiatric nursing researchers, and because it was important in the development of the design and method of this study.

Understandings of psychiatric nursing prior to Altschul (1972): American sources

Work on American nursing is held by some British authors (Cormack, 1976; MacIlwaine, 1980; Altschul, 1980) to be of moot relevance to British psychiatric nursing. However, it is relevant to understanding key themes in the British discourse. It forms part of the background to understanding British psychiatric nursing and this monograph. British psychiatric nursing researchers use terms from American nursing discourses, if only to dispute them. The themes I will note are the privileging of theoretical knowledge over common sense, psychiatric nursing over lay approaches to helping patients, and deliberate talk over haphazard communication.

Theme: the privileging of nurses' presence and language in communication with patients, and development of common understandings

Peplau's (1952) *Interpersonal Relations in Nursing* is a classic text in nursing. Its recent republication in Britain marks its continued relevance. Peplau (1952) defined nursing (including psychiatric nursing) as an interpersonal, interpretive process and she stressed the importance of treating the meaning of behaviour to the patient as the basis of nursing action (1952, p. 226). The nurse's feelings and actions, as well as the patient's, had to become 'the focus of inquiry', because the patient was considered to be acting in relation to the situation including the nurse in the situation, and vice versa. She (p. 283-4) outlined the role of the nurse:

> The nurse is a participant observer in most relationships in nursing. ...All nursing judgements in practice grow out of participant-observation...*nurses* - like other human beings - *act on the basis of the meaning of events to them, that is, on the basis of their immediate interpretation of the climate and performances that transpire in a particular relationship.* At the same time, the patient will act on the basis of the meaning of his illness to him. *The interaction of nurse and patient is fruitful when a method of communication that identifies and uses common meanings is at work in the situation.*

The aim of nurse-patient communication is 'common understanding', accomplished through the nurse's 'ever increasing' awareness. In Peplau's discourse, 'awareness' is privileged over 'intuition'; 'responsible' talk over 'ad hoc' or 'haphazard' talk. The main themes of subsequent discourse are present in Peplau's (1952) work.

Peplau (1960, p. 964) wrote about 'talking with patients':

> Social chit-chat is replaced by the responsible use of words which help to further the personal development of the patient. It is this complexity which distinguishes the verbal part of the professional nurse's work from the verbal approach a layman might use toward a sick person.

In this discourse, lay and professional talk are demarcated in terms of 'awareness', 'responsibility' and 'productivity'. 'Responsible use of words' is privileged over 'chit-chat'; nursing talk over lay talk; 'productive' over unproductive talk.

Introducing a theme important to this monograph, Peplau (1978, p. 44) defined psychiatric nursing in relation to the definition of mental illness and the 'work' the patient had to do:

> The definition of the nature of 'mental illness' is in effect the definition of the work which the patient is to do in order to change himself into a more fully functioning person. The role of physician and nurse flows out of the definition of the patient's work. The question of who will decide the patient's work is another matter.

The theme of privilege in 'definition of work' will be discussed below. In Peplau's discourse the definition of work is legitimated in terms of the aim of getting the patient 'to change himself into a more fully functioning person'.

The report by The Committee on Psychiatric Nursing of the Group for the Advancement of Psychiatry (1955, p. 2) on 'Therapeutic Use of the Self - a Concept for Psychiatry' also advocated a participant observer role for psychiatric nurses. It promulgated 'psychiatrically oriented concepts' as the basis for interpreting patients' behaviour:

> The understanding of these concepts should offer a basis for communication among the various participants in patient care. It is only through such communication in the hierarchy of personnel that consistency and direction can be brought to the total therapeutic regime.

The common theoretical language is seen as necessary in order to coordinate the nurse's role in the 'therapeutic effort'. In this report definition of psychiatric nursing is accomplished through delineation of its borders with lay and psychiatric discourses (p. 10).[1] The Committee's report promoted the value of psychiatric nurses' relationships with patients:

> Cogently directed patient-nurse relationships are therapeutically effective...The nurse can become aware of the meaning and significance of her very presence in relationship to the patient.

The Committee's discourse established psychiatric nursing knowledge in a zone between psychiatric understanding and common sense. The nurse was privileged in relation to the patient through the concept of the 'therapeutic use of the nurse's self'. The theme of 'presence' is important to this monograph. The nurse's privilege lies in her very 'presence', which gives her access to meaning and the possibility of effectiveness.

Hays and Larson (1963, p. 2) emphasise the presence of the nurse:

> *Every comment* the nurse makes to the patient or within his hearing can be evaluated as having therapeutic or non-therapeutic value, i.e. it either contributes to his emotional growth or it reinforces his illness.

The value depends on the nurse's awareness of the meaning of what she says.

'Awareness' is necessary for the 'purposefulness' which Travelbee (1969, p. 25) sees as necessary for psychiatric nursing:

> ...many aspects of the (nurse-patient) interpersonal process are reciprocal...The difference hopefully lies in the purposefulness of the nurse's activities, as well as in the theoretical or content background she draws upon to understand, plan, give and evaluate results gained in the interpersonal process.

Travelbee claims (cf. Peplau, 1952) that both patient and nurse change and learn through the 'interactive process'. The oppositions established in this discourse, with privileged terms first, are: 'purposeful' nurse and 'non-purposeful' patient, 'observation' and 'failure to observe', 'interpretation' and 'taking things at face value', 'interaction' and 'non-interaction'.

Travelbee (1979, p. 1) defines nursing in terms of the patient as potential agent. Privileged terms are 'nurse', 'agent', 'independence', and 'experience put into words'. Language (an 'instrument') is central to Travelbee's definition of nursing:

> (The nurse) cares for the suffering person through the medium of words...The nurse and the patient must put the experience into words and then examine, analyze and clarify their meaning in order to understand one another.

The complete privileging of the nurse's presence is seen in Travelbee's (1979, p. 9) claim that with Peplau 'the nurse became the therapy'.

Psychiatric nursing as interaction

The works discussed above emphasised the nurse-patient relationship and the process of communication. The following texts define nursing in terms of interaction. Diers and Leonard (1966, p. 226) reviewed 'interaction analysis in nursing research':

> ...there appears to be a need to clarify the term *interaction*. The term is generally used to refer to the study of actual behavior, not attitudes or role definitions. Nurse-patient interaction is not identical to nurse-patient *relationship*, and the connection between nurses' attitudes and their interaction with patients is a research problem, not something to be assumed.

Diers and Leonard (pp. 227-8) claim, though not on the basis of empirical evidence, that 'the nurse-patient interaction...(is) a distinct kind of communication between people, guided by a theory unique for the purpose to be accomplished'; and argue for appropriate 'measuring devices'.

Among American interaction studies from this period were those of: Caudill et al (1952), who found the role of the psychiatric nurse in relation to neurotic patients in an admission ward vaguely defined; Carter (1959), who used the critical incident technique to study patients' perceptions of 'therapeutic patient-patient interaction' on a psychiatric ward; and Conant (1965), who used Bales' (1951) interaction process analysis to study nurse-patient interaction[2]. Manaser and Werner (1964) provided various 'instruments for study of nurse-patient interaction'. Hargreaves and Runyon (1969) examined differences in interaction patterns between psychiatric patients and high and low ranked nurses.

This brief review of American nursing literature is not intended to be exhaustive, but rather to introduce some of the themes and 'voices' which form a background to later British work.

Definition of psychiatric nursing in British work prior to Altschul (1972): lay-person versus professional, and interaction as gossip

In addition to the American work noted above, two empirical British studies on the work or role of psychiatric nursing are relevant to understanding Altschul (1972) and the themes continued in this monograph. The Joint Committee of the Manchester Regional Hospital and the University of Manchester (1955) used 'general observation and common sense as well as statistical analysis' to study 'the work of the mental nurse'. They considered that 'observation of tasks' missed the 'qualitative aspect', the 'heart of the job' (p. 120). The authors introduced a claim that the work of the psychiatric nurse centres on the personality of the nurse rather than any other more clearly defined features of 'role' - a claim repeated in later British nursing discourse (cf. Shanley, 1988). Nurses were seen as involved in a sort of 'moral' treatment, 'teaching' patients to be 'socially conscious' and 'responsible'.

John (1961) found that there was no clearly defined role for psychiatric nurses and that '"lay" outlooks' were common (p. 115). She claimed that nurses generally did not know diagnoses (p. 35), and that this created 'problems in building relationships' and generated 'gossip' (p. 118). Nurses blamed patients rather than searching for causes of behaviour and attempting to 'cure' these. John (1961, p. 129) found that:

> The lay attitude was...illustrated by the day-to-day connotation of the word 'neurotic' rather than the use of the word with its medical interpretation. As a result, one frequently heard comments that neurotics were just in 'to dodge responsibility'...or 'You don't know how much of the illness is genuine and how much imaginary' or they were 'too pampered'. This was particularly astonishing in view of the obvious handicaps under which certain patients were placed by their illness, e.g. fear of being left alone, or even of stepping outside their own front door. These attitudes, however, were interesting in light of the amount of sympathy which was extended to patients with evidence of 'tangible illness', e.g. vomiting.

John drew 'attention' 'to the neurotic whose distress is intensified by being dubbed spineless, imaginative or pampered' (p. 130). The oppositions which structure John's discourse are: 'diagnosis'/'gossip', 'psychiatric nursing'/'lay', 'ill'/'not ill', 'obvious handicaps'/'what the nurses considered imaginary', 'sympathy'/'blaming', 'neurotic'/other patients. The oppositions accomplish an irony: the nurses appear 'interesting', 'astonishing'.

The nurse's interaction with the neurotic patient is focused on in subsequent British psychiatric nursing research discourse, reviewed below.

Altschul's contribution: the theme of common sense

Altschul's (1972) work was one of the main reference points for this study in three ways. Her work introduced into the British context the terms of the American discourse, in particular the distinction between 'common sense' and theoretically guided practice based on 'deliberate, purposeful talk'. I will note below Altschul's findings on neurotic patients. I drew on her recommendation about method, discussed below. In this summary of her (1972) work I will discuss issues of theory and method relevant to this study.

Altschul wanted to know whether nurses and patients had therapeutic relationships. She (1972, p. 30) hypothesised that relationships would depend on number and duration of interactions, and that reciprocal relationships would be experienced as therapeutic. She justified her search for therapeutic relationships by reference to American claims that these are the 'core' of psychiatric nursing (Peplau and Leininger, cited in Altschul, 1972, pp. 23-24).

Altschul justified her study of interaction[3] as a means of investigating relationships on the basis of an assumption that the interactions might 'contribute to' relationships (p. 30). However, she does not clarify the conceptual relationship between interaction and relationship. She noted that it was not possible, due to the constraints imposed by confidentiality, to ask 'psychotherapists' what patients told them about their 'experience of involvement' with nurses (pp. 25-26). Hence, she sought 'another way' of investigating nurse-patient relationships. This methodological difficulty indicates that rights to ask, to know and to share knowledge reflected structures of interest and power in the psychiatric setting. I will review Altschul's method and argument and return to the problem of adequate conceptualisation.

Altschul's method involved participant observation in different wards to enable observation of interaction. Having observed (but not participated in) an interaction, she asked the nurse 'what it was about'. In subsequent interviews she asked patients about the help they got from nurses, and which nurses they remembered. She analysed the frequency, duration and direction of interaction; and did a qualitative and quantitative analysis of interview data.

There is a tension in Altschul's analysis which reflects a tension in her theoretical perspective. Altschul drew key concepts from different discourses. The concept of relationship was drawn from psychodynamic discourse, while interaction was defined in terms of 'factors' such as duration and frequency, the relationship of which to meaning or quality of interaction from the points of view of the participants is left unclarified.[4] On the one hand, the implication is that nurses 'respond' to patients' 'stimuli' (p. 137). On the other hand, she refers to Ogden and Richards' (1949) understanding of meaning, and is interested in the quality of interactions and relationships. Altschul acknowledges limits to the inferences she could draw regarding therapeutic outcome on the basis of her interaction data, but implies that 'control of other treatment variables' and 'independent criteria' would permit one to 'establish' therapeutic effect (p. 22).

The lack of clarity about the theoretical perspective is reflected in her method. She quotes Kendall (cited in Altschul, 1972, p. 54):

> Observability of the behaviour of any group is a precondition for exercising social control over that group.

Altschul claims: 'The relevance to this study is clear: observability of patients is a precondition for nurses exercising any influence on patients' (p. 54). It could be argued that Altschul's method was also a form of observation for the purpose of exercising (professional) social control or influence[5] over nurses. Her method can be construed as establishing a second-order 'observability' of interaction, through access to the nurse's point of view and through inference by Altschul about the patient's point of view.

Altschul's aim to understand interaction from the point of view of the patient as well as the nurse was only partly accomplished. Nurses' views were privileged, in that only they were asked what happened in interaction. Patients were asked about help they got from nurses, and what they would have wanted nurses to have done had the nurses had more time. 'Availability' and 'time' are common-sense terms used by Altschul as both resources and topics of investigation. Structuring enquiry through these terms may have limited the scope for understanding of how patients understood interaction. Altschul's method and analysis can be construed as privileging the researcher's (professional) point of view.

'Common sense' versus 'identifiable perspective': the tale of three returns

Altschul (1972) discusses a theme central to this monograph: 'common sense'. Her method involved asking nurses she had observed in conversation with patients to tell her what they had talked about. Nurses claimed that what they did was 'common sense'. Altschul framed the nurses' use of the term 'common sense', giving examples of what she construed as 'very different approaches' to patients returning to a ward after absences. She argues that 'all three patients received different "common-sense" approaches from these three nurses' (p.146). Consecutive interactions between different nurses and the same patient were also held by Altschul to be 'contradictory' and evidently ineffective. She argues, on the basis of examples, that while nurses were 'satisfied' with their 'responses', her interpretation of later accounts indicated that their interventions were 'unsuccessful', the patients still anxious or 'not satisfied' (pp. 147-8). She found (p. 150, quoting Hays and Larson, 1963) evidence of 'non-therapeutic interpersonal techniques':

> Whether their effect was non-therapeutic is however open to doubt. It would seem to the observer that some of the nurses' responses were non-effective, because based on insufficient knowledge or because they were inappropriate in the circumstances, rather than because they were non-therapeutic in themselves.

She notes that she found it difficult to follow the logic of the nurses' explanations for why they 'gave attention' in different situations; that, while nurses' tone of voice indicated that their action was 'self-evident', their action did not appear to her to have been based on 'decisions' made on the basis of 'general principles' (p.164).

Altschul's analysis thus raises questions about the nurses' use of the term 'common sense' in accounting for their work. Because critique of Altschul's analysis is important to the argument of this monograph, I will construe the meanings and interpretations of the term 'common sense' as used by the nurses and by Altschul. What I am arguing is that the 'first order' meaning of the term 'common sense', that is, the meaning of the term to the nurses, is not clarified by Altschul. Instead, the term is brought uninterpreted into her 'second order' (researcher's or professional) discourse, where it is opposed to 'identifiable perspective'.[6] The consequence is that the nurses' perspective is left unclarified. The status of 'common sense' as a form of rationality in nursing practice is largely unexplicated and undetermined.

In her ('second order') analysis, Altschul distinguishes common sense from a kind of rational decision-making based on general principles. It could be argued that the issue as defined by Altschul was not whether the nurses practised on the basis of common sense, but whether they practised consistently, on the basis of an 'identifiable perspective' or general principles. However, I argue that the issue in either case is the same. The issue is whether the researcher accepts the nurse's ('first order') definition of her own work; including the frame of meaning provided by the nurse, that is, the frame of meaning 'common sense'.

I thus find in Altschul (1972) the central problem in the definition of psychiatric nursing: the contradiction between psychiatric nursing as it makes sense to nurses in practice; and psychiatric nursing as it could or should be, as seen by the nursing researcher.[7] This contradiction is based on two other contradictions. One is the set of contradictions Altschul locates in the nurses' discourse, and the other is that between her discourse and theirs. In effect, the nurses' claim that their action was (implicitly) accounted for by reference to 'common sense' is 'contradicted' by Altschul through a discourse which juxtaposes the nurses' accounts with Altschul's observations or with later accounts. However, Altschul does not address the issues involved in her 'contradiction' of the nurses' justification of action by their claim of 'common sense'. Instead, she locates the contradiction in the contrast between what she saw as 'different' nurses' actions, and their claim that what they did was 'common sense'. There is no possibility of remedy on the nurses' part for this interpretation of the contradictions in their work. The contradiction as it appeared to Altschul was not resolved through discussion with the nurses in the setting; for example, by exploring with them the meaning of 'differences' or whether 'common sense' would 'cover' differences in approach. Her method, which invited the nurses to tell about interaction, stopped short of full dialogue.

My interpretation of this problem in Altschul's analysis does not establish the meaning of the term 'common sense' in the nurses' discourse. However, it does suggest possible interpretations of that meaning. One possible reading is that 'common sense', as the term was used by the nurses, referred to a body of tacit knowledge (Polanyi, 1967) drawn on by nurses in interaction. Nurses referring to 'common sense' in this way may have intended to demonstrate the (accountable) grounds for action. Secondly, 'common sense' may have referred to the form of the rationality the nurses displayed in interaction: not 'What did you know?' but 'How did you know?', or common sense as a way of thinking and acting (cf. Garfinkel, 1967).[8]

In Altschul's discourse, the concept 'common sense' is contrasted with theory-guided rational practice. Like John (1961), Altschul privileges in her discourse the terms opposite to those she found privileged in the nurses' discourse. Altschul (pp. 191-192) disagreed with some nurses' claim that 'all psychiatric nursing is "common sense"', suggesting that an alternative might be based on 'an identifiable perspective':

> ...nurses did not have any identifiable perspective to guide them in their dealings with problematic situations. Their own insistence that all psychiatric nursing is 'common sense' would appear to support this belief.

Thus Altschul (e.g. 1972, pp. 168, 169-197) develops a discourse with oppositions between 'common sense' and 'identifiable perspective', 'intuitive action' and 'reasoned, self-conscious, deliberate' action (cf. Peplau, 1952; Hays and Larson, 1963; and Travelbee, 1969). What the contents of these sets of terms might be is unclear. However, it may be inferred that the latter terms in the pairs are related to diagnosis, personal and situational circumstances, since these are the terms Altschul used to code nurses' answers (p.138). The privileged terms were not derived from the setting of practice, but rather were brought in from outside, and reflected the American discourse. The former terms in the pairs denote nursing as anybody would do it, and might be equivalent to lay approaches (p. 194):

> The intuitive nature of interaction resulted in contradictions in the approach of different nurses to the same patient or to different patients with the same problem. Though this may be no more harmful than the lay approach which the patient had encountered prior to admission, it was wasteful of therapeutic opportunities.

The question of how practice was organised in the absence of an 'identifiable perspective' is not addressed. Altschul's critique of the nurses' use of the concept 'common sense' can be interpreted as a critique of its inadequacy in explanation; as a complaint that 'common sense' functions in the nurses' discourse as the main category in the explanation of nursing interaction, while in Altschul's analysis it is rendered a 'residual category'[9], residual to action guided by an 'identifiable perspective'. My argument is that the concept 'common sense' is rendered a residual category in Altschul's and other nursing researchers' accounts of nursing interaction and knowledge, the non-privileged term counterpoised to the privileged terms.

I noted two possible 'readings' of the nurses' use of the term 'common sense'. These imply a third. Nurses may have used the term to define the limits to Altschul's enquiry, to resist it. When Altschul (p. 41) visited the study site:

> An explanation of the study was given and it was stressed that little was known about the kind of relationships nurses formed with patients, or about the kind of relationships which it might be therapeutic to form. At least some of the sisters...felt that the investigator should know, and that the investigation was aimed at finding out if they were doing the right thing; that this was obvious, and that the questions did not seem to make sense. However, all...said that they would gladly cooperate.

And later, 'The nurses by their intonation indicated that the reasons (that they gave attention) were self-evident' (p165).[10] These remarks suggest that the nurses, however cooperative, were responding as practitioners engaged in practical concerns who treat it as a matter of course that 'insiders' will recognise the rationality of what they do (Garfinkel, 1967). This proposal is discussed below.

'Common sense' and 'waste of opportunities'

According to my analysis, Altschul does not distinguish between 'common sense' (as a resource) and use of the term 'common sense' (as a topic). It is therefore unclear on what basis she sees as problematic the nurses' claim that what they did was common sense. In the passage noted above (Altschul, 1972, p. 194), 'intuitive', (possibly) 'harmful' and 'wasteful of therapeutic opportunities' are aligned with 'common sense', in contrast to the privileged terms 'reasoned, self conscious, deliberate', and 'helpful' or 'therapeutic'. Altschul commands the distinction between 'same' and 'difference' which underpins these other distinctions. That is, the claim that the nurses did the 'same' thing in 'different' circumstances is based on Altschul's determination of similarity and difference. The appearance of the 'problem' is a product of her analysis and interpretation.

The problem defined but not resolved here is how to appraise Altschul's difficulty in accepting the nurses' claim that their interaction was (or was justified by a claim that it was) 'common sense'. An alternative way of reading Altschul's example of different accounts by three nurses of 'the same sort' of interaction, is that the rule according to which something was said to accomplish the shared agreement was the rule of invoking 'common sense' as an explanatory and justificatory concept (Garfinkel, 1967). It is possible that Altschul has identified a use, by nurses, of 'common sense' which functions like Garfinkel's 'common understanding' (see below). Both may function unproblematically in practice, as resources for recognising and understanding practice and communication that occurs in practice. Competent members use common sense to do their work; reflexively, their work accomplishes the appearance (to them) of common sense. Common sense should be evident and require no explanation, especially to a nurse.

Thus the 'problem' of common sense may be a theoretical problem, not a practical problem. Altschul sees the nurses' use of the term as problematic because it does not indicate to her a set of contents ordered without contradictions, as she implies would be expected in a practice guided by theory, or based on 'identifiable perspective'. There are two 'mismatches': Altschul and the nurses did not make a 'common sense'; and 'common sense' did not 'match' what might have been, an 'identifiable perspective'[11]. However, it is possible to argue that a 'match' of contents would not be expected. Garfinkel (1967, p. 282) distinguishes between theoretical and common-sense rationalities and advises that 'Instead of the properties of rationality being treated as a methodological principle for interpreting activity, they are to be treated only as empirically problematic material.'[12]

The problem with Altschul's critique of 'common sense' is that she has to use common sense as a resource (her understanding of what made each interaction 'different') in considering the topic of nurses' common sense. Readers are required to do the same: to draw on their common sense to warrant Altschul's critique of the nurses' common sense. The question that arises from Altschul's work is how to understand the nurses' rationality. This will be a theme in the discussion in Chapter 5 of nurses' and patients' knowledge.

Themes in Altschul's (1972) work relevant to subsequent British psychiatric nursing discourse

In Altschul's (1972) text can be seen the key features of subsequent British psychiatric nursing discourse. First, the distinction between theoretical foundation and common sense is established. A theoretical perspective is privileged. What is valued in her discourse is psychiatric knowledge and evidence of therapeutic relationships. What is left over as not making sense is the nurses' common sense. Common sense as a 'residual category'[13] may be seen as an artefact of Altschul's method of analysis. The categories for content analysis are drawn from outside the settings in which the action was constituted as accountable (see Garfinkel, 1967, discussed below).

What is established in Altschul's analysis is a 'hierarchy of credibility' (Becker, 1967, see below) conjoining terms from the discourse of American theorists with the discourse governing empirical British psychiatric nursing practice. The 'hierarchy of credibility' is mediated by Altschul's knowledge. The hierarchy is seen in Altschul's claim that nurses 'missed opportunities'. The perception of opportunity was brought in, from outside, through the researcher.

Thus understanding of the interaction between the nurses and patients was mediated through the researcher's understanding in ways that cannot be accounted for. The nurses' accounts were searched for evidence of action meaningful in relation to categories that did not arise from the actors' subjective understandings or the contexts of action.

The methods used to investigate the interaction, and the method of analysis limit the validity of conclusions about the nurses' understandings of interaction. Altschul's intention of getting some 'indication of the nurses' conceptualisation of the meaning of the interaction' (p. 137) is translated into a categorisation based on 'level of knowledge or understanding' (p. 138). Altschul acknowledges the limits of this method of analysis. The point that is important to the argument of this monograph is that Altschul's interpretation of interaction is mediated by interpretive principles derived from outside the context of interaction. The meaning of the interaction to the nurses and patients, that is, the meaning of the action in the setting of its occurrence, remains largely uninterpreted, residual.

Further work by Altschul and summary of themes

In publications since 1972 Altschul has developed some of the above concepts and arguments. Though not reports of research they are relevant to this argument. Altschul (1978, p. 335) recommended a 'systems approach to the nursing process', arguing that existing models of nursing had 'signally failed to represent either the patient's, the nurse's, or the institutional reality'. She claimed that documentation of what nurses do is not useful since 'the chief instrument the nurse uses is her own personality'. She argued that care plans would not be suitable because 'it is such activities as the exercise of responsibility, authority and decision-making which may be disordered' in psychiatric patients and no 'simple nursing plan' could 'remedy' these. She explored the notion that the nurse may be inside or outside the patient's system in various ways, and concluded that 'if she found herself inside', the nurse would have to decide when the patient was discharged whether to 'accompany the patient into the much larger system of the real world' (p. 340). Altschul (1978, p. 348) introduces concepts of inside-outside, the patient's disorders of responsibility, and the patient's experience of 'the hospital stay...as an episode during which the subsystem of illness, treatment and recovery was sharply put into focus' (p. 340); all of which will be seen as relevant to the argument of this monograph. Altschul (1980, p. 650) considered that the emphasis in the American literature on 'therapeutic use of self' was possibly 'arrogant', if it implied that this was an exclusively nursing function; and that the benefit of use of this 'tool' was uncertain. She argued that nurse-patient interaction often centred on 'everyday responsiveness' and the patient's recovery of ordinary social skills. She advised against persistent questioning as patients would resist 'probing'. This advice, seen as having 'universal applicability', was contrasted with the specific 'styles' of interaction dictated by the more general theoretical approaches in the settings: medical (formulating diagnosis), sociological, or psychotherapeutic. Altschul (1984a, p. 38) addressed the problem of identifying the object of nursing practice if the patient were not regarded as mentally ill, and concluded that:

> psychiatric nurses must identify their specific contribution with reference to the principles underlying the treatment of mental disorders, and not with reference to some principles which are currently referred to as 'nursing theories'.

Unable to identify 'what good practice is in psychiatric nursing', she concluded that:

> Being a good psychiatric nurse is like being a good mother or a good friend - it is what you might do, not what you are in fact doing.

Altschul (1984b, p. 50) discussed some of the pitfalls in the 'search for principles to determine what psychiatric nursing is about', and criticised the principles of assessment of 'health needs' and the search for those the nurse could 'most effectively' meet. She argued that to attempt to base nursing action on the principles of nursing theory, without taking account of the 'total system of beliefs and practices surrounding health care' (including the patient's 'ideology') was 'futile'. Summarising issues related to four 'models' of nursing practice in different settings, she concluded (p. 51) that:

> ...whatever the mode of treatment, the patient's own task is to examine his lifestyle...During his period of treatment the patient tries to learn better ways of behaving, adopting better social skills, and better ways of dealing with his fellow human beings.

Thus in more recent work, Altschul has addressed issues of theory and practice in somewhat different ways than in Altschul (1972). It could be argued that in dismissing the claims of 'nursing theories' as adequate sources of principles for practice Altschul has revised her understanding of the relationship of theory to practice, and that she has advanced the grounds for interpreting the common sense of psychiatric nursing. However, the later views on practice are not based on empirical research. There has been no attempt to address the question of who is to define that common sense, and how it is related to 'specialist discourse'. Moreover, the theoretical perspectives provided by the 'principles of treatment of mental disorder' remain 'privileged'. These later articles could be read as implying that there are two 'strata' in nursing practice, one based on 'common' activities and social relationships, and addressed to what may be considered 'common' problems of responsibility, and the other based on theoretical understandings rooted in the discourses of medicine and the social sciences. There is thus a tension in Altschul's work between the claim that the practice of psychiatric nursing depends on the 'kind of person' the nurse is and the claim for the priority of specialist discourses in determining the basis for practice.

I will note in Chapter 8 the relevance of this later work to the present empirical study. However, I consider that the analysis presented above of the issues of common sense and evaluation of practice in Altschul (1972) is valid, and that subsequent research in psychiatric nursing can be interpreted in relation to that work. The limits of the theoretical development in Altschul (1978) may be related to the lack of a theoretical basis for relating 'common-sense' understandings of practitioners to the privileged 'identifiable perspective'. These limitations are related to methodological limitations. It may be argued that Altschul's (1972) method and analysis limited the nurses' ability to elaborate the 'reasons' for their action. There is neither theoretically nor methodologically any means of accounting for the interpretations which form the basis for judgements on the legitimacy (accountability) of the nurses' actions. The 'hierarchy of credibility' is established on an insecure base, as it omits the views of the patients involved in the interaction and limits the nurses' opportunities to dispute Altschul's interpretation. These theoretical and methodological issues will be pursued in Chapters 3 and 4, and I will return later in this chapter to a discussion of Altschul's recommendation that 'accounting' be used to 'increase observability'.

In the following sections I will consider the main themes of the discourse as these appear in British nursing research since Altschul (1972).

Relevant nursing literature after Altschul (1972)

British general nursing literature on interaction and communication: the drive to observe interaction and talk: search for 'actual conversation' as the basis of determining appropriate care; surveillance and personal responsibility

The themes outlined above, of 'inappropriate'[14] practice and nurses' inability to account for practice, continue in the nursing discourse, usually in the context of patient assessment or information giving. A number of researchers have studied verbal interaction in general nursing and found it 'inappropriate'. They tried to increase objectivity, to get at 'actual conversation' through various methods of surveillance of nurse-patient interaction. Faulkner (1979) monitored nurse-patient conversation in medical wards, using a tape recorder attached to the nurse. She found that conversations were generally brief (2-3 minutes), and that nurses 'avoided' answering patients' questions, regardless of topic. On the basis of a rationale that appropriate nursing care depends on good assessment, and that good assessment depends on 'communication skills', Clark (1981) used audio and video recordings, observations and field notes to study 'communication skills' in interaction between nurses and surgical patients. Interactions were found to be brief and task oriented, with nurses 'controlling' and 'blocking' communication and paying patients' emotional needs only 'lip service'. Nurses were found to be wanting in their 'professional responsibility'.

Clark (1982, p. 200), describing the same study, reported her attempts to develop a 'data base of real-life nurse-patient interaction'. The study:

> was concerned with the general question of what actually takes place when nurses and patients communicate by talking to each other.

This attempt to capture 'what actually takes place' failed in its own terms, as, in one phase of analysis, the decontextualised data from recorded interactions could not be reliably coded (p. 149).

British psychiatric nursing literature since Altschul (1972): observation and interview and the concern with role

The main focus of psychiatric nursing research since Altschul (1972) has been on the role of the nurse in different settings. Those studies relevant to the methods or aims of the present study are reviewed. A theme that runs through the literature is 'lack of a recognisable body of knowledge'.

Sladden (1979), in a study of community psychiatric nursing, noted that participant observation studies are limited in their capacity to reveal actors' purposes, perspectives or ideology. Using a method based on self-recording by CPNs and on interviews, she found a 'lack of specificity in nurses' definitions of their own functions and of the objectives of nursing care' (p. 138). She echoed John (1961) and Altschul (1972) in finding 'opportunities' missed by nurses. She contrasted the 'appropriateness' of nurses' technical language used for clinical functions with the (by implication less appropriate) use of 'lay' language for 'interpersonal aspects'. Noting (p. 139) a 'haphazard collection of intuitive insights and individual experience', she found that the nurses had:

> difficulty in defining situations...in terms of general concepts...as a basis for a rational selection of methods of care and for the evaluation of results...

She concluded (p. 139) that the nurses' practice was:

> essentially a non-professional kind of practice; depending on personal aptitude rather than on the application of a body of knowledge by reference to explicit principles.

Cormack (1976) used participant observation to study the work of psychiatric charge nurses. He found (p. 82) that the interaction content in one-to-one verbal interaction:

> ...gave no indication that the nurse was consciously attempting to influence the mental health of the patient by her own personal endeavour.

In Cormack's discourse, 'consciously attempts to influence' echoes Altschul's notion of 'deliberate' attempts to influence (cf. Leininger, cited in Altschul, 1972, pp. 23-24), and is opposed to 'assessing change'.

Cormack (1983, pp. 185-6) noted the 'increasing realisation of nurses' inability to describe the nature of nursing'.[15] His descriptive study of psychiatric nursing was undertaken (p. 1) in light of:

> the general responsibility which any professional group must have to possess a knowledge of its own function, in other words, to know and *be able to describe what the professional role involves.*

Cormack (1983, p. 24) reviewed the 'prescriptive literature' on the role of the psychiatric nurse, concluding that the:

> descriptive literature fails to identify actual nursing practice as being the same as that prescribed in much of the contemporary nursing literature.

Cormack (1983, p. 33) used Flanagan's (1954) critical incident technique, arguing:

> One major strength of the critical incident technique is that it usually results in a specific description of what nurses actually do, rather than in a description of what respondents think they do or what they should do.

Cormack thus tried (like Clark, 1982) to get at what 'actually happens' in nurse patient interaction. However, he did not conceptualise practice adequately. His analysis stripped nursing action of the subjective meaning and context that might have enabled understanding of the critical episodes as interaction. The result is a proposal for what amounts to total surveillance of the patient (and, by implication, of the nurse) through a system of assessment of every patient's 'potential need' for a vast array of nursing actions.[16]

Reynolds and Cormack (1982, p. 236)) studied clinical teaching of nurse learners and concluded:

> Learners have great difficulty in analysing the nurses' verbal and non-verbal behaviour, that is, describing *how* the nurse performs an activity, rather than *what* she does...The reason for this difficulty may be that many nursing responses are intuitive and unstructured.

The 'problem' with understanding is located in the learners, in their inability to explain nursing action. Reynolds and Cormack (1982) do not consider that their methods, which involved asking the learners to explain 'how' the nurses did what they did, may have required the learners to perform an impossible hermeneutic task (cf. Garfinkel, 1967). The oppositions in Reynolds and Cormack's discourse on psychiatric nursing's 'problems' are: 'intuitive'/'unstructured' v. 'conscious'/'analysed'; 'task orientation' v. 'work with individual patients'; 'practical' v. 'theoretical'; with the latter terms privileged. The proposed remedy is 'objective recognition' of 'needs' and reporting of 'observed behaviour'. What is missing from the authors' analysis is any sense of the processes of interpretation involved in 'recognition' of needs.

I have highlighted the theme of observation in studies of nurses. Carr (1980) described the 'role of the nurses working in a district general hospital psychiatric unit'. He found that nurses emphasised the importance of 'observational skills', and he claimed (p. 281) that:

> it was vital ...that patients should be unaware that they are being watched...There must be daily reporting in depth on patients' conditions in order to permit any deviations from the norm to be detected.

The opposition of 'watcher' and 'watched', with the 'watcher' privileged, recalls the discourse on 'awareness' discussed above. Carr defines a discourse which privileges that which nurses do not privilege: the 'role as social interaction'.[17]

A summary

The main points from the above writers may be summarised as they are relevant to the argument of this monograph. The main themes in the discourse of British psychiatric nursing research literature are: the lack of a clearly defined role (John, 1961; Joint Committee, 1955; Altschul, 1972; Cormack, 1976; Sladden, 1979; Barker, 1982; Carr, 1980); the lack of a defined body of knowledge; nurses' inability to tell what they do; and haphazard and intuitive rather than ordered and rational practices.

Remedies are sought for these problems. The nurse is called into a professional discourse through the device of a system of 'objective' determination of need, or otherwise is subjected to remedial discourse through mechanical or conversational devices enabling surveillance of talk.

Thus there is a gap between what nurses say they do and what is recognised by researchers as adequate or appropriate description and explanation. While some authors distinguish between prescriptive and descriptive nursing literature, descriptive literature is also prescriptive. In the discourse which articulates the above themes the psychiatric nurse appears as someone unable to tell, satisfactorily, what he does. He appears indistinguishable from a lay person in talk and action. His failure lies partly in his attribution of his action to common sense rather than to an identifiable perspective (Altschul, 1972). He does not give objective views (Cormack, 1983; Reynolds and Cormack, 1982). He acts without deliberation.

The image of the psychiatric nurse

I have read the literature as a discourse in which certain terms are privileged. The nurse 'present' (that is constructed as desired) in the discourse of nursing researchers and not 'present' (empirically) in practice is the deliberate practitioner, referring to a body of knowledge and professionally responsible. The nurse opposite to this is the one 'present' in practice, said to be indistinguishable from a 'layman'. However, the 'layman' is never actually present, and instead has to be supplied by the nursing researchers who draw on their own common sense as a resource in understanding or failing to understand the nurse. The 'layman nurse' is never present to ask how he manages to do the work of the psychiatric nurse. What is missing from the discourse is the nurses' common sense in practice.

The discourse produces a set of contradictions which privilege the researcher's view by locating the contradictions in the nurse or among the nurses. The appearance of the 'lay nurse' or the 'self-contradicting' nurse may be an effect of the methods of production of knowledge about psychiatric nurses in interaction with patients. All of the above nursing studies were characterised by analytic and methodological individualism. When observation was done in wards, accounts or interview, responses given by nurses were dislocated from the social context of their production. This focus may be related to the role research plays in a professional discipline; the role of locating (or constituting through the methods of the research) the accountable individual practitioner and devising remedies for 'absence'. Analytic and methodological individualism diverts attention from the social context on which nurses draw and which they sustain through their interaction with the patients. What is 'absent' is understanding of the subjectivity of the nurse, interpretation of her interpretation and her role in the construction of the practice context. Before exploring work which addresses these issues I will describe the literature on nursing of neurotic patients, which focuses some of the themes discussed above and forms the background for the study reported here.

The literature on patients diagnosed as neurotic focuses the main themes from the wider literature on psychiatric nursing

To frame the present study I will outline how the themes in the psychiatric nursing literature relate to the literature on psychiatric nursing of patients diagnosed as neurotic.[18] I have discussed above the problem of the definition of psychiatric nursing. Nursing researchers' and writers' definitions of the people involved in psychiatric nursing - nurses and patients - are privileged in public discourse. Those definitions are linked to the definition of psychiatric nursing, as in Render (1947). For example (p. 2):

> The study of psychiatric nursing pivots around pathological behaviour.

and (p. 153):

> Unwholesome attitudes are seen best in the psychoneuroses (neuroses).

and (p. 154):

> A helpful attitude toward the patient with symptoms of these illnesses (neuroses) is an appreciation that you and he do not look upon the world from the same point of view.

Psychiatric nursing of neurotic patients is thus defined through construction of the patient as other. The nurse's way of seeing is 'clear cut logical' compared to that of the patient, who is 'tied up emotionally'.

The British literature can be construed as two conflicting accounts of nurses' work with neurotic patients. One line of literature portrays psychiatric nurses as able to assess and help neurotic patients. The other line portrays the interaction of nurses and neurotic patients as problematic.

Neurotic patients are helped by nurse therapists and community psychiatric nurses

Marks (1977) reported an experimental programme of education and training which trained psychiatric nurses to be behaviour therapists able to treat adult patients diagnosed as neurotic as effectively as psychologists and psychiatrists. Marks (1985) reported that a nurse therapist (trained in the above programme) effectively helped neurotic patients in a general practice setting. Treatment was cost-effective even without taking into account the patient's subjective sense of improvement. Paykel et al (1982) reported a controlled trial comparing 'supportive home visiting by a CPN' (Note: 'CPN' is 'Community Psychiatric Nurse') and 'routine outpatient psychiatric care' for chronic neurotic patients. There were no significant differences in symptoms, social adjustment and family burden; and patients were more satisfied with CPN treatment. The results were held (p. 580) to 'support the role of such nurses in the after care of neurotic patients'. Paykel and Griffith (1983), reporting more fully on the same study, described the results of content analysis of CPNs' sessions with the chronic neurotic patients. The authors noted (p. 81) that CPNs were slow to regard their 'supportive contacts' as the 'main specific therapy', but as they developed relationships with patients:

> they were able to encourage examination and self understanding. They began to see their role as more interpretive.

Tilley and Weighill (1986) reported on nurse therapists' methods of assessment and case management of alcohol and sedative use by patients (mainly 'diagnosable' as neurotic) referred for behaviour therapy.

Thus there is a body of literature which attests to the ability of psychiatric nurses, some with special training in behaviour therapy and some practicing as CPNs, to assess and help or treat patients diagnosed as neurotic.

Neurotic patients get the worst from psychiatric nurses

I have noted above John's (1961) comments on nurses and neurotic patients.

Altschul (1972) found that the rate of interaction between nurses and patients varied with diagnosis.[19] Nurses interacted less often with (the few) patients with a main diagnosis of 'neurosis' than with patients with other diagnoses. Altschul (1972, p. 80) noted that this difference was only slightly less for patients with a secondary diagnosis of 'neurosis':

> It would appear that the label of neurotic disorder did act as a disincentive to interaction, but that positive encouragement would be needed if nurses intended to interact in a more prolonged way with neurotic patients. Absence of diagnostic label is not enough to encourage interaction.

Altschul accounted for the lower frequency of interaction by citing American sources, rather than the nurses' reasons.[20] She argued that clarification of nurses' aims with these patients was needed, and that doctors should be asked if nurses have a role to play with neurotic patients.

Cormack (1976), too, found that neurotic patients[21] were involved in proportionately fewer interactions than those with other diagnoses (p. 53). Cormack (p. 53) cites remarks by two nurses:

> One nurse said 'I don't like talking to neurotic patients, they are less ill than the psychotic patients. Neurotics are out to gain something. They seem to take a loan of nurses.' Another said 'Neurotic patients don't really need nursing, they can look after themselves.' Hofling and Leininger (1960) were of the opinion that more rather than less attention and time be given (Note: *sic*) to the neurotic patient.

The order and content of Cormack's discourse exactly parallels Altschul's (1972, p. 54). (See also John, 1961.) In what may be regarded as an ironic discourse, the nurse's judgement is juxtaposed with an 'authoritative' American author's opinion.

MacIlwaine's thesis: 'inappropriate' nursing of neurotic patients

MacIlwaine (1980)[22] studied the process of 'the nursing care of female neurotic patients in psychiatric units in general hospital' to determine its 'appropriateness'. Her work is chiefly relevant to this monograph because it is the major British empirical study on non-specialist nurses' care of neurotic patients in admission wards. I will review aspects of the theoretical perspective and method in order to distinguish MacIlwaine's approach from that taken in the present study. Some more detailed analysis of aspects of the method is included in footnotes.

MacIlwaine's thesis can be summarised: a) nurses and neurotic patients differ in their perception of what nurses do for these patients; b) nurses do not understand the experience of neurotic patients, do not see them as ill, and underestimate their suffering; c) to the extent that a) and b) are true, nurses adopt an inappropriate role in relation to neurotic patients; d) nurses avoid these patients partly because they do not understand their needs or cannot meet them and partly due to the demands other patients make on their time; e) for these reasons nurses are ineffective in their interaction with neurotic patients.

MacIlwaine's methods included devising and use of a scale to measure 'perceptions of nursing of neurotic patients'; and a 'direct observational study of the nursing of 24 female neurotic patients', using a radio microphone worn by the patients (cf. Faulkner, 1979; and Clark, 1981 and 1982), with content coded on the basis of categories derived from interviews. She noted but did not explore the 'psychiatric ideologies' of the four wards studied and nurses' involvement in ward activities. Nurses and patients rated patients' anxiety and depression and their ratings were compared.

Her conclusions (pp. ii-iii) on how nurses and patients perceived the nursing of neurotic patients were that:

> (Nurses) had a clear perception of themselves as giving emotional support, coordinating services, administering wards, and saw themselves as highly relevant to treatment. Patients agreed that nurses provided some emotional support, but saw them mostly in terms of administrative functions and quite irrelevant to their treatment.

Nurses consistently rated neurotic patients' distress lower than the patients did. However, the latter finding cannot be clearly interpreted as no comparison group was used.

MacIlwaine also examined a number of texts on nursing practice and found that the role prescribed for nurses was one of giving emotional support, perhaps also acting as 'agents of behaviour change', but not 'giving insight'. She concluded that nurses acted in accordance with these prescriptions in giving emotional support and not giving insight, while their role in behaviour change was limited.

MacIlwaine concluded that nurses lacked 'any real knowledge of the patient's condition...(and) had difficulty recognising even obvious and important psychiatric symptoms'. They 'construed (neurotic disorders) as the layman would' (p. 272). She proposed (p. 274) to remedy the deficiencies in nursing practice by education[23]:

> If nurses had a clearer understanding of psychiatry and the implications of a medical diagnosis, it might enable them to make more accurate observation, move quickly, and avoid a great deal of wasted hospital time.

MacIlwaine's thesis thus reiterates the oppositions noted in previous nursing discourse, with privileged terms first: professional knowledge versus lay; apt use of time versus wasted time; 'real knowledge' of the patient's condition and point of view versus ignorance; 'accurate observation' versus inaccurate.

Critique of the thesis MacIlwaine's thesis may be criticised on methodological and theoretical grounds. There are weaknesses in the study design and methods. The questions asked of nurses and of patients in interviews used to devise the questionnaire differed[24], and different responses may have reflected the different questions rather than the nurses' and patients' different views. Similar criticisms could be made of MacIlwaine's questionnaire.[25] The second problem is that questions used in the interview which provided categories for the questionnaire were somewhat forced, with choices related to 'nurses doing for' the patients, for example. Third, lack of weighting in analysis of responses meant that key understandings could have been underrepresented in quantitative analysis. Moreover, the statements from tape-recorded interaction were decontextualised and lack power to inform about the process of interaction. This problem was reflected in large 'residual categories' when the data were coded.

Since the strength of MacIlwaine's thesis depends on maintenance of the line of argument, from interview to questionnaire to recorded data analysis, these questions of validity are crucial. Correlation between nurses' and patients' 'support' for the categories she supplied, based on the interviews; and correlation between the rank order of 'support' and data from tape recorded interaction, are crucial to her arguments about 'appropriateness'.

The central problem in MacIlwaine's thesis is not the methodological problems I have noted, though these are sufficient to impair the study in its own terms. The central problem is theoretical and relates to the issue of 'appropriateness'. If appropriateness is the suitability of means to ends, then the ends must be known.[26] MacIlwaine's problem, shared with other nursing researchers, is that the ends of psychiatric nursing have not been defined. This is usually taken to be an issue of outcome - since no definition of 'therapeutic' is generally accepted, or therapy may not be the aim of nursing practice, it is not possible to evaluate the appropriateness of interaction. The conceptual shortcut of claiming that, in the absence of consensus on the ends of nursing, appropriateness should be judged by agreement with what is expected, does not solve the problem. It avoids the issue of justifying appropriateness: can one judge the nurses' practice to have been inappropriate on the grounds that the patients and nurses differed in their view of what the nurses did; or, can one judge it to be inappropriate on the grounds that the nurses did not do in interaction what, in interview, they said they did? Because the practical, expressive and moral enterprises (cf. Harré, 1979; see Chapter 3 below) involved in the interaction of nurses and neurotic patients are not defined, we do not know what is the appropriate behaviour for the accomplishment of acts in the furtherance of those enterprises. The issue relates to one of the main themes of this literature review: what is the basis of legitimation of practice?

The issue of appropriateness cannot be resolved by fiat. If the issue is the grounds for warranting of action in a setting, then the debate about appropriateness centres on whether the question will be settled in the setting and with the actors involved. The theoretical and methodological issues implicit in this claim are explored in Chapter 3.

Gender and diagnosis MacIlwaine does not develop an analysis of the problems of research based on diagnosis or gender. She justifies her work by indicating that if nursing of neurotic patients is problematic, it is a sizeable problem[27]. She cites her own and others' experience to suggest that nurses deprecate neurotic patients. Referring to claims about variation in diagnostic practices, she used as an operational definition of 'neurotic' any patient whose formulation[28] included terms which indicated 'neurosis'. This method of patient 'selection'[29] is based on a number of assumptions. Firstly, she accepted ward medical staff's formulations as unproblematic. Furthermore, there was no basis for thinking that the nurses considered the patients in the study as 'neurotic', or that the implications of that term were relevant to their interaction with the study patients. There was no basis for thinking that her meaning of 'neurotic', as indicated in the method of patient selection, coincided with the doctors' and nurses' 'working' usages. MacIlwaine thus relied on unexplicated background understandings to 'create' a category of patients, to whom she then applied interpretations based on largely unexplicated ordinary, psychiatric and nursing discourses. That MacIlwaine assumes the relevance of the meanings conveyed by psychiatric diagnosis is indicated by her assumption that increased knowledge of symptomatology would improve nurses' understanding and care of neurotic patients.[30]

MacIlwaine (1980) does not address the implications of gender as the basis for patient selection in her main study, beyond citing the greater frequency with which women are diagnosed as neurotic. There is no a priori ground for claiming that she should have considered the analytic significance of gender.[31] However, gender and diagnosis meet in the common-sense notion of the 'neurotic woman'. There is already an unacknowledged and unaccounted for 'dialogue' between common-sense understandings and those of the researcher, in that MacIlwaine calls on the reader to recognise what she means when she says that the nurses' understandings were those of a 'layman'. MacIlwaine thus used common sense and lay knowledge as resources in lieu of further analysis of them as topics.

The problem I am highlighting here is that in the absence of paradigmatic theoretical knowledge, common sense is the resource shared by nurses, nursing researchers and consumers of psychiatric nursing research. It is the common sense of psychiatric nursing that is always, implicitly, being debated in the literature. However, MacIlwaine, like the other researchers noted above, failed to account for the problematic character of common sense (cf. Billig et al, 1988; Garfinkel, 1967). Instead these researchers have treated language as if under the right conditions it could provide a window onto what is 'actually' being done. MacIlwaine chose to use 'objective' measures of anxiety and depression to gauge the 'accuracy' of nurses' perceptions of distress, but did not attend to the processes of interpretation which shaped the nurses' participation in the social reality of interaction.

MacIlwaine's thesis and the themes of the discourse The problems with MacIlwaine's thesis reflect problems in researching a topic the language concerning which is loaded with implications for personhood and social valuation. The very impossibility of asking neurotic patients how nurses treat 'neurotic patients' rather than 'the patients' reflects the analytic significance of the social construction of reality through language. My criticism of MacIlwaine's (1980) thesis is thus based on theoretical and methodological grounds. The two are closely connected. MacIlwaine tried to judge 'appropriateness' of nurse-neurotic patient interaction using a method based on theoretical assumptions about the relationship between face to face interaction, expressed view about a category of patients, and implications of the theoretical constructs 'anxiety', 'depression' and 'neurotic'. The consequence of decontextualisation of the data on the nurses' practice, and of omission of their interpretations of what they did in interaction, is that it is impossible to draw conclusions relevant to the practice of face to face interaction with patients. MacIlwaine's (1980) recommendations for policy changes based on her research therefore cannot be regarded as justified. I will return, when considering alternative methods, to the implications of this critique.

This critique of MacIlwaine's (1980) work recalls the discussion of studies reviewed above. Research on nursing of neurotic patients has reflected the problems and issues already discussed. The problems centre on defining the basis on which nurses act and on legitimating what nurses do as something different from what 'the layman' would do. Researchers have questioned the practice of nursing with these patients in terms of knowledge (it is just common sense), efficacy (nurses miss opportunities to help the patient) and moral quality (nurses treat these patients less well than others and judge them as lay people do).

The British researchers generally have not addressed the implications of using language to research a topic in which use of language is construed as part of the problem. Nursing researchers have routinely 'policed' the boundaries of discourse, common or lay and professional and medical, marking out the boundaries (see Robinson, 1985; and Chapman, 1987, below). They have not investigated how the nurses and patients themselves interpret talk in interaction; nor how they police the boundaries, locate themselves subjectively within the discourses, and locate each other for purposes of social construction of reality. These will be the main themes of this monograph. Before indicating the methods I chose to explore those themes, I will review literature, mainly published during the period of this research, which addresses the issues of language and discourse in nursing practice, the problems of subjectivity and interaction, and the theoretical and methodological relevance of context.

The above critique may be summarised as a claim that British psychiatric nursing literature is a discourse, or a set of discourses, in which echoes of American discourse resonate. The researchers' discourse(s) relate(s) problematically to the largely unexplicated discourses of psychiatric nursing practice. The problem of knowledge in British psychiatric nursing is not, on the basis of the above analysis, only or primarily a problem in practice. Rather, it is a problem of the theoretical stance towards and methods of investigating practice.

A review of studies which take account of language, interpretation and the context of interaction

The researchers whose works have been discussed thus far have generally decontextualised interaction, either taking accounts of interaction out of context, or focusing on individual nurses' reasons as data on interaction. Nurse-neurotic patient interaction remains largely undescribed and unexplored. I will describe in Chapter 3 the theoretical perspective of this monograph, according to which interpretation of interaction is based on understanding the intentions of the actors and the acts they intend to accomplish through their interaction, in relation to the context of interaction. From this perspective, the adequacy of researchers' 'second order' understandings depends on adequate interpretation of the actors' 'first order' understandings. In my analysis of the literature above I argued that 'common sense' was treated by researchers as a 'residual' category, used to explain what could not be accounted for as 'appropriate', 'deliberate' or theoretical understandings. The role of common sense in interaction remained unarticulated. The nurses' and patients' (and researchers') subjectivity, intersubjectivity and interpretations were not adequately taken into account. The social construction of the reality of psychiatric nursing was unexplicated, while researchers had to resort to interpretations imposed on the phenomena of interest, or to consigning the nurses' knowledge to 'common sense' construed as a residual category.

The work now to be discussed is characterised by attempts to understand interaction in terms of its meanings for actors, or as discourse, and in relation to the contexts the interaction reflexively constitutes. I will briefly review some of the key features of this literature as they are relevant to the argument of this monograph. The work will be reviewed in terms of themes of 'interpretation' and 'context'.

Interpretation and subjectivity

Kasch (1986) argues that an adequate account of nursing action is needed to link theory and practice, and advocates a symbolic interactionist stance. She considers that nursing action is related to interpretive processes and contextual factors. Kasch argues that nursing competence is a function of 'person knowledge', and using the metaphors 'nurse as implicit social scientist' and 'nurse as communication strategist' elides the distinction between practising nurse and social scientist. The nurse's definition of the situation and pursuit of goals are linked in this conception of action.

Clarke (1986) describes Shotter's 'theory of person action' and advocates its potential for development of practice.[32] Clarke uses her analysis of Shotter to advocate 'constant self monitoring' by nurses, and development of power to give explanations on different levels.[33]

Points of view I noted the limits of previous psychiatric nurse researchers' investigations of nurses' and patients' understandings. Davis (1984, p. 78) argued that 'the nursing process is pre-emptive in that it views the interaction or relationship from the point of view of the nurse...'. Wilson-Barnett (1988) criticised the emphasis in psychiatric nursing research on the nurse rather than the patient. I will review work which has added to understanding of the importance of taking account of different views of interaction in trying to describe the social reality of interaction structured by participants on the basis of their interpretations.

Kennison (1983) investigated differences in oncology nurses' and patients' understandings of the 'clinical reality of sickness'. Nurses' 'exclusion of self' cost them their tacit knowledge (cf. Polanyi, 1967). Kasch (1986) argued from an interactionist perspective that nurses and patients work to support each other's identity in interaction. Sugden (1980, p. 124) concluded that his study of psychiatric nurse-patient 'contact' should have included the 'participants' views of the process of psychiatric care'. In an American study, Vidoni (1984, p. 105) investigated 'nursing staff's recollection of the patient's behaviour prior to the seclusion episode (and) the patient's recollection of his feeling state prior to the seclusion episode'. Ruffing-Rahal (1986) advocated use of 'personal documents' on the grounds that nursing practice development depended on taking the patient's experience into account.

New understandings of context Webb (1989) critiqued narrow methodological strategies which yielded 'inadequate pictures' of social action, and advocated action research grounded in 'participant comprehension' (Collins, cited in Webb, 1989) to produce research useful to actors in changing their lives. Wooldridge (1971) argued that nursing researchers have a responsibility to develop practice theories of nursing.[34]

Clinton (1985) found that context (ward or classroom) was relevant to the kind of knowledge displayed by student nurses. He discussed the social power involved in definition of patients' needs and nursing action, and determination of 'what constituted a knowledgeable and skilled approach to nursing care' (p. 139). Bunch (1985) developed a grounded theory of how nurses in their talk with schizophrenics 'balanced the mandates' of therapy prescribed by the profession against the institutional requirement to '(conduct) business as usual'. Heyman and Shaw (1984) interpreted terms of conflict between nurses and patients in terms of ambivalence rooted in the nature of the work, rather than individual nurses' problems of communication.[35]

I have noted the theme, persistent in the literature, of nurses' 'missed opportunities'. There are two objections to this claim. Because researchers have, through their methods, decontextualised the interaction, the validity of their perception of opportunities 'missed' by the nurse cannot be evaluated. More importantly, I will argue in this monograph that the interpretation of the actor in the situation in part determines what is to count as an 'opportunity',[36] and that the claim of 'perception' made by anyone not involved in the practical setting cannot claim priority. Fielding (1982) used an ethogenic methodology (cf. Harre and Secord, 1972) to study student nurses' accounts of talk with patients. She acknowledged that she decontextualised interaction by presenting to students 'snippets' of their conversations with patients and asking them to account for their part in the interaction. She noted that understanding of the episode, crucial to ethogenic understanding because crucial to the actors in their interaction, was thus compromised. The value of these caveats is reduced when Fielding nonetheless concludes that nurses 'missed opportunities'.[37]

Benner (1984) distinguished between 'know how' and 'know that' and recommended research designed to produce 'interpretive descriptions of actual practice'.[38] She argued (p. 6) that:

> Common meanings become apparent when narrative accounts of diverse clinical situations are given with the intentions, context, and meanings intact.

Benner's (1985) phenomenological perspective emphasises the necessity of interpreting the 'background understandings' which partly constitute the phenomena of nursing. Benner's position recalls Peplau's (1952) quest for 'common understandings' through processes of self-and-other interpretation by nurse and patient. She reasserts the importance of taking account of subjectivity and interpretive practices in understanding nursing practice.

These researchers' perspectives justify making the common sense of nursing the focus of interpretive investigation: the need is to understand the common understandings of nurses and patients, not to look for congruence with a theory or criterion derived from outside the situation of interaction.

The social context of nursing practice

The work on psychiatric nursing reviewed in the first part of this chapter did not adequately take account of the social context in which interaction took place. A claim of the main theoretical perspective of this monograph is that the social context includes knowledge of the social context. The social context of nursing practice and knowledge has been addressed by recent nursing writers. Hagell (1989) argues that knowledge is related to its experiential base; and that nursing knowledge, women's knowledge founded on the experience of women in nursing practice, is devalued. She argues for a reversal of the 'hierarchy of credibility' which privileges men's scientific knowledge. Webb (1981) uses Bernstein's concept of 'framing' to refer to the 'penetration of (teachers' and pupils') everyday community knowledge' into educational knowledge. She uses the concept to discuss changes in production of nursing knowledge through the nursing process. Grypdonk (1987) has discussed, on the basis of an empirical study, the potential for loss of knowledge when nurses are required to organise their practice through writing rather than talk.

Common sense and typification work

One of the main themes in the literature on psychiatric nursing with neurotic patients is the construction of the patient as a 'type' familiar from everyday life: the 'neurotic woman'. Nurses' moral judgements and interaction were attributed to their 'inappropriate' use of lay understandings and judgement; or use of 'inappropriate lay concepts'.[39] One of the main critiques of nurses' treatment of patients diagnosed as neurotic is that they fail to acknowledge the patient's illness (John, 1961, MacIlwaine, 1980). Nursing researchers' concerns with commonsense versus professional judgement may thus be construed in terms of nurses' 'typification work'.[40] A number of researchers have investigated aspects of nurses' typifications (Kappeli, 1987), their relationship to common sense, and their role in the organisation of nursing work.

Belknap (1956) found that the day to day life of patients in an American state mental hospital was determined by (untrained) aides' classifications of them, and that work was guided more by hospital administrative classification systems than by psychiatric diagnosis. Stockwell (1972) examined nurses' identification of and behaviour towards 'popular and unpopular' patients in general wards. Kappelli (1987) argued that nurses' classification of patients determines the patients' care, 'sick' patients being seen as 'legitimate'. Pollock (1989, p. 143) found that 'how the nurses viewed and described patients affected their work'. Jeffery (1979, p. 297) observed that in a casualty department 'good' patients are seen 'in terms of their medical characteristics...whereas disvalued patients...were subject to more blatant, commonsense, moral evaluations' .

Kelly and May (1982) reviewed literature claiming that 'neurotic' patients were among those said to be typified as 'bad' patients, and claimed that the literature on 'good' and 'bad' patients was characterised by 'analytic individualism'. They proposed an 'alternative framework' which would 'view the nursing role from an interactionist perspective' (p. 154); suggesting that the attribution of the labels 'good' or 'bad' to patients may be the outcome of a process of interaction involving mutual legitimation of nurse by patient and patient by nurse (or non-legitimation). May and Kelly (1982) examined nurses' informal typifications of psychiatric patients - 'chancers, pests and poor wee souls' - and the dynamics of their attributions of responsibility and blame. Their claim (p. 291) is that 'it is more difficult for nurses to reject patients whose behaviour is attributable to their illness - hence the reluctance to define disvalued patients as irresponsible.'. They discussed Bott's (1976) analysis of hospitalisation as a form of 'control and care', and the power of patients to control others. They argued that 'in categorising some patients as "bad", nurses not only pronounce on patient performance, they reaffirm their own professional and personal values, and reinforce the functional solidarity of their group' (p. 281). They claimed (p. 292) that:

> the issue of the problem patient is bound up with the nurses' sense of professional identity...(To) acknowledge that one might actually dislike particular patients, or find some unpleasant or difficult to manage, is in essence to deny one's professionalism, since the touchstone of psychiatric nursing lies in the ability to understand, accept and manage the most bizarre, irritating or downright obnoxious behaviour.

They noted (p. 295):

> ...(The) therapeutic skills and competencies to which (the psychiatric nurse) lays claim are, at the very least, difficult to identify...(Nurses)...appeal to rather nebulous personal qualities, rather than to specific professional skills. As one staff nurse put it, 'I think psychiatry is about seventy-five percent commonsense and empathy'. This is rather an uncertain basis on which to rest claims to competency, since the possession of such qualities is all too open to dispute, or to competition from other persons or groups.

In a sociological investigation of psychiatric nursing, Towell (1975) found that nurses' work was structured differently in different settings, e.g. geriatric wards and admission wards. He found (p. 130) that:

> work-salient denotations of patients' behaviour and characteristics used by staff were more salient for daily activities...than particular diagnostic classifications.

Towell (1975) explored the relationship between definition of behaviour as action, judgement of responsibility for the action, view of patients as responsible agents, and sanctions. He argued (p. 197) that an interactive process was involved in psychiatric nurses' responsibility ascription: 'it was only with behaviour assumed to be self-willed that expressions of disapproval and reaffirmation of normative conduct could serve as means of control...'. The thrust of Towell's (1975) and May and Kelly's (1982) arguments is that legitimation (or non-legitimation) of the nurse cannot be divorced from legitimation (or non-legitimation) of the patient.

Simm (1978) analysed aspects of the social construction of the reality of psychiatric nursing, including nurses' use of the concept 'insight' and their appraisals of patients' common-sense theorisings. 'Insight' was construed (p. 258) as:

> a categorisation device employed to locate persons with respect to their capacity to engage in rational common-sense theorizing about their problem.

and (p. 261):

> The patient who is ascribed insight is one who is at least aware (and this is the necessary condition) of the rules of the social order of hospital life, which both subsist in and are infused with common-sense knowledge of the community at large.

He argued (pp. 218-219) that:

> We should regard ward order as that sense which nurses methodically seek, create and maintain through their socially organised perceptions, inferences and constructions of 'what is happening' on the ward, rather than that sense which we as social scientists impose through our own assumptions and methods.

Simm found that nurses rely on 'personal typifications' and understandings of 'normality', and analysed psychiatric nursing observation as 'scenic interpretation' on the basis of which 'time and attention are allocated'. Simm stressed nurses' dependence on 'background knowledge', acquired through socialisation, to do their work (cf. Dingwall, 1977; and Melia, 1981). His sociological analysis stands out as different from psychiatric nursing research, in its emphasis on the need to understand nurses' and patients' interpretations and common sense because these are the basis of production of the practical settings of interest to the researcher. Simm's thesis emphasises the need to understand the nurses' language-in-use in the production of the sites of practice. He argues (p. 305) that 'a sensitivity to the socially constructed nature of reality' enables 'consideration of psychiatric nursing as a corpus of practical knowledge (which) adds a new definition to our understanding of the hospital'.

Allen (1981) studied nurses' and other staff members' talk about patients in a psychiatric day unit, examining its 'function in maintaining the social structure of the unit and meeting the personal needs of the staff'. She concluded (p. 355):

> This appears to be of particular importance against the background (common to many psychiatric settings) of staff-patient and interdisciplinary role ambiguity, high patient chronicity, and the absence of many of the structural and symbolic 'props' of a conventional hospital.

Context, role and ideology

Pollock (1989) addressed the issue of typification and individual care. She discussed CPNs' difficulties in realising their 'expressed ideology of providing "individualised" care' in a context characterised by finite resources. She analysed how nurses used an ideology based on assessment and treatment to manage the contradictions in their work. Pollock argued (p. 128) that the ideology of individualised care, in conjunction with a rationale based on not fostering dependence, allowed nurses unwittingly to 'fit' patients to resources.

Chapman and non-normative nursing research: ownership of discourse, construction of subjects

Chapman's (1987,1988a) articulation of the concept of discourse and its role in the constitution of reality distinguishes her work from previous nursing researchers. In an empirical study of a therapeutic community, Chapman (1988a, p. 256) investigated how:

> utterances, talk and text form part of professional discourse; the set of meanings, beliefs and ideas which nurses...bring to their everyday professional activities.

The nurses' talk and records were 'viewed neutrally with respect to professional appropriateness' (p. 256).

Chapman (1988b, p. 16) argues that nurses participate in a discourse based on the inducement of patients to speak, surveillance and a 'grid of observation'. They 'act on the boundaries of a professional discourse which they do not control' (p. 19).[41] Chapman (1987, p. 151) found that nurses were not 'independent practitioners able to define a particular reality both in the language of observation and description and the language of explanation'. Like others who found that nurses' 'ideological' statements depended on the setting in which they practiced (cf. Strauss et al, 1964; Cormack, 1976, 1983; Towell, 1975), Chapman found that nurses in the therapeutic community were dependent on psychoanalytic theory and language. Indeed, only the nurses' 'intimacy' with psychoanalytic language distinguished them from the patients in the 'lived reality' of the setting. While they did the 'same' things (e.g. cooking), the nurses' role was construed as 'work' and the patient's in terms of 'problems' (p. 152). The nurse and patient were constructed as different kinds of person through the discourse: the nurse as rational adult, the patient as more childlike; the nurse as 'surface', there to work; the patient as having deep rooted problems.

Chapman's work opens the way in nursing research for understanding of talk in terms of location of nurses and patients as subjects in (subject to) discourse(s).[42]

Robinson and the social construction of nursing knowledge

There is a thread running through much of the work that I have reviewed: the appropriation of language. Nursing researchers take language from the producers and sites of production and subject it to an analysis or interrogation as a result of which the practising nurses' language appears 'inappropriate'. The knowledge that language is inappropriate is produced through this process of appropriation and transformation. The process of appropriation and transformation reaches its apogee in the claim that by recording conversation, correlating the recorded material with the researcher's observation of behaviour, and analysing the conversation in terms of structure, the researcher is getting 'actual conversation' (Clark, 1982). This method decontextualises interaction, freezing it for positivistic analysis. It omits analysis of power in interaction, and the 'background understandings' which constitute the meaning(s) of interaction.

Robinson (1985) addressed the issue of ownership of knowledge, in discussing the social construction of health visiting knowledge as a form of occupational knowledge.[43] She noted that occupational knowledge is 'knowledge in use', and that '(there) is little known about the relatively private articulation of professional knowledge in practice' (p. 163). She discussed (p. 169) the articulation between the occupational knowledge and the health visitors' background knowledge:

> (Health visitors in training) are...receiving tuition in the area in which commonsense lay knowledge is itself predominant, that is, social life and social relationships...(They) use their existing commonsense theories to accept, reject or modify the new knowledge.

She discusses the divergence between health visitors' knowledge and clients' knowledge in terms of 'conflict and negotiation where each perspective is presented as the only "real" view' (p. 172). She notes (pp. 183-4) that claims that knowledge is 'special' are also claims to remove from debate the question of whose knowledge is better. Thus Robinson construed the problem of nursing knowledge as a theoretical problem and a methodological problem. The theoretical problem is the social construction of nursing knowledge. The methodological problem is one of studying nurses' language in use. Robinson provides the basis for a theoretical understanding of the grounds of rationality for a practice discipline (cf. Diers, 1979; Kasch, 1986; Clarke, 1986), and for methods of research 'appropriate' for generating knowledge for a practice discipline.

The need to bring the background to the foreground

May and Kelly (1982) noted that sociological researchers had found, in general hospitals and casualty wards, that psychiatric patients were seen as 'problem patients'. However, May and Kelly caution (p. 281):

> By treating psychiatry as a residual category that substitutes for explanation we are deceived into thinking that all that is at issue is the threat to nursing routines. This is not only unfair to nurses, but glosses over a much more complex relationship...

A similar argument can be made with regard to use of the concept 'common sense' in psychiatric nursing. My argument based on this review of the literature is that there are two 'glossings' of the term. The first is the gloss by the nurses themselves in accounting to researchers for their practice. Nursing researchers regarded that gloss as unsatisfactory, on the grounds that the term is insufficiently explanatory and because claims based on reference to 'common sense' do not display what the researcher regards as the grounds of professional competence (see Altschul, 1972; Sladden, 1979; May and Kelly, 1982).

The second gloss is the researchers' labelling of the nurses' explanations as 'lay' or 'common sense'. If nurses use common sense as a residual category, so too do nursing researchers. The category is used to accommodate whatever is not 'identifiable perspective', 'professional', 'theoretical'. However, use of the category by nursing researchers is inadequately explanatory. The very vulnerability of practising nurses' claims made on the basis of 'common sense' (see May and Kelly, 1982) applies to the claims of nursing researchers as well. The difference is: practitioners gloss practical reasoning and action through reference to common sense, in a setting in which such glosses are normally legitimated; while researchers gloss theoretical explication of the nurses' practical reasoning. What is missing from the British nursing literature is an adequate theoretical account of the place of common-sense reasoning in practice, and empirical exploration of nurses' common sense. In Chapter 3 I will discuss theoretical perspectives which enable a start on work on these problems.

Recommendation of use of accounting to observe and remedy

In this chapter I have defined the body of knowledge in which the present study is located. I defined Altschul (1972) as a central work in that body of knowledge. The main terms of the discourse are present in her work. From the point of view of this study, Altschul (1972) was important in another way. She concluded her study (p196):

> In the case of this study only one aspect of psychiatric nursing was examined and the theoretical background was found to be absent.

She proposed a remedy (p.196):

> If nurses were asked to account for their interactions, junior nurses by senior nurses, and all nurses by doctors, if senior nurses were encouraged to make explicit what at present is being done without insight, a great deal of existing skill would become observable, and some lack of skill would be remedied. There seems to be an urgent need for a deliberate and conscious effort to increase communications and to increase observability of patients by nurses, of nurses by each other, and between nurses and doctors. Only then can the necessary theoretical background for effective interaction with patients become available.

The reader will recall that 'observability' was regarded as a 'precondition for exercising control over that group' (Kendall, cited in Altschul, 1972, p. 54). Altschul's suggestion can thus be read as a recommendation for greater social control of patients by nurses, and of nurses and doctors by each other.

The outcome of Altschul's analysis was that theoretical 'background' was missing and foreground 'common sense' could not be interpreted as meaningful. Accounting would be the means of remedy. However, it is unclear in what way 'theoretical background would become available' through accounting. It may be inferred that the 'theoretical background' may be located in the knowledge of senior nurses and doctors. Altschul's (1972) perspective may be contrasted with that of Benner (1984, 1985); and Benner and Wrubel (1989). Benner construes background knowledge as practical knowledge embedded in various forms of knowledge in practice. The distinction is important. Altschul may have been calling for the tacit to be made explicit, the intuitive and haphazard to be made conscious and deliberate; for greater realisation of the 'presence' of what is privileged, through increased observability.[44] However, without an adequate understanding of the distinction between practical and theoretical knowledge, it may be assumed that production of accounts would reproduce the problem of Altschul's (1972) work: how to interpret the accounts in the absence of shared background understandings?

Summary

In this chapter I have reviewed literature on psychiatric nursing, in particular that related to nursing care of neurotic patients. I have construed the central problem, the problem of the definition of psychiatric nursing, in terms of two closely related problems. The first is the problem of defining a practice-based discipline. The second is the problem of 'orders' of interpretation: the researchers' use of nurses' 'first order' constructs ('common sense') in another, 'second order', theoretical or professional discourse. The problem is that the meaning of 'first order' terms is uninterpretable after their translation from one discourse to another. This is related to the methodological problem of defining what people do in interaction (when that includes the meanings they attach to actions) on the basis of decontextualising observation or categorisation. The 'problems' of inefficacy, haphazardness, and inappropriate moral judgement may thus be interpreted as problems of practice as interpreted from certain theoretical perspectives and using certain social scientific methods.

Altschul's recommendation of accounting can be read as a call to continue in the tradition of defining psychiatric nursing as a process of observation and discipline,[45] intended to produce and reproduce a privileged theoretical discourse. Alternatively, the recommendation of accounting may be heard as a call for a reconceptualisation of nursing practice and of methods for understanding it; and a call to understand nurses' methods of making common sense through their practices. I read the recommendation in the latter sense, and this monograph is my response. The theoretical basis for this response is established in Chapter 3.[46]

Notes

1 Cf. Chapman (1987) and Robinson (1985), reviewed below.

2 Conant (1965) gathered data on 'satisfaction and the meaning of the interaction' by playing back material from interaction in separate interviews with nurse and patient, asking each for her interpretation of 'what was happening', her own and the other's feelings.

3 Altschul (1972, p. 12) cites Diers and Leonard's (1966) definition of interaction (see above).

4 It could be argued, for example, that very high rates of aversive interaction would not be expected to yield therapeutic relationships.

5 The topic of influence with reference to rhetoric (Burke, 1969a and 1969b; Szasz, 1979) will be discussed more fully below.

6 The terms 'first order' and 'second order' taken from Schuetz (1943) are explained in Chapter 3.
7 See below for discussion of Altschul's later work as it bears on this question.
8 See Garfinkel (1967); reviewed in Chapter 3.
9 Asquith, personal communication, indicated the possible usefulness of the concept 'residual category' in understanding processes of sense-making.
10 This whole problem can also be interpreted in terms of Altschul's critique of (what she saw as) the nurses' claim that their reasons were 'self-evident'. This would involve an argument about the limits of the nurses' 'self' or the authority of the nurses' 'self' in the context of critique of practice.
11 The only 'identifiable perspective' available is that provided by Altschul.
12 See also Chapter 3.
13 'Residual categories' function to account for what cannot be accounted for by other means (Asquith, personal communication).
14 The attempt to increase visibility through surveillance, in the interests of evaluating patient care, may be read in the context of a wider discourse (Clark, 1988) generating terms of accountability and judgements on appropriateness of care.
15 He did not note that nursing research constructs that 'realisation'.
16 Recourse to the concept of 'potential need' is a consequence of circular reasoning evident in the research design. The research (Cormack, 1983, p. viii) was based on '..the belief that nursing practice is designed to meet patients' nursing needs...This study starts from dual and interdependent points...by identifying patient needs by means of describing what nurses do'. This reasoning assumes the objectivity of needs. The resultant system of objectification through surveillance is a consequence of failure to take into account subjectivity and context in the nurses' work with patients.
17 Carr's comments recall Nightingale's (1924) remark that skilled nurses, who acted as observers and reporters, observe so well that patients are unaware of being observed. The role of observation is central: '...it is observation only that makes experience' (Nightingale, 1924, p. 141-142). Nightingale introduced the metaphor of 'reading patients': 'The very alphabet of a nurse is to be able to read every change which

comes over a patient's countenance, without causing him the exertion of saying what he feels.' (p. 141). Here non-verbal communication between nurse and patient is privileged over verbal communication to such an extent that Nightingale notes 'a good nurse scarcely ever asks a patient a question' (p. 147). The major shift in later nursing writers is not from privileging of observation, but toward privileging of verbal communication as the medium of observation.

18 As noted below, the terms 'neurotic patient' and 'patient diagnosed as neurotic' are used at different points in this monograph; the implication in the case of either usage being that diagnosis is regarded as problematic.

19 See below for a discussion of the problems of evaluating the reliability of diagnosis, treated as relatively unproblematic by previous psychiatric nursing researchers.

20 Altschul (1972, p. 84) followed John (1961) in suggesting that nurses preferred to care for those patients who were physically ill rather than those, among them neurotic patients, who were not.

21 He found this as well for depressed, hypomanic and paranoid patients.

22 Aspects of the study are summarised in MacIlwaine (1981) and MacIlwaine (1983).

23 She also recommended video feedback to the nurses of their interaction with these patients on the grounds that that would help them 'to begin to understand the impact of their behaviour patterns upon neurotic patients' (pp 273-4).

24 The patients were asked 'What do the nurses do for you?', not 'What do they do for you as neurotic patient?'. It is unclear whether 'you' could have been interpreted to mean all patients, the individual patient, or patients diagnosed as neurotic; while in the nurses' version the reference was clearly to 'neurotic patients' as a category. There is thus a potential lack of fit between nurses' responses (based on a categorisation of uncertain relevance to their practice), and patients' responses. It could be argued that even to consider asking the patients what the nurses did for them as 'neurotic patients' highlights issues related to the sociology of knowledge and to the fit between nurses' practice and researchers' interests. The problem relates to the avoidance of use of a term with has a pejorative connotation in everyday talk. This in turn reflects the pervasiveness of commonsense understandings by researchers

and subjects alike on this topic. The problem of psychiatric nursing of neurotic patients epitomises the problem of discourse in psychiatric nursing. It is the point where issues of language and power become acutely focused, in the policing of boundaries between psychiatric discourse and ordinary discourse.

25 The nurses' and patients' versions of the questionnaire differed. Examples of differences include: nurses' version: 'Neurotic patients don't get much satisfactory treatment here'; compared to the patients': 'Things aren't very well run here.'. A second example: nurses' version : 'The nurse is like the onlooker who sees more of the game'; and patients': 'Nurses are good to talk to because they aren't involved in your problems.'. A third example: nurses' version: 'Nurses make sure patients get their tablets on time'; and patients': 'Patients see the nurses mainly when they receive their tablets.' (pp. 374-381).

Since nurses and patients were asked different questions, grounds for arguing that their perceptions differed based on their differing responses are invalid, and all arguments depending on these data are weakened. The conclusions regarding different construction of interaction are specifically weakened. A similar conceptual problem arises in MacIlwaine's claim that the respondents 'support' the categories. Their agreement with questions selected from a set of categories devised by the researcher is not equivalent to supporting the category; rather, it is used by the researcher to support claims about the category.

The fact that the reliability of the questionnaire could not be tested because the nurses did not take it seriously and answered all questions the same also casts doubt on its validity.

The categories from interview were inadequate for analysis of recorded interaction, and when categorised in an expanded system the recorded material differed significantly from what would have been predicted on the basis of the interview and questionnaire responses. Given the doubts about the latter, however, any conclusions about the meaning of this difference must be treated with caution.

26 MacIlwaine's method yielded contradictions between what the nurses said they did and what the patients said the nurses did. This contradiction may be an artefact of the methodology, which imposed judgements of 'agreement' on statements made in different contexts for different purposes. This was a consequence

of the privileging of the researcher's position and voice over those of the respondents. The researcher had the last word. The contradiction lies in that last word.

MacIlwaine criticised Altschul's (1972) emphasis on relationship formation, on the grounds that British nurses would not be expected to base their practice on that end, since they were not trained to do so. She instead nominated communication as the main role: 'It was decided to define the nursing of neurotic patients in terms of the interaction they had with the nurses, since the nurse's role with this group of patients is largely one of communication' (p170). Her choice is no less a priori than Altschul's.

MacIlwaine focused on verbal interchange on the grounds that 'the main channel of communication in man is verbal' (Hinde, cited in MacIlwaine, 1980). This definition of the aim of nursing with these patients is not well founded, however, for it overlooks Altschul's finding that communication with them is singularly lacking, and the possibility that 'the main channel of communication' in neurotic patients may differ from that of other folk. Moreover, it overlooks the argument (cf. Robinson, 1985), that disagreement (or agreement) may be more a matter of conflict (displayed or deferred) than communication.

27 Neurotic patients comprised 18% of admissions to general hospital psychiatric units, according to MacIlwaine.

28 The formulation is the statement made by a doctor after assessment which details the grounds for diagnosis.

29 In effect this is patient 'creation' since these formulations might not have been reliably correlated with diagnosis.

30 A position antithetical to that implied by MacIlwaine's (1980) logic can be found in Kennison (1983), a thesis comparing the views of oncology patients, oncology nurses, and oncology patients who were nurses, regarding the patients' illness. The divergence of MacIlwaine's and Kennison's views reinforces the conclusion that diagnosis should be regarded as problematic in nursing research concerned with nurses' and patients' points of view.

31 However, the question of relationship between gender and diagnosis may be relevant to investigations of interaction between patients and health workers (cf. Roberts, 1985).

32 She cites Vygotsky's (1978) thesis that action develops from spontaneous behaviour to the recognition of it by another as action (action through another's agency), to making the action

one's own. This forms the basis for her advocacy of Shotter's programme to derive theory from practice and feed it back to develop practice. Shotter is said to counter analytic and methodological individualism, claiming that the grounds of responsibility for action do not lie with the individual: action depends on intelligibility to others; thus action has to be capable of being shown to accord with shared criteria. (See a related argument in Chapter 3 below.)

33 This is only one way of reading the potential usefulness for nursing of a theory of 'language acquisition' through accounting in and for practice, and I will return at the end of this monograph to discuss an alternative possibility.

34 Dickoff et al (1968) in an influential work on theory for a practice discipline, construed theory as 'a conceptual framework to some purpose' and discussed four levels of theory relevant to nursing: factor isolating, factor relating, situation relating and situation producing. They argued that nursing research should aim to be situation producing.

35 Compare this to Menzies (1970) on nurses' social defences against anxiety; and Melia's (1981) arguments about contextual factors and nurses' communication.

36 See Dreyfus (1983), reviewed in Chapter 3.

37 A main theme of this monograph is the question of the ontological status of a 'missed opportunity'

38 She suggested as strategies the investigation of: 1) graded qualitative distinctions, 2) common meanings, 3) assumptions, expectations, and sets, 4) paradigm cases and personal knowledge, 5) maxims, and 6) unexplained practices.

39 It could be argued that the objection is to their 'appropriate' use of a lay concept (that is, they mean by the term what a competent lay speaker would mean) in an 'inappropriate' context (that is, a competent nurse should not use a lay concept in that context).

40 MacIlwaine's (1980) thesis may be seen as an attempt to investigate the typification of neurotic patients, and to contrast perceptions based on this with evidence of the patient's subjectivity.

41 See also Bloor and Fonkert (1982); reviewed in Chapter 3.

42 See notes on Foucault, Chapter 3 below.

43 Occupational knowledge is defined by Robinson (1985, pp. 181-182) as 'specialised theories produced by practitioners to account for their work and their problems'.

44 Compare Melia's (1981) argument that background and context may not be observable, hence actors' understandings are required.

45 Discipline might involve the scrutinising of nurses' accounting practices to ensure their adherence to an 'identifiable perspective', through a hierarchical system of observation by accounts, a sort of 'moral panopticon' (Asquith, personal communication - see Foucault, 1979, on 'discipline' and the 'panopticon').

46 A concern shared by Robinson (1985) and Chapman (1987) is the question of ownership of discourse. This articulates with the concerns related to psychiatric nursing generally and to nursing of neurotic patients in particular. The issue of 'common sense' and the constant effort to distinguish the psychiatric nurse from the layman should be seen in the context of attempts to claim and defend a discourse justifying the claim to professionalism. Chapman (1987) introduces an opposition between ownership of discourse and borrowing of discourse, with ownership privileged. Ownership of discourse is a vital concern in a context, such as that current today in psychiatric nursing, in which knowledge is a resource in a 'free market economy'. The individual nurse is valued as a resource in relation to his or her accountability for knowledge, power and place in a moral order. In effect, the patient is valued in terms of his or her participation in the nurses' legitimating discourse. It may be argued that much of the nursing research summarised in this section marks the researchers' policing of the boundaries of nurses' discourse with lay discourse on the one hand and psychiatric discourse on the other.
This review of the literature by and on nurses was written after the empirical work and analysis had been completed. The review is an attempt to locate this monograph in relation to nursing discourse. The view of nursing I have elaborated above is the view *post hoc*. When I set out to follow Altschul's suggestion on accounting, I thought it might lead relatively unproblematically to discovery of the *langue* of psychiatric nursing through understanding the nurses' and patients' *paroles*. What I did not know, but discovered through the empirical work reported in Chapters 5, 6 and 7, is that understanding the *parole* of psychiatric nursing depends on understanding nurses' and patients' common and uncommon senses. In Chapter 3 I outline the case for considering the

accounts by nurses of their talk with patients diagnosed as neurotic, their knowledge in use, as articulations of nurses' 'working knowledge' (Harper, 1987), marked by the occasions of their production.

3 Theoretical background

Introduction

In Chapter 2 I highlighted nursing researchers' problems in understanding interaction between psychiatric nurses and neurotic patients. To appraise those problems, and to develop better methods for investigating nurse-neurotic patient interaction, I drew on theoretical and empirical work in the interpretive tradition; in particular, on theoretical understandings of accounts, interpretation and the social construction of reality. Theoretical perspective and methods are inextricably linked. In this chapter I will introduce a discussion of the theoretical background to this study by describing the shift from construing accounts as methods of 'observation' and control, to seeing them as 'tools' for work on understanding social reality. The shift in perspective can be seen by comparing two passages. The first was the passage from Altschul (1972, p. 196) (see end Chapter 2 or footnote[1]). The second is from Harré (1979, p. 186):

> If rough passages in social action are smoothed over by accounting, then lack of skill in accounting is sure to lead to a troubled life for the individual with that deficit. Perhaps one of psychiatry's functions is to provide more powerful accounting material as well as a measure of improved skill in using it. It may be that psychiatry could be a more potent technique if its practitioners made more deliberate efforts to amplify both resources for and skill at accounting.

There are similarities between the two passages. Both authors recommend 'deliberate' efforts by practitioners.[2] However, there are important differences. Accounting in Altschul's recommendation can be regarded as a means of increasing observability in line with the existing 'hierarchy of credibility', juniors accounting to seniors. The assumption underlying it is that the purpose of accounting is to 'make available' the 'theoretical background' necessary for effective practice, as a 'remedy' for practice without a theoretical perspective.[3]

Harré's concept of 'rough passages in social action', on the other hand, conjures up an image of accounts as devices for managing problems in social life. Harré talks about development of skills in accounting, indicating that accounting is itself a social practice shaped by and shaping interaction. Accounts in Harré's view are practical devices, not conduits of theoretical knowledge[4]: devices for 'smoothing rough passages'. Harré suggests possibilities for accounting as a method of developing understandings, rather than theoretical knowledge.

Below I will clarify that in Harré's view (Harré and Secord, 1972; Harré, 1979) accounts, as commonsense devices used by actors as resources for solving problems in social interaction, can be used by the social scientist as topics for analysis in developing theoretical understandings. It is possible that such a project is implicit in Altschul's (1972) suggestion. However, I juxtapose these two passages to emphasise that accounts may be construed as practical devices, and that accounts of accounts (as the psychiatrist's might be) may be of a different order. Harré's (1979) view represents a step toward understanding the theoretical and methodological issues involved in interpreting accounts, construed as practical understandings, from a theoretical perspective.[5]

I found in the work of Harré and others in the interpretive tradition ways of understanding both accounts as practical devices, and the problems of interpretation in social science. I also found what I had not found in the nursing literature: adequate concepts of action[6], the person and agency, and interpretation; and a sense of what nurses and patients might be doing in giving accounts. The most important ways in which the theoretical perspective informed this research can be summarised by explicating the use in the interpretive tradition of the concept 'account', including the distinction implied, in use of the term, between ordinary practical and theoretical understandings. In this chapter I will review some understandings of accounts, then describe aspects of the interpretive tradition, in particular the work of Harré (and Secord), Schutz, and Berger and Luckmann.

Accounts as interpretations

To understand interaction between patients and nurses I needed concepts that would enable me to 'see' it more clearly, in the sense of interpret it more clearly. What I needed in order to 'see' better were not better means of 'observation', but better conceptual lenses.[7] To introduce the main concept, 'account', as used in this thesis I will outline how the term has been used in relevant theoretical sources.

Harré and Secord's (1972) 'new paradigm' for social science was based on a 'realistic' view of science; that is, a science interested in knowing what is really responsible for the empirically observed phenomena of the world.[8] Power ascriptions locate responsibility for a phenomenon (p. 186). In scientific explanation 'conceptions of the natures of things are part of our theories of their behaviour' (p. 187). Observing is the 'kind of perceiving...described metaphorically as "reading the world"' (p. 195). The role of theory in science is to inform us about the real world by means of analogy (Harré et al, 1985).[9] This conception of theory (p. 22) is the 'first shift' toward a 'new paradigm' of social science:

> The Second Shift (from the old Paradigm) concerns the nature of the entities that are being studied and their mode of action. Conceiving of human beings as people, and their mode of action as social beings to be self-monitored rule-following, means that very different models of the processes which generate social behaviour must be used.

Conceiving of people as self-monitoring and rule-following, Harré and Secord (1972, p. 9) established a methodology based on accounts of social action given by the actors and interpreted by researchers familiar with the settings of action:

> If we follow the paradigm of non-positivist science, explaining behavioural phenomena involves identifying the generative 'mechanisms' that give rise to the behaviour. The discovery and identification of these 'mechanisms' we call *ethogeny.* We believe that the main process involved in them is self-direction according to the meaning ascribed to the situation. At the heart of the explanation of social behaviour is the identification of the meanings that underlie it. Part of the approach to discovering them involves the obtaining of accounts - the actor's own statements about why he performed the acts in question, what social meanings he gave to the

> actions of himself and others. These must be collected and analysed, often leading to the discovery of the rules that underlie the behaviour. The explanation is not complete, however, until differing accounts are negotiated and, further, put into the context of an *episode* structure. Greater precision of meaning through such procedures is analogous to greater accuracy of measurement in the physical sciences.

Thus accounts, from the ethogenic perspective (Harré and Secord, 1972), reveal the (social) cause of social behaviour, locating it in the intentions of actors, regarded as agents.[10] Harré (1981) defined 'accounting' as talk which renders action and speech 'intelligible and warrantable; that is, transparent as to meaning, and justified as occurring at the place it did' (p. 50). Accounts are 'interpretations and justifications' (p. 77).

'Accounts' render action meaningful (interpretable) in a moral order, as motivated action (cf. Burke, 1969 a). Vico (cited in Shotter, 1984, p. 131) argued that action in the social world is to be understood in terms of the projects and motives of the actors, in terms of knowledge *per caussas*; 'cause' in the social world referring to the agency of the actor, the motive. To understand someone's action, 'Why not ask them?' (Harré and Secord, 1972). The narrative responses are the proper subjects of a 'science of narration' (Vico, in Shotter, 1984).

A note on meaning

The concept of meaning which underlies the ethogenic notion of account is found in Marsh et al (1978, p. 25):

> Human behaviour enters social reality in so far as it can be given a meaning...(The) meaning of an action is the social act which the performing of the action brings about... We, as members of a culture, interpret a light kiss on the cheek as a greeting...the act is a greeting, the action is a kiss, that is a brushing of the cheek by the lips as an intended action. The act is a social entity; the action is a physical contact interpreted with respect to a certain intention, namely to greet. Thus the intention of the actor is to perform the act, and local knowledge provides him with the means to achieve it...The very same act may be performed through very different actions in other cultures.

The aim of ethogenic research (see below) is to grasp the behaviour-action-act structure underpinned by and underpinning interpretation and convention, and thus social order.

Implicit in the view that the 'local knowledge'[11] of the culture which provides the actor with the means (the meanings of his behaviour interpreted as action) to accomplish socially constituted acts is a claim for the primacy of the social over the personal: we are 'born into the conversation'.[12]

Other conceptions of accounts

In Harré and Secord's (1972) understanding of accounts can be seen some of the key meanings of the term. Actors use accounts in action or in commentary on action to interpret what was done. Thus accounts are devices used in the social construction of reality.[13] They convey something of the actor's subjectivity as well as a view of him as an agent. I will briefly discuss other meanings of 'account' used by other social scientists before turning to consider how accounts function in interaction in ways relevant to understanding this monograph.

Hammersley and Atkinson (1983) claim that accounts given by fieldwork informants can be read for information and perspective. In accounts, participant knowledge is both topic and resource. Potter and Mulkay (1985) construed accounts as 'products of (interview) participants' contextualised interpretive practices' (p. 265). People in interviews could operate two different 'accounting systems', with 'actions and beliefs flexibly characterised in terms of different accounting systems in differing interpretive contexts'. Bloor and Fonkert (1982) studied the role of accounts in processes of social construction and de-construction in therapeutic communities. They construed the systems of account-giving as socialisation processes in which the giving, hearing and negotiation of accounts was the therapy. Llewelyn (1985) studied psychotherapists' and patients' accounts of therapy and concluded that psychotherapy is essentially a process of negotiation.

The term 'account' is particularly significant in the work of ethnomethodologists (as will be discussed more fully below). Garfinkel (1968, p. 17) claims that accounts make features of settings 'seeable and reportable, i.e. accountable' for practical purposes. Talk is a constitutive feature of what is done. Wieder (1974, p. 172) argues that through a 'documentary method' an account makes the occasion of constituting the account and the normative moral order behind it:

> ...observable and reportable as patterned, recurrent, and connected instances of motivated actions in socially standardized situations. Accountings-of-social-action...are methods of giving and receiving embedded instructions for seeing and describing a social order.

Self and setting are reflexively[14] elaborated through accounting.

Accounts as practical not theoretical devices

Shotter (1984) argued that accounts are primarily practical devices, and distinguished between accounts and theories.[15] Accounts enable perception of events in the flow of time as something familiar (p. 3). They name things as what they are for practical purposes, not in theoretical terms[16]. Because accounts are practical devices, authority on what they mean rests with the author of their meaning, the account giver; with exceptions to be discussed below.

Another aspect of accounts is important for this argument. Shotter (1984, p. xi) argues in the 'social accountability thesis' that social competence lies in the ability to account for how one makes one's actions 'conformable to common sense'. Thus self expression and social accountability are linked; practical accounting being the production and hermeneutic interpretation of 'warrantable understandings from within a frame of reference' (p. 115). Like Mair (1987) and Giddens (1976), Shotter (1984, p. 218) argues that social life is both structured and structuring: 'systems of accountability speak us'.

Accounts thus function to order interaction by ordering the perception of social reality. I found it useful to think of this with the help of an example. If in bumping into someone I say 'Excuse me, it was an accident', I am giving an account which tells what the social action and act were: accident, not assault. I declare that I had no intention to bump into the person, and make a claim to be absolved from responsibility for the action. I order the action, bringing it into the frame of meaning 'ordinary accident'; and I 'order' the other person to see it for 'what it was' and to take part in ordering the subsequent interaction: acceptance of apology, rather than calling the police.

Accounts as part of decision-making processes

One feature of accounts was especially relevant in the context of this study. In accounts, actors name social actions as what they are and in doing so attribute responsibility for action. Lyman and Scott (1970, pp. 112-113) defined 'account':

> By an account, then, we refer to a statement made by a social actor to explain unanticipated or untoward behaviour - whether that behaviour is his own or that of others, and whether the proximate cause for the statement arises from the actor himself or someone else.

Because accounts can be interpreted as devices for attributing responsibility (Lyman and Scott, 1970) they play an important role in decision-making processes. The role of accounts in formal decision-making processes has been investigated by various writers. Accounts are used in processes of judgement and labelling. They may take any of the forms which Garfinkel (1967) and others (for example Baruch, 1981; Hughes, 1980) see as embodying the rationality of commonplace activities: stories, metaphors, analogies, ironies.

These devices, in particular story, enable people to grasp those features of situations (e.g. responsibility, agency, motive) necessary for the making of social judgements; and can therefore be used in formal processes of judgement, e.g. jury trials (Bennett and Feldman, 1981). The discourse of law intersects ordinary discourse through the medium of stories (Bennett and Feldman, 1981). The ability to construct accounts which 'count' as claims to value in a moral order depends on the capacity to interpret one's own and others' action and to express the interpretation in the form of accounts which accord with recognised discourse principles (Bennett and Feldman, 1981; Harré, 1983).

Accounts, deviance and diagnosis

Accounts enable judgements of deviance[17] and illness (Smith, 1978). Judgements of responsibility hinge on attribution of motive conveyed through accounts and stories. McHugh (1968) has analysed the commonsense concept of deviance, which involves judgement that the person knew what he was doing and could have done otherwise.

Goffman (1967) interpreted psychiatric symptoms as violations of social order. Accounts are called for when there has been some violation of public order (Goffman, 1967; Lyman and Scott, 1970). The understanding of diagnosis as a form of accounting is based on understanding that failure to play one's role as agent is grounds for requiring an account, given by oneself or another. The rights to give certain kinds of account are reserved to professionals (e.g. accounts of illness based on diagnosis are reserved to doctors). Hence professionals are involved in the maintenance and repair of social order; that is, in practices of social control (Parsons, 1951; Turner, 1987).

Accounts may mediate ordinary judgement and professional judgment, and convey the ordinary judgement without which professional judgement could not be accomplished (Hughes, 1980). Commonsense judgements have been found to underlie medical and nursing judgements of illness through the mediating concept of excuse from responsibility (Hughes, 1980, 1988a; Turner, 1987).

To claim that responsibility is established through diagnosis (or through 'objective' testing: MacIlwaine, 1980) is inadequately explanatory, for two reasons. Firstly, diagnosis may follow from successful attribution of responsibility or non-responsibility (cf. May and Kelly, 1982, and the empirical data presented below in Chapters 5 and 7). Secondly, the practical meaning of diagnosis depends on the interpretation of the diagnosis in the practice setting.

Accounts, accountability and moral reasoning

Because accounts are devices for determining responsibility, through explanation, justification and excuse (Lyman and Scott, 1970), they play a vital role in the social processes through which social work, medicine and nursing are accomplished. They provide the occasions and the means of moral reasoning. The concept of accountability is closely tied up with issues of discretion in provision of care (Adler and Asquith, 1981; Hughes, 1988b). Accounts are means of doing work in 'common sense situations of choice' (Garfinkel, 1967). They may display the accordance of action with practice ideologies.[18]

Accounts may provide occasions for and devices for negotiation of responsibility. I will present findings in Chapters 5, 6 and 7 indicating that, empirically, interpretation (and in some cases negotiation and determination) of responsibility was a main part of the 'work' in interaction between psychiatric nurses and neurotic patients. Accounts were the devices through which the 'work' on responsibility was reflexively accomplished.

Accounting and accountability

Because the method of this study was based in part on accounts, the concepts of accounting and accountability are important for understanding the argument of this monograph. Accounting entails, for nurses and patients, the problem of accomplishing acceptance of oneself as best authority on the reasons for one's actions. Clark (1988) argues that this problem is a central one in determination of nurses' accountability.

The concept 'accountability' as used in this monograph has two senses. In the first, accountability means the capacity and obligation, if one is called on, to display one's action as action which is socially sanctioned and in accordance with the local discourse principles (this sense being basically the same as that of Garfinkel, 1967; Harré, 1979; and Shotter, 1984). In the second sense, accountability is the obligation to display to specific others in a socially organised setting the rationality and appropriateness (in relation to the 'discourse principles' of the setting) of one's action. The first sense covers the case of a person's ordinary accountability as a member of the wider social community, and the second sense covers, for example, accountability in work settings and professional accountability (Thompson et al, 1983). Garfinkel (1967) indicates that empirically the two senses of accountability are closely related in settings organised for the accomplishment of practical purposes. Empirically, this was the case in the two psychiatric admission wards in this study.

Accounts and competence

I will discuss below the ethogenic claim that accounts can be used to investigate the competence of local actors. Harré (1979) argues that people realise social projects through action and accounts. Social settings can be understood by analysis of either, and preferably both. Accounts will only in 'the long run' give a full picture of the structures of the setting. They derive from representations in the actor of the stock of social knowledge. Accounts can be interpreted to develop competence theories, not performance theories of social action. Competence in accounting is itself a form of social competence.[19]

The meaning of 'account' in this monograph

In this monograph accounts are construed as interpretations of social action which accomplish the attribution of or relief from responsibility for social action and thus realise social acts. They are tools for defining, maintaining and repairing social reality (Berger and Luckmann, 1967); tools used to define situations and require compliance with the implications of the definitions.[20] Accounts may thus function as claims about responsibility for appearances; and, as forms of knowledge, they may be refuted. They may function in negotiation of social reality.

The methodological implications of this conceptualisation of accounts will be discussed in Chapter 4. In getting accounts from patients and nurses I intersected the 'hierarchies of credibility' (Becker, 1967) in the study sites. The stance taken in this study was that social reality is a process of interpretation and negotiation in which people act on the basis of their definitions of reality as perceived from their positions; and in which no final version of reality, no 'true' account, is possible.

The logic of this monograph in relation to the problem of nursing knowledge: accounts and rationality

I have noted above that nursing researchers called into question nurses' accounts of their interaction with patients. I construe this, using Schuetz' (1943) term, as their calling into question the nurses' rationality. To be considered as warrants that the speaker is a rational, responsible person accounts must accord with discourse principles (Harré, 1983). It can be argued on this basis that the nursing researchers' discourse principles differed from those of the practitioners.[21]

The logic of this study was that I could discover the discourse principles which structured nurses' accounts by interpreting the accounts with their speakers and in the sites of their production. The assumption was that it is in the local setting that the terms of discourse are used to do the work of the setting. I had to go into the local worlds to learn the local knowledge, reasons and reason.

Understanding common sense

In saying that the logic of this study centred on finding the nurses' discourse principles I am framing the problem of this monograph in relation to the problem I saw in the nursing literature. The issue concerns the relationship between common-sense understandings and theoretical understandings, or understandings from within a practice setting and those from outside it. The problem may be construed in terms of two rationalities.

The problem of rationalities is a problem on two levels. Schuetz (1943), Garfinkel (1967) and Harré and Secord (1972) discuss the theoretical problem of the relationship between ordinary and theoretical rationalities. I will show in this monograph that the problem of 'rationalities' was an empirical problem for nurses and patients, and will interpret the empirical problem of rationalities in light of Berger and Luckmann's (1967) analysis of the social construction of reality.

Nursing researchers did not address adequately the theoretical problem of the relationship of practical knowledge to theoretical knowledge, and of common sense to theoretical knowledge. The problem is that the order of previous nursing research has been wrong. The researchers interpreted the nurses' practical action in light of theoretical interests or concerns brought in from outside the sites of practice; rather than interpreting interaction from the nurses' and patients' own perspectives. There was little sense of the nurses' and patients' worlds and of what interaction in the intersubjective world meant to the actors. It was as if a residue of unshared 'common sense' rendered the nurses' practice opaque to the researchers.[22]

I concluded that what was missing from previous nursing research in this area - what accounted for the researchers' 'missing'[23] nurses - was adequate consideration of the problems of interpretation. The problem was one of ordering interpretations and rationalities. Nursing researchers interpreted the nurses as misinterpreting the patients and argued that nurses did not account for their own interpretations. However, the nursing researchers likewise did not account for their interpretations. More importantly, they did not account for the problems of interpretation faced by nurse and patient, and for the problem of interpreting the interaction of nurses and patients structured through their interpretations. The present study was an attempt to understand and explore these issues more fully.

To better understand what it might mean, methodologically, to interpret an already interpreted world, I turned to the literature on the social construction of reality. I found in the theoretical literature a conceptualisation of talk as a process of mutual interpretation through which reality is negotiated for the actors' mainly practical purposes.

Accounts, the interpretive paradigm and the social construction of reality

Construing accounts as linguistic devices which function to clarify what is happening by attributing responsibility is based on understandings about man and society. These views will be elaborated briefly. The views are broadly those which reflect the interpretive paradigm in studies of social life (see, for example, Wilson, 1970; Giddens, 1976; and Denzin, 1989).

Within the interpretive paradigm investigation of social life is concerned with understanding social action. Understanding of action is accomplished by a hermeneutic process of interpretation of a pre-interpreted reality.

In the interpretive paradigm both actors' and researchers' interpretations are construed as 'interpretive descriptions' (Wilson, 1970), though of different 'orders' (cf. Schuetz, 1943; Kaplan, 1964[24]; and Harré and Secord, 1972). Interpretive descriptions are not 'intersubjectively verifiable in any strong sense' since they depend on negotiation of 'a common social reality' (Emerson, and Scheff; cited in Wilson, 1970, p. 704).

Language and reality construction: the role of accounts

The interpretive perspective centres on the view that the social world is constructed through interaction mediated by people's interpretations of the shared, intersubjective world (Denzin, 1989; Schutz and Luckmann, 1974; Harré, 1979). These interpretations are structured by the discourse which shapes both subjectivity and the sense of 'reality' of the 'objective' world. Accounts are events in the discourse which interpret the situation and order action in it. Accounts shape social reality in part because they regulate others' view of the person and therefore the view the person has of self (cf. Mead, 1934). The discourse in which accounts have their social effect is primarily talk, conversation. People enter the discourse and the intersubjective social world by taking their places in the conversation. The conceptual links between subjectivity, intersubjectivity and the construction of social reality are of central importance to this study. The link is through language. The theoretical position on which this study was based maintains that social reality is an intersubjective reality sustained through interaction, mainly talk.

Social construction of reality, and the process of interpretation

The theoretical perspective that reality is socially constructed and that language is the main medium for construction of social reality was derived from several sources (Schutz and Luckmann, 1974; Harré, 1979 and 1983; Berger and Luckmann, 1967; Giddens, 1976). Social scientists' understanding of social life is understanding of a form of life which is already interpreted by the actors involved in it in light of their pragmatic purposes, structured to meet their expressive and practical ends (Harré, 1979). Social science is thus based on a 'double hermeneutic' (Giddens, 1976), involving interpretation of an already interpreted reality. The self is part of the already interpreted reality, interpreted by others (Mead, 1934; cf. Schutz, 1968).

The conception of human nature

The methodology of this study of nurses and patients in interaction implies a conception of human nature drawn from various sources (Schutz and Luckmann, 1974; Harré, 1983; Mead, 1934). People are construed as agents capable of self-direction to realise their projects. Beings with selves which are forms of social interaction (Mead, 1934), people inhabit a reality which they experience as intersubjective. They draw on common stocks of knowledge, and self-monitor to act appropriately. They are capable of reflection, ongoingly in self-monitoring of action, and retrospectively. The image is of an ongoing process of exchange, mediated by processes of interpretation, between objective and subjective reality. Thus Harré (1983) speaks of the 'thoroughgoing reciprocity of the personal and the social'. Personal being is an 'appropriation and transformation of social resources, including the local theory of selves' (Harré, 1983, p. 257). This reciprocity is a process of hermeneutic interpretation.

Subjectivity and intersubjectivity

Discourse structures subjectivity by subjecting the individual (marked by 'I' in the conversation) to the implications of discourse (Foucault, 1979, 1980, 1982; Harré, 1983; Bakhtin, 1984). Accounts are devices used to manage the appearance of the subject in the discourse and the subject's part in action structured by the discourse.

Personal being is appearance of person and self in the discourse, managed through accounts (Harré, 1983). Subjectivity is structured by the forms of subjectivity available in a society, self being a 'theory of the person' (Harré, 1983, p.26). Thus:

> I can change my personal being only if I can come to believe a theory of self derived from the concept of a person current in another and different society.

Discourse mediates the objective world and subjectivity.

The theme of a discourse which shapes the world and subjective being appears in the work of Foucault as the understanding that identity as subject/object of knowledge is constituted by or in relation to (in resistance to) a discourse which operates as knowledge/power. Foucault (1982) discussed 'ways a human being turns him or herself into a subject'. The term 'subject' in Foucault is double-edged, meaning (p. 212):

> subject to someone else by control and dependence, and tied to his own identity by a conscience or self-knowledge.

He defined a 'pastoral power' 'linked with the production of truth - the truth of the individual himself' (p. 214). Foucault saw resistance as a catalyst, bringing out the features of power, and recommended that the study of power be based on the study of resistance to power. Foucault (1979) described the link between power, knowledge and subjectivity in his analysis of the 'disciplinary society', in which people in institutions are constituted as subjects of forms of knowledge (e.g. prisoners as subjects of the knowledge of the warder and the penologist) through being subjected to the discipline of the institution.[25]

Accounts and the moral order

The notion that accounts are occasions for interpretation of self and world, and the appearance of the subject in discourse, can be construed in terms of Harré's analysis of moral order. Harré (1983, p. 245) claims that a moral order exists when people have a set of public rituals for marking respect and contempt, treat actions as displays of character, and make 'moral commentary'[26] on action to interpret and warrant it. He notes that in a moral order the rights to perform these actions are differentially distributed. Personhood and selfhood as moral statuses are achieved in moral orders, for example by showing that one is an agent capable of directing one's own action. Accounts are thus implicitly claims about personhood and selfhood. They are spoken from places in a moral order and interpreted in a shared discourse. They shape the intersubjective, shared world.

The 'thoroughgoing reciprocity of the personal and the social' (Harré, 1983, p. 270) is based on reflexivity:

> The gift of reflexivity creates personal being...(R)eflexivity and the maintenance of personal being (are) the core of...the moral orders of honour and of 'will', of personal standing and personal (as opposed to social) power.

Persons with the 'gift of reflexivity' are capable of reflexively realising the reality of social order through participation in interaction.

Harré draws on Mead's (1934) analysis of the development of responsibility and selfhood. Mead claimed that a person becomes responsible by taking the part in interaction which enables him to participate in the 'game'. Responsibility is the process of interaction in which the person takes account of the other's interpretation of self and social act and acts accordingly. This social process is internalised as the self, the interaction between the person's 'I' and their 'me'. The internalisation of the process of social interaction as self is the basis of intersubjectivity.

Harré and Secord's (1972) ethogeny

I drew on Harré and Secord's (1972) concept of 'ethogeny' in devising methods for investigating the social world of nurses and patients. The ethogenic assumption is that social life is possible as it is empirically observed because the cognitive resources of the community (ethnography) are 'represented' in community members.

Harré (1979, p. 111) states the ethogenic principle: the 'structure of the collective is represented in the cognitive resources of individual competent members'. Both actions and speeches come from a single set of social resources, a set of social skills comprising rules of action and interpretive principles (p. 163). This hypothesis justifies using analysis of action and of accounts to attribute knowledge to actors competent in the society. One can get access to the social resources through observation, and to the individual's personal meanings through analysis of accounts he gives. Empirical research is then guided by use of an analytic model which construes social action in terms of a behaviour-action-act-episode structure; and analytical concepts for study of accounts.

The methodological problems for the ethogenic researcher are: 1) grasping the structure of the social world within which the interaction takes place; 2) understanding how that world is understood by the participants in it; 3) discovering the resources they have for action, and their performances. These will be discussed more fully in the next chapter. Ethogenic research seeks to understand a reality already constituted through ordinary 'theorising'. Harré et al (1985) suggests that the aim is thus, for example, to make the 'implicit psychologies of everyday life explicit, and then, in the light of that understanding, (apply) the techniques of *theory-guided* empirical research to develop, refine and extend the body of knowledge and practice'[27]. He examines how commonsense understandings can be made both resource for and topic of understanding.

A central point of this monograph should be emphasised here. From the ethogenic perspective, social life has two aspects: action and talk. Both produce social reality; both are practical and expressive. This structure provides the researcher with two means of 'access' to understandings of social action: through observation and through interpretation of accounts.

From the ethogenic perspective people are construed as acting toward the 'achievement' of showing 'that we "willed" our actions' (Harré, 1979, p. 168, citing Mishima). Accounts play a part in this by showing that one's 'acting rightly in the right circumstances', or competence, is rooted in cognitive resources which represent the local ethnography (p. 182). Accounting is a skill. Accounts 'smooth rough passages in social life' by clarifying the meaning of action and justifying or excusing it. The adoption of an 'agentive' view is, Harré argues (p. 267), a moral rather than an empirical or philosophical issue; yielding a set of consequences for how one views, investigates and adopts policies toward others. Harré claims that 'part of what it is to have a place in a social order as a personal being is to be able to contribute to the conversation...some disclosure of thoughts and feelings that are uniquely ours' (p. 283).

The method of ethogenic analysis will be discussed in Chapter 4. Harré (1981, p. 150) recognises that accounts 'gloss' action: 'attribution passes through impression management' (cf. Garfinkel, 1967). Account analysis is only 'unproblematic' as a competence theory, not as a performance theory.

A key ethogenic principle is Vygotsky's maxim that investigators should not adopt methods of analysis that destroy the property of the structure being investigated (Harré, 1978, p. 52). The essential property of social life is that it is created by actors related through intersubjectivity and interested in producing and reproducing the world for their purposes. Methods which destroy important aspects of this structure, for example, by imposing methodological or analytic individualism on 'subjects', are inappropriate for illuminating important aspects of social reality. In the following section I will explore some theoretical understandings related to understanding the 'paramount reality' (Schuetz, 1943) of the intersubjective 'lifeworld' and commonsense understanding. One of the main conclusions of this monograph (see Chapter 8) is that the most important property of the structure of social life in psychiatric admission wards is its character as the paramount reality of everyday life.

Schutz

Because one of the main problems faced by previous researchers was understanding the common sense of nurses, I drew on Schutz' (Schutz and Luckmann, 1974; Schutz, 1968) phenomenological understanding of the ordinary world of day to day life. His work enables understanding of the basis of commonsense knowledge, and forms the backdrop for two other lines of thinking which informed the perspective of this study: the 'social construction of reality' argument, and ethnomethodology.

Among the themes from Schutz' work important to the argument of this monograph is his distinction between commonsense understanding and scientific theorising. He rooted this distinction in a phenomenological analysis of the 'attitudes' and 'interests' of ordinary life and science. From a phenomenological viewpoint, these different interests and perspectives constitute different 'provinces of meaning'.[28]

Schutz and Luckmann (1974) describe 'orders of reality' constituted not through 'ontological structures of their objects' but through the meanings of actors' experiences. The actor understands and acts in his world, construing it from the point of view of its relevance to his projects. Ordinary life is experienced as a succession of typical experiences, for dealing with which the actor has a stock of mainly pre-theoretical knowledge. In pre-scientific thinking, typifications 'depend upon my problem at hand for the definition and solution of which the type has been found' (McHugh, 1968, p. 16).

Schutz and Luckmann elaborate the 'rationalities' that constitute knowledge in the different 'orders' of reality. Ordinary life is the 'paramount' order of reality, the order governed by the 'natural attitude'. The natural attitude in ordinary life is characterised by an assumption of intersubjectivity and a suspension of doubt that the world is as it is perceived and understood by the actor in the world. In the natural attitude, the knowledge that suffices is common sense, the knowledge that enables one to find his way in the primary reality.

Schuetz (1943) argued that scientific and practical rationalities are based on different 'interests'. Practical action, ordinary action in 'the lifeworld' is based on typification and the use of 'cookery-book knowledge'.

Scientific rationality is distinguished from practical rationality; e.g. it requires that statements be logically consistent. The differences between the rationalities are explicable in terms of the differences between the ontological conditions under which the actor lives in the natural attitude and the scientist lives in the theoretical attitude. The scientist constructs 'puppets' which represent real actors, but are not subject to the ontological conditions of the lifeworld.

Schuetz (1943, p. 147) argues that because the natural attitude is primary, the test of adequacy of social scientific description of social life (the 'postulate of adequacy'; cf. Harré) is that it should be 'reasonable and understandable for the actor himself, as well as for his fellow men'. The principal aim of social science research is to interpret those meanings that constitute the reality of ordinary life, and to explain social action, taking account of the meanings given it by actors (cited in Bernstein, 1976, p. 139):

> It is (the) thought objects of (men) which determine their behaviour by motivating it. The thought objects constructed by the social scientist, in order to grasp this social reality, have to be founded upon the thought objects constructed by the common-sense thinking of men...Thus, the constructs of the social sciences are, so to speak, constructs of the second degree, that is constructs of the constructs made by actors on the social scene, whose behaviour the social scientist has to observe and explain in accordance with the procedural rules of his science.

In the theoretical attitude, doubt that the world is as it is perceived is a methodological principle, but in the natural attitude that doubt is suspended.[29]

The concept of 'adequacy' casts light back onto the nursing research which consistently found nurses' accounts 'inappropriate'. The inadequacy, in terms of social scientific explanation, may lie in the second order understandings of researchers, insofar as they do not enable understanding from the perspective of the actors.

Understanding, not truth as the aim of interpretive research

The aim of ethogenic and other interpretive research is not truth but understanding. Harré and Secord (1972, p. 236) argue that:

> ...the demand for final, absolute, unrevisable *truth* cannot be met (in the physical sciences or ethogeny). In ethogeny it is not even viable as a theoretical ideal. The possibility of endless reinterpretation must remain and it must always be admitted that each interpretation has some explanatory power.

The process of interpretation and negotiation of understandings is hermeneutic (Ricoeur, 1971). If accounts are seen as representations of the meaning systems of those who give them, then veracity is not the crucial issue.[30] Discrepancies of meaning are guides to locating the positions of account givers in relation to each other and to the researcher within the larger social field.

Social construction of reality

I drew on two lines of theoretical development which flowed from Schutz' work - Berger and Luckmann's 'social construction of reality' thesis, and ethnomethodology.

I interpreted the nurses' and patients' accounts of conversations and my empirical observations of the construction of the 'reality' of the sites, using Berger and Luckmann's (1967) ideas on the sociology of knowledge and the social construction of reality. Berger and Luckmann argue (p. 27) that:

> The theoretical formulations of reality...do not exhaust what is 'real' for the members of a society. Since this is so, the sociology of knowledge must first of all concern itself with what people 'know' as 'reality' in their everyday, non- or pre-theoretical lives. In other words, common-sense 'knowledge' rather than 'ideas' must be the central focus for the sociology

> of knowledge. It is precisely this 'knowledge' that constitutes the fabric of meaning without which no society could exist. The sociology of knowledge, therefore, must concern itself with the social construction of reality.

They construe the social construction of reality as a dialectic process. People in expressing themselves produce objects ('externalisation'). These products, now social products, are regarded as part of objective reality: they are 'objectivated'. They are apprehended as part of reality (but not as socially constructed) and internalised during socialisation. They thus become subjectively real. Thus: *'Society is a human product. Society is an objective reality. Man is a social product.'* (p. 79). Part of the reality that is objectivated is knowledge that knowledge is socially distributed; that there are experts; and that one is oneself a different kind of person as understood in the terms of a different kind of knowledge. To understand the dialectic process it is necessary to gather data on all three aspects of the process: ideology, subjective understanding and action.[31]

Language

Berger and Luckmann argue (p. 84) that:

> Knowledge...is at the heart of the fundamental dialectic of society. It 'programmes' the channels in which externalization produces an objective world. It objectifies this world through language...It is internalized again as objectively valid truth in the course of socialization. Knowledge about society is thus a realization in the double sense of the word, in the sense of apprehending the objectivated social reality, and in the sense of ongoingly producing this reality.

Language enables people to typify the acts and the actors which constitute 'institutions'. Routine, typical action requires no further interpretation. Non-typical situations are handled through interpretation in terms of something else in the repertoire of the actors. Knowledge is used to 'maintain and repair' the social order. Accounts are forms of repair, clarifying what is responsible for the disruption to reality and indicating the required remedy.

Knowledge is thus essential to the production, reproduction, maintenance and repair of social order. But Berger and Luckmann (1967, p. 83) argue:

> theoretical knowledge is only a small and by no means the most important part of what passes for knowledge in a society...The primary knowledge about the institutional order is knowledge on the pre-theoretical level. It is the sum total of 'what everybody knows about' a social world.

From the interpretive perspective, conversation is to be understood as social construction of reality through talk.

Knowledge of knowledge: legitimation

Berger and Luckmann (1967, p. 110) describe 'legitimation' as the use of 'second order' objectivations of meaning to highlight the objectivity of first order objectivations and make them subjectively plausible. Legitimations confirm that things are what they are and are as they ought to be. The highest form of legitimation involves construction of 'symbolic universes'. In these, experiences belonging to different systems of reality are ordered in the same universe of meaning. The principal symbolic universe is the one which orders all spheres of meaning in relation to the paramount reality of everyday life (p. 116). I will argue in this monograph that the paramount reality for psychiatric nurses and patients is that of the common sense of the community. The creation of a symbolic universe, claim Berger and Luckman, puts everything 'in its place' and provides a site to which 'strays' from the primary reality can return. The symbolic universe confirms the correctness of objective reality and is internalised to confirm subjective identity.

Reality construction, maintenance and repair

Berger and Luckmann (1967) argue that reality maintenance procedures will include methods for dealing with alternative symbolic universes: 'conceptual machineries of universe maintenance'. The reality will include experts in reality definition. Their methods include the process of 'therapy', or applying legitimating apparatuses to individual cases. A system of therapy needs a theory of deviance, a diagnostic apparatus and a conceptual system for the 'cure of souls' (p. 131). An alternative to 'therapy' is 'nihilation', in which the alternative reality is symbolically (or literally) annihilated.

Subjective reality maintenance

The 'other side' of the construction of reality thesis is that subjective identity is formed through internalisation of objectivated reality.[32] Berger and Luckmann (1967, p. 172) argue that routine maintenance and repair of subjective reality is accomplished through conversation:

> The most important vehicle of reality-maintenance is conversation...It is important to stress...that the greater part of reality-maintenance in conversation is implicit. Most conversation does not in so many words define the nature of the world. Rather, it takes place against the background of a world that is silently taken for granted.

In interpreting the empirical data of this study I used Berger and Luckmann's thesis for understandings of the process of legitimation and maintenance and repair of reality, both objective and subjective.

Ethnomethodologists

I drew on the work of ethnomethodologists to understand features of the relationship between knowledge, language, reality and accountability. The ethnomethodologists used Schutz' analysis of the difference between scientific and everyday rationalities to investigate how people organise their actions in practical settings to make the actions accountable as features of the settings. More broadly they offer understandings of the methods by which realities are constructed and ordered, and the moralities associated with maintaining the paramount status of everyday life.

I took from the ethnomethodologists ideas on: 1) how nurses organise practical settings[33]; and 2) how they maintain the common sense of the lifeworld.

Since maintenance of the order of common-sense reality depends on background understandings which are never fully interpretable ('hermeneutic circle') the ethnomethodologists take as the primary task of the sociologist the investigation of the methods through which background understandings are drawn on to produce common understandings. Since those methods work to maintain the flow of interaction and constitute reality, studying them involves investigating breakdowns in reality, forms of 'trouble' (Garfinkel, 1967).

Some themes from the ethnomethodologists: indexicality, documentary method

I took from the the ethnomethodologists some concepts useful for interpreting features of everyday interaction. To maintain ordinary interaction and the reality of everyday life, ordinary actors in practice use language to make sense within the flow of action and experience. 'Indexical' expressions or actions are those the meaning of which is tied to the situation of their production. Examples are terms like 'I', 'there', 'today'; the meaning of which on any occasion of use depends on understanding of the situation of use. The meaning of the terms depends on 'documentary' interpretation which takes account of background understandings and other features of the situation. Reflexivity refers to the characteristic use of language to refer to and constitute certain features of the settings and hence render them 'accountable'; that is, to be taken into account in understanding the setting as what it is. Reflexivity is an essential feature of practical rationality.[34] Reflexivity refers both to the characteristic of the self, that it is both a subject and an object in the world; and to the characteristic of features of objective reality, that they are constituted as known through the process which recognises them as features of reality. Language mediates the reflexively known self and the reflexively known world.

Garfinkel (1967) argues that members of practical settings are morally obliged to use common-sense understandings to maintain the reality of everyday life and the definition of the situation.[35] The work of interpretation is accomplished using the 'documentary method' (attributed to Mannheim)[36]. Interpretation is based not on matching sets of content, but on an 'inner-temporal course of interpretive work' (p. 24), involving understanding how the speaker was speaking as well as that he was speaking and what was said. I will use the concept to interpret aspects of nurses' and patients' 'work'.

I drew on Garfinkel to illuminate understandings of the 'mutual work' done by nurses and patients in psychiatric admission wards. Interpretive work included the elaboration of meaning of indexical statements about what 'reality' was and whether 'I' could do something, and an 'inner-temporal course of interpretive work'. Accounts of practice, including records, are part of the operations of the setting, and do not unproblematically reveal it.

Accounts as data for understanding rationalities

The theoretical understandings outlined above led me to use accounts as data on the rationalities of the sites. In accounts nurses and patients used concepts like 'reality', 'illness', 'problems' and 'responsibility' to constitute these features of practical life. Garfinkel (1967, p. 34) notes:

> In exactly the ways that a setting is organized, it *consists* of members' methods for making evident that settings' ways as...rational conventions...*consists* of methods whereby its members are provided with accounts of the setting...as accountable events.

The theoretical problem in understanding practical settings is how to make sense of how the members make sense. The ethnomethodologists argue that because common-sense understandings depend on shared interpretive work, they cannot become available for theoretical investigation unless their properties are revealed through breakdown or through the investigator becoming 'a stranger to the "life as usual" character of everyday scenes, or (becoming) estranged from them' (Garfinkel, 1967, p. 37).[37]

Mutual work of rationality as moral work

Garfinkel (1967, p. 53) argues that the 'mutual work' participants in practical settings perform to maintain the settings as accountable is moral work:

> Common sense knowledge of the facts of social life for the members of the society is institutionalized knowledge of the real world...in the manner of a self-fulfilling prophecy the features of the real society are produced by persons' motivated compliance with these background expectancies.

I will argue from the data that the nurses are mainly interested, not in a scientific attitude, but in enforcement of the 'paramount' reality. I will argue that nurses maintain the sites as 'institutionalised knowledge of the real world', and in doing so they depend on 'common sense facts of social life'.

A conception of narrative useful for understanding nurses' work

I have discussed the concept 'account'. In interpreting the data of this study I also drew on understandings of 'narrative' and 'story' to interpret nurses' and patients' accounts as forms of what 'passes' for knowledge in practice. I drew on work by Burke (1969a), Bennett and Feldman (1981), and Mair (1987, 1989) in understanding narrative, metaphor and story, as well as accounts.

Burke's (1969a and 1969b) work highlighted links between narrative and agency in the microprocesses of discourse. Burke (1969a, p. xv) asks 'What is involved, when we say what people are doing and why they are doing it?' and claims that the answer lies in the attribution of motives, accomplished through use of the 'dramatic pentad' of dramatism: act, scene, agent, agency, purpose. These correspond to the classical categories of who, what, when, where, why and by what means. In answering the question, one tells a story. In telling the story one makes claims about reality. The 'ratios' between the terms of the pentad determine the meaning of narrative. People in telling stories create the conditions for ordinary ethogenic interpretations of social reality, what is responsible for an event (cf. Harré, 1970). Through narrative they establish episodes, acts, actions, actors and their motives. I will explore in this monograph the function of narrative and interpretation of narrative in attribution of responsibility.

Bennett and Feldman (1981, p. 4) analysed the function of stories ('capsule versions of reality') in the administration of justice in American jury trials:

> (F)ormal justice procedures...must engage some parallel form of social judgment that anchors legal questions in everyday understandings...(A) particular everyday judgment and communication device, the story, fits into a formal scheme of legal judgment...The story is an everyday form of communication that enables a diverse cast of courtroom characters to follow the development of a case and reason about the issues in it.

I am arguing that stories are used in a similar way in the 'social judgement' processes which comprise assessment and treatment of the patients in this study. Stories provide the means for recognising violations of social order (Erikson, 1968; Smith, 1978), and for relating these to categories enabling psychiatric nursing judgement and response (cf. Scheff, 1966).

I will explore the usefulness of construing narrative as understood by Burke (1969a), and story, metaphor and accounts, as bases of nurses' knowledge, description and explanation of their interaction with patients. To anticipate the argument of this monograph, nurses' practice is seen as forms of response to two questions: 'Why is she here now?' and 'What do we have to do for her?'. The responses to these questions may be narratives or action guided by metaphors, both of which display the meanings of action for interpretation by other actors.

Narrative and cognitive-emotional understanding: feelings and emotional reality

Denzin (1989) uses analysis of narrative and hermeneutic interpretation to define an 'interpretive interactionist' perspective suitable for understanding 'cognitive-emotional' reality. His analysis is relevant to interpretation of accounts of interaction between psychiatric patients and nurses. Berger and Luckmann (1967) theorise that disruptions of subjective reality will be accompanied by disturbed affect. Harré (1979) has investigated the social construction of emotion. Hochschild (1983) discussed the 'signal function' of feelings, the role of feelings in apprehension of reality; and the interaction between feelings and perception of reality. She articulated the concepts of 'emotional labour' and 'emotional work', the hidden work people do on their feelings in order to function socially or in paid labour.[38]

Accounts and personhood: of agency and patienthood

It is now necessary to draw together some of the key arguments of this chapter. I have discussed accounts, and how they may function in a 'new paradigm' realistic 'account' of social interaction. I have discussed the distinction between first and second order interpretations and the relationship of common sense and theory. I used these understandings in devising methods and forms of analysis suitable for understanding the empirical data of this study (see Chapter 4 below).

I have discussed some understandings of accounts, including their role in enabling actors to attribute and determine responsibility. Harré and Secord's (1972, p. 84) 'motto' for a 'realistic' social science was 'for scientific purposes, treat people as if they were human beings'; that is, as the kinds of being they are with the kinds of powers and potentials human beings have. Harré and

Secord (1972) and Harré (1983) explicate the concept of human powers in terms useful for understanding nurses and patients in interaction. According to Harré and Secord (1972, p. 246):

> One who has a generic power is an agent; he is one who initiates his own performances, that is explanations of their genesis terminates with such items as the wants, needs or intentions of that individual.

They say (pp. 247-8) regarding patienthood (characterised by 'succumbing to a liability'):

> There is nothing mysterious about being an agent. It has to do with the balance between and changes in external and internal, intrinsic and extrinsic conditions in the accounts that are given of the genesis of action...One who is an agent must figure as the source of his action in his or our account of it, while he who succumbs to a liability may either have 'only himself to blame', as we say, or it may be that in accounting for the manifestation of the liability, we look for the source in circumstances external to himself.

Accounts that make 'not acting' intelligible include (p. 243):

> 1. 'Not wanting' is the back-stop which preserves our status as an agent when we fail to act when the enabling conditions have been fulfilled. 2. 'Not being able to bring oneself to' claims the complementary status of a patient, but preserves the conceptual system intact. 3. All those items, the non-obtaining of which prevents the exercise of powers in action, but which lie outside the person, we lump together as circumstances.

The concept 'account' links the concepts 'agent', 'patient' and 'power'. The facility to give accounts demonstrating agency is one mark of an agent, entitling the agent to respect in a moral order in which agency is valued (Harré, 1983).

A note on rhetoric

In discussing aspects of what may be involved in regarding accounts as 'demonstrations' of agency, I will argue in later chapters that nurses' and patients' talk may be construed as rhetoric. Burke (1969b, p. 46) explored aspects of rhetoric, which he construed as: 'the art of persuasion, or a study of the means of persuasion available for any given situation'. He claimed (p. 43) that:

> ...(Rhetoric) as such is not rooted in any past condition of human society. It is rooted in an essential function of language itself, a function that is wholly realistic, and is continually born anew; the use of language as a symbolic means of inducing cooperation in beings that by nature respond to symbols.

The interpretation of rhetoric as persuasion has been echoed more recently by Szasz (1979). Szasz (1979, p. 12) construed rhetoric as 'a certain kind of conversation'. He cited Entralgo's view that 'the persuasive word could heal or harm depending on the intentions of the user' (Szasz, 1979, p. 13); and Aristotle's argument that rhetoric is 'concerned with such things as come within the general ken of all men and belong to no definite science' (Aristotle, cited in Szasz, 1979, p. 13). Szasz noted the distinction between the noble and the base rhetorician, the latter mis-portraying the world by depicting 'cause without consequence or consequence without cause, acts without agents and agents without agency (thus blocking) definition and cause-and-effect reasoning' (Weaver, cited in Szasz, 1979, p. 20).

An ideology of work

I have described the interpretive perspective as one which emphasises attending to the social context of interaction. The reflexive relationship between interaction and institution is a key concern of all of the main theorists on whose work I have drawn. A main conclusion is that understandings of social reality in practical settings should be based on actors' interpretations, among other sorts of data, including understandings available to the researcher through interaction in the social reality.

The concepts discussed in this chapter - accounts, interpretation, subjectivity, the social construction of reality - can be drawn on to argue that the problem with previous nursing research into interaction between nurses and neurotic patients was that the researchers did not adequately interpret nurses' and patients' accounts in the settings the nurses and patients reflexively realised through their interaction. The problems arose in using accounts to interpret interaction, when the accounts could be construed as devices for attributing responsibility for what really happened. Previous researchers did not interpret the interaction as a form of social life, realising a social world.

Previous nursing researchers have not shown empirically how the nurse, who did not draw on theoretical knowledge, managed to work with patients. I will argue on the basis of empirical data that the nurses' and patients' 'work' was a form of accounting and making sense; and that the rationality of the nurses' work with these patients consisted of the way that claims of agency and patienthood were managed in practical settings.

I used the concepts to investigate the practical 'work' of the nurses and patients as interpreted through their accounts and through fieldwork. Peplau (1978) laid the grounds for the interpretation of the 'work' of psychiatric nurses through her claim that mental illness is the work the patient needs to do to get better, and that the nurses' work depends on the patient's work (cf. Altschul 1978; Altschul, 1980; 1984a and 1984b).

I will argue that the concepts of 'work' and the 'working relationship' were elements in a working ideology mediated by accounts, stories and metaphors, structured by and structuring the administrative practices of the sites (cf. Smith, 1980).

I will argue that the metaphors, stories and accounts had as their topic and served as resources for the accomplishment of responsibility in interaction between nurses and patients. These devices functioned to link the experience of the patient to the processes of practical judgement and decision-making in the sites (cf. Denzin, 1989). They linked narratives of 'troubles' to the administrative processes of assessment and treatment (cf. Bennett and Feldman, 1981).

The ability to construct reality through attribution of responsibility is not one-way. I will emphasise that access to patients' accounts opens the door to alternative constructions of responsibility. Nonetheless, the power to make accounts 'stick' (Giddens, 1976; Mair, 1987) is unequally distributed. The realisation of patients as patients (patients, not responsible) and nurses as nurses (responsible agents) is a dynamic accomplishment.

I explored the empirical data on determination of responsibility, in the first instance a practical matter, using these theoretical concepts. I focused on how the determination of 'powers' was accomplished through practices of accounting, the 'microphysics' of power (Foucault, 1979, p. 139) exercised at the 'capillaries' of the institution (Foucault, 1980, p. 96), in face to face interaction in which 'will' was negotiated and contested.[39]

I will argue that responsibility is something not only negotiated, but shaped by nurses in their interaction with the patients, and that this is indeed the work of nurses and patients in the sites. Accounts were the main devices through which the work of the sites was reflexively accomplished. I will interpret the 'rationality' of that 'work', construed in the sense defined by Harré (1983, p. 271):

> Only within moralities of honour and reflexive power can we give an account of person-making as a moral activity...To be rational is to display one's actions as being in accord with some socially valued discourse principle...To display oneself as rational is to make a sustainable claim to worth...

and Harré (1983, p. 272):

> Value accrues to human beings just in so far as they are seen to be intentional actors because by that alone they can lay claim to personhood, to a place in a moral order. This is not because they are then seen to be responsible for good actions, but because of the respect due to beings who are capable of planning and acting...

Accounts as devices for maintenance and repair of social reality

If intentionality and responsibility are the webs that hold action together as meaningful action, rather than just behaviour, then the importance of accounts for the maintenance and repair of reality is clear. Accounts are the devices through which people accomplish their appearance as agents or patients when this is called into doubt.

I intend the term 'appearance' to recall the 'dramatist'[40] notion that narratives and accounts enable people to play their parts in social life through processes of symbolisation. Thus I will argue that the appearance of patients in one site as characters in stories in which they were helped to a certain point but then had to help themselves accomplish some process of development or progress, may be compared with the accounts in another site which focused on deliberation on questions of responsibility.[41] The two primary questions from which practices sprang - 'Why is she here now?' and 'What do we have to do for her?' - occasioned different responses in different settings.

Accounts name behaviour as action and thus render it interpretable in the local system of meaning. They function to maintain the local setting by calling into play interpretations based on local knowledge. When such interpretation fails, legitimating accounts are called for that order systems of meaning, rendering an account in one system interpretable in another; for example, an account of inability interpreted as a sign of illness. This is the role of accounts in maintaining and repairing reality. By rendering things -

people, action - intepretable they bring them 'into play' linguistically and otherwise symbolically.

Accounts thus 'smooth rough passages in social life' (Harré, 1979). In terms of the narrative metaphor, the smoothing of the rough passages allows the story to proceed. Accounts restore the sense of the story, the rationality of life. I will argue that nurses used knowledge of the methods of maintaining and repairing mutual understanding, that is, knowledge of accounts and accounting practices (including calling on patients to participate in 'my (Note: the nurse's) reality'; using stories and metaphors), to cultivate (practical) rationality or to investigate troubles with rationality.

Summary

In this study I looked at interaction from a 'social construction of reality' perspective. The concept 'account' is a lynchpin of the method and argument of this monograph. Accounts are spoken in people's voices, in inherited language,[42] from the centres of their worlds. They interpret the world, define reality from that perspective.

Subjective reality as well as objective reality is constructed. People are 'grown' (Harré, 1983; Shotter, 1984). Individuals, sites of subjectivity, are effects of power and vehicles of power (Foucault, 1979, 1980, 1982). The subjectivity of individuals reflects the social construction of reality. The implication of this perspective for the argument of this monograph is that the microcosm of nurse-patient interaction can be taken as reflecting the broader world of nursing and the broader social reality. Subjective and objective reality are ordered through knowledge conveyed mainly in talk.

People draw on knowledge to order interaction. When problems arise, they use accounts to interpret social reality and negotiate intersubjective reality. Accounts, too, are ordered.[43] Accounts by 'experts' may be used to solve social problems e.g. the account of a doctor accomplishing relief from an obligation to work. Accounts by experts may 'order' realities: interpreting something as 'illness' rather than 'one of those things'. The hierarchy of credibility of knowledge is associated with power to interpret and order reality, to shape and create social reality. Some accounts count more than others. Professional and scientific accounts may be privileged in construction of reality. The adequacy of accounts in accomplishing order, 'smoothing rough passages in social action' (Harré, 1979) is a matter for empirical investigation.

I began this chapter by claiming that previous empirical work by nursing researchers into interaction between nurses and neurotic patients had not addressed adequately the question of the relationship between theory and observed practice. I construed the problem in terms of 'orders' of interpretation. The theoretical perspective outlined in this chapter justifies a study aimed at understanding interaction between nurses and patients diagnosed as neurotic through interpretation of the accounts given in their voices, from the centres of their worlds, illuminating their perspectives on the social reality they create in their interaction. This is one way to understanding, not truth.

Notes

1 Altschul (1972, p. 196): 'If nurses were asked to account for their interactions, junior nurses by senior nurses, and all nurses by doctors, if senior nurses were encouraged to make explicit what at present is being done without insight, a great deal of existing skill would become observable, and some lack of skill would be remedied. There seems to be an urgent need for a deliberate and conscious effort to increase communications and to increase observability of patients by nurses, of nurses by each other, and between nurses and doctors. Only then can the necessary theoretical background for effective interaction with patients become available.'

2 Harré's focus on psychiatrists does not preclude applying the same analysis to psychiatric nurses.

3 This emphasis can be found in Altschul (1972, p. 193): 'Ordinary human relations of liking and disliking are bound to occur and their existence needs to be acknowledged. Understanding and control of such relationships, and their conversion into therapeutic relationships can only occur, as Kendall points out, if they are observable. Not all psychiatrists would wish to exert control over nurse-patient relationships, their psychiatric orientation might not include a belief that nurse-patient relationships are relevant to treatment.'

4 The distinction I make here is somewhat simplified, since I will note below that the research programme of Harré's ethogenics (Harré and Secord, 1972) is based on use of accounts to generate material for 'second order' theoretical interpretation.

5 See below, the discussion on 'first order' and 'second order' interpretations.

6 An exception in the nursing literature is Kasch (1986).
7 Harré (1970) claims that in a realistic science, 'precision of concepts corresponds to accuracy of measurement'.
8 Harré's (1970, p. 185) argument is that scientific descriptions are 'power attributions', not attributions of qualities. He acknowledges Kenneth Burke's influence.
9 Harré et al's (1985) argument is that in a realistic or explanatory science, analytical models enable observation of patterns. Boyle's use of an analogy - air can be compressed like a spring - enabled observation of pressure-volume correlation. Source models are used to describe the source of patterns observed through use of analytic models. Darwin's theory of natural selection, for example, drew on the source model of domestic selection (gardening).
10 I will return to a fuller discussion of Harré and Secord's (1972) understanding of the role of accounts in determining agency and patienthood.
11 Previous nursing researchers using methods and analyses which decontextualised action and talk could not provide a sense of nurses' 'local meanings', the basis of 'common sense'.
12 I have tried to locate the source of this phrase, considering that it might be Harré, Shotter or Mair. I have found it in none of my sources. Mair (personal communication) thinks it could be his phrase or mine. It is unattributable at present.
13 See below for fuller account of the 'social construction of reality' thesis.
14 For a definition of the meaning of 'reflexivity' see below.
15 The justification for the methodology of this study was that the primary aim in nursing research is to understand practice. Investigation of the 'theoretical background' to or in accounts (Altschul, 1972) must be deferred until understanding of accounts as practice has been accomplished.
16 A problem with previous nursing research was that it treated accounts as if they were meant to be theorisings, interpretable in terms of scientific rationality (see Schuetz, 1943, discussed below).
17 The role of accounts in legitimation can be seen in studies of deviance construction, largely within the symbolic interactionist tradition (McHugh, 1968; Scheff, 1966; Rubington and Weinberg, 1987).

18 See for example Smith (1980) in social work; and Towell (1975) and Pollock (1989) in psychiatric nursing settings, on how practice ideologies articulate with practices of need assessment.

19 See the discussion at the beginning of this chapter.

20 People are able to use accounts to do this because the structure of situations is known collectively, intersubjectively (Schutz and Luckmann, 1974).

21 Accounts, being reflexively related to discourse principles, cannot be the grounds for determining the validity of discourse principles.

22 See the critique of Altschul (1972) in Chapter 2 above.

23 Nursing researchers looked for and did not find 'responsible use of words'; found 'missed opportunities'. They found, not nursing, but 'lay' practices; but did not interpret these in relation to other 'lay' practices. They did not interpret the moral orders of the settings of nurse-patient interaction in relation to other moral orders. Previous studies of nurse-neurotic patient interaction emphasised what was absent or 'inappropriate'. Schuetz's (1943) concept of 'rationalities' enables interpretation of the literature on psychiatric nursing of neurotic patients as a dispute about reality. This dispute was mediated through language. The dispute about the reality of nursing of neurotic patients can be construed as a dispute between or about discourses, or as a slippage between discourses - a gap - through which the view of the 'real' nurse gets lost.

24 A note is needed here on the 'order' of interpretation and meaning. Decontextualised, an actor's first-order meanings may feature in second-order theoretical schemes. Kaplan (1964) draws the distinction between 'acts' (like Harré's 'behaviour'), 'act meanings' (meanings to the actor), 'action' (the act with its meaning as interpreted by the scientist) and 'action meanings' (how that action is understood in the theoretical scheme). Harré's 'behaviour-action-act' and Kaplan's 'acts' and 'act meanings' are conveyed by Schuetz' (1943) notion of 'first order' constructs, used by social actors to understand what they are doing. Kaplan's 'action meanings' are what is conveyed by 'second order' constructs, used by the social scientist to elaborate theoretical understandings of social action.

25 This understanding is compatible with Berger and Luckmann's (1967) understanding (see below) that conception of self and world is a product of socialisation into a socially constructed reality. The theoretical positions of Foucault and of Berger and

Luckmann coincide in arguments that the grounds of knowledge, the conditions of knowing, are linked to systems of power, with 'therapy' or other forms of resocialisation functioning to construe and correct deviations from normal understanding.

26 For example, an account - 'it was an accident' - might also mean 'I am not a thug'.

27 It could be argued that this is also the intention implicit in Altschul (1972). However, the emphasis there seemed to be on bringing already existent theoretical knowledge to bear on nurses' accounts of practice.

28 Researchers going into different sites are going into different provinces. If they go in with imperialistic designs they are in danger of seeing only what is not, not what is of value in the setting (Asquith, personal communication).

29 An example of Schutzian analysis is Baruch's (1981) study of the 'two realities' of parents and health professionals.

30 See also Schuetz (1943, p. 149): 'But to one who is not satisfied with such guarantees and asks for greater reality, I want to say that I am afraid that I do not exactly know what reality is...It is a misunderstanding of the essential character of science to think that it deals with reality if we consider as the pattern of reality the world of daily life. The world of both the natural and social scientist is neither more nor less real than the world of thought in general can be. It is not the world within which we act and within which we are born and die.'

31 See Smith (1980) for an empirical study based on Berger and Luckmann's 'social construction of reality' thesis, aimed at exploring the social construction of need.

32 The child knows the world and its place in the world through language, especially talk. Berger and Luckmann's (1967) analysis of the internalisation of subjective identity follows that of Mead (1934) (cf. Harré, 1983). The child takes on the roles of significant others and internalises them as part of self, as the 'me'. The self is thus a reflexive (Mead, 1934): the self is both what one is addressed as, an objective entity in the objective world; and what is experienced as subjective identity. As the self takes on the role of the 'generalised other', identity and reality 'crystallise'.

33 Cicourel (1976) explored the ordinary commonsense understandings drawn on by police in order to make the 'formal legal and clinical categories...work' (p. 111). He formulated an

'articulation between procedural rules and observable referents, joined by a theory of action' (p. 121). Cicourel (1964) in a critique of traditional methods emphasised the necessary and unaccountable role of common sense in social scientific method and measurement.

34 Garfinkel (1967, p. 8) claims: 'With respect to the problematic character of practical actions, and to the practical adequacy of their enquiries, members take for granted that a member must at the outset 'know' the settings in which he is to operate if his practices are to serve as measures to bring particular, located features of these settings to recognizable account. They treat as the most passing matter of fact that members' accounts, of every sort...are constituent features of the settings they make observable.'

35 The theme of the morality of everyday life is pursued by Goffman (1969, 1967).

36 Garfinkel (1967, p. 78) claims that: 'According to Mannheim, the documentary method involves the search for...an identical homologous pattern underlying a vast variety of totally different realizations of meaning. The method consists of treating an actual appearance as "the document of", as "pointing to", as "standing on behalf of" a presupposed underlying pattern. Not only is the underlying pattern derived from its individual documentary evidences, but the individual documentary evidences, in their turn, are interpreted on the basis of "what is known" about the underlying pattern.'

37 This interpretation cuts two ways. Patients could be interpreted as having through illness become estranged from everyday life, and as having to interpret the new reality they found themselves in (see Chapter 5 below). Nurses then are kinds of ethnomethodological tutors. Also, I became 'estranged' from nursing in order to understand it differently. See also Schutz (1944) on 'the stranger'.

38 See Smith (1988) and Darbyshire (1990) on the relevance of these concepts, for nursing.

39 The concept 'microphysics' of power is elaborated in Foucault (1979, p. 139). Likewise the concept of power exercised at the 'capillaries' (Foucault, 1980, p. 96) is a theme that can be traced in various of Foucault's works.

40 See Burke (1969a); on whom Harré (1979) has drawn.

41 The former process can be likened to Foucault's (1979) 'economy' of power. I will elaborate how nurses practiced an

'economy of respect and contempt' expressed in terms of allocation of time: 'the usual five minutes' being an example of a calibrated allocation of 'attention' in response to a 'demand'. This will be related to Foucault's (1982) notion of 'pastoral power'.

42 See Bakhtin (1984) on using words that have passed through the mouths of others.

43 This notion can be related to ideas in Schutz and Luckmann (1974) and Berger and Luckmann (1967).

4 Methods, analysis and description of the sites

Section 1: Methods

Introduction

The aim of this study was to understand interaction between neurotic patients[1] and psychiatric nurses from their points of view, and to situate their understandings of the interaction in the contexts of the admission wards in which it took place. No previous research had specifically sought the views of both nurses and patients on their conversations together, and none had tried to relate the understandings of the participants to the context in which it took place and which it reflexively realised. The aim was thus to advance the debate, to add to the 'conversation' described in Chapter 2. The study was small-scale and the advance claimed is a slight development of understanding of the complexity of the issues involved in making sense of nurse-neurotic patient interaction. The complexity was addressed by devising methods of investigating the subjective understandings of the nurses and patients as well as features of the institution that impacted on and were shaped by the interaction.

In this Chapter I will describe the design, methods and modes of analysis in the study, and address questions of reliability and validity. The design of the study involved: preliminary conceptual analysis and development of methods; a 'trial of methods'; in depth investigation of the interaction of patients and nurses in one site; analysis of the data of this site; and in depth investigation of the interaction of patients and nurses in a second site. The methods and analysis were qualitative, intended to produce description of interaction and contexts, and understanding of meanings.

The plan of the chapter is: in Section 1 I discuss the evolution of methods; in Section 2 I discuss the mode of analysis and issues of reliability and validity; and in Section 3 I present an overview of the sites and the patients, including a discussion of the problem of diagnosis in this study. In Chapters 5, 6 and 7 the main themes and understandings that form the 'findings' of the study are elaborated. Chapter 8 comprises conclusions and recommendations.

Introduction to methods

In Chapters 2 and 3 I discussed Altschul's (1972) recommendation that nurses should be asked to account for what they did, and developed the theoretical justification for use of accounts. I construed accounts as occasions for interpretation and devices for reality maintenance and repair, and argued that they could be used to develop practical knowledge. In this chapter I will describe the methods I used to develop understanding of interaction between these nurses and patients. The choice of methods was based on a developing theoretical understanding of interaction. Construing interaction from an interpretive perspective, I needed a methodology which would enable me to gain access to the meanings of interaction for both nurses and patients.

Burton (1978) analysed the relationships between theory, method and substantive topic, in a discussion of issues related to participant observation. A brief summary of his argument will serve to relate the theoretical perspective and the methodological and empirical concerns of this monograph. Burton argues that there are three methodological issues related to participant observation as a method of generating data in sociological investigation: fact versus researcher's value judgements; the effect of observer presence on the phenomenon of interest; and the question of post-factum explanation. He claims that these three problems relate to a core problem - the stages and processes of becoming an insider. This problem in turn is construed (p. 171) in terms of a theory of data:

> This theory of data can be treated as the stages and process by which the researcher became cognizant with the social worlds that he is studying. A documentation of the passage of becoming an insider correctly conflates theory and methodology. It attempts to link explanatory claims with the process by which they were arrived at. Methodologically the

> theory of data is an account of the author's socialization into his respondents' society.

Burton (citing Cicourel and Schutz) discusses the 'translation problem' involved in grasping the 'pre-interpreted world' of the people he is interested in, in terms other than the researcher's ('sociologist-as-man''s) own 'set of pre-theoretic meanings'. He claims (p. 171-172) that 'the statement of how an author becomes socialised into the world that he is studying requires a theory of the translation problem, a theory of data':

> Yet this socialization problem is exactly the theoretical purpose of the study. Theoretically the author is interested in the model of the actors' world (the social consciousness)...By explicating the grammar and syntax of the actors' social world the researcher is stipulating both the content of that world (the theoretical base) and *how* that world presented itself to the researcher (the methodological problem)...It is the interplay, between the ordering of the empirical world through theory and the emphasis that the theory is explanatory of the empirical world, that constitutes a theory of data. (Note: italics in original.)

This analysis highlights some of the features of the 'documentary method' discussed in Chapter 3. The main point relevant to the argument of this monograph is that the choice of methods is determined on theoretical grounds. In the case of the present study, participant observation and accounts were chosen because I assumed on the basis of my theoretical perspective that nurses' and patients' participation in their interaction is based on their interpretations of a socially constructed reality. The methods used were intended to enable entry into the structures of meaning that shape that reality. The methods were those by which the researcher becomes aware of the 'social meanings in that world' (Burton, 1978, p. 173).

Silverman (1985) summarised a key argument which links the theoretical perspective of the interpretive tradition, and the kinds of methods used in this study. The central point of the interpretive tradition is that adequate description is adequate scientific explanation, insofar as description elaborates the methods by which meaning is accomplished. The logic of this position is based on the claim that 1) understanding is accomplished by grasping concepts used by actors to conduct their social life, and 2) this is also the method of explanation. I argued that 'adequate' second-order description and explanation had to be based on actors' first order description and explanation (Schuetz, 1943). The aim of interpretive research is broadly that of ethnography: 'grasping and comprehending the culturally appropriate concepts through which actors conduct their social life' (Halfpenny, cited in Silverman, 1985, p. 97).

The methods used to generate adequate descriptions (participant observation, interview and accounts) and the kinds of data

The three principal methods I chose to generate adequate descriptions were participant observation, interviews and accounts.[2] The data were: 1) field notes; 2) interview notes of various sorts, including notes on nurses' 'conceptual systems' derived through a process of 'conceptual sorting' (Brown and Canter, 1985); and 3) text transcribed from audio tape recordings of the interviews with nurses and patients in which they gave accounts of their interaction with each other.

An ethogenic methodology for this research

In Chapter 3 I discussed the ethogenic conception of social action. From the ethogenic perspective, the problems faced by the researcher who wants to understand and describe interaction are: grasping the 'episode' structure of the social world within which the interaction takes place; and discovering actors' resources for action, and for accounting for their performances.

By what means can the structure of the social world be known? To the extent that the researcher participates in this world, the availability of his commonsense knowledge of it may be problematic. Schutz and Luckmann (1974) explored commonsense understanding as the basis for participation in the world. Garfinkel (1967) argued that because the social scientist shares commonsense understandings with those he studies, it is necessary to devise methods which render research settings 'anthropologically strange'.[3]

The unit of analysis: the episode Argyle et al (1981) argue that the key to understanding the ethogenic method is understanding that it takes the episode as the principal unit of analysis and meanings. Harré (1982, p. 86) argues:

> To understand an episode we have to try to find out what projects the actors might have, so that our study can be directed to the way actors go about realizing their aims and plans...what Goffman (1969) called the 'strategic' aspect of an interaction.

Harré's language is shot through with metaphors based on the dramatic model, one of his principal analytic and source models.[4]

Once the structure of episodes has been understood, participants' accounts are interpreted to yield understandings of how they directed their action so as to be seen as competent in playing their parts in the episode. Accounts are data for analysis of the participants' understandings of situations and their resources for socially effective action.

Participant observation as a method for understanding the episodes of interaction: the definition of the situation

I chose participant observation as a method for understanding the sites in which accounts of interaction would be given. Participant observation is grounded in the theoretical understandings of symbolic interactionism (Rock, 1979; Blumer, 1969) and the tradition of ethnographic fieldwork (Silverman, 1985). The method involves learning the language and participating in the daily life of a people, and asking questions of informants until the researcher understands the culture from the inside. Language and other symbolic systems are considered the means of access to the lives of others.

Language and participant observation The central point in the symbolic interactionist perspective is that people act in the situation as they define it. Language is the main set of symbols used to define the situation. What matters is the meaning of the symbols to the participants. The meanings can be grasped by the researcher in the situation seeing how people use the symbols to organise and take part in interaction. Understanding of the meaning can be 'checked out' by the researcher when he uses the symbols and sees how they work to define situations in interaction with the actors.

My rationale for participant observation was that I wanted to understand contexts in which nurse-patient interaction occurred and in which accounts were given. Participant observation provides one means of understanding a setting through participation in it, relying on the development of a shared capacity for symbolic interaction. The rationale was also based on Harré and Secord's

(1972) recommendation of participant observation as a means of discovering the structure of episodes which partition social life. 'Definition of the situation' (Blumer, 1969) in symbolic interactionism corresponds to understanding of 'episode' in ethogenics. My understandings based on fieldwork and accounts constituted local 'ethnographies' (Harré and Secord, 1972). The development of understanding through interaction was thus both the method of this study and its topic (cf. Burton, 1978).

The form of participant observation is often defined using Gold's (1958) continuum of observation and participation: observer; observer as participant; participant as observer; and participant. I found that my role in the situations of this research could be construed in radically different ways. I could be construed as a participant in the situations in the wards, or I could be construed as participating in the definition of nursing through the research.[5] I could be observing the situation in the ward, or other nurses. In different situations I was called on to play one or another role - for example, a patient asked me to switch on a radio, and I asked myself whether I was being put into a nursing role. I knew the role I was being called on to play in part by my response to the call. Because the research was intended to describe a practice discipline of which I was a member, I was defining a category of which I was a member, regardless of my claim to be acting in a 'student' or 'observer' role.[6]

The concept 'participant comprehension' (Collins, in Webb, 1989) conveys the points I have made. I comprehended aspects of nursing through participation in dialogue with nurses and patients intended to further understanding of nurse-patient interaction. My participation and comprehension, as well as the participation and comprehension of the nurses and patients, were two aspects of the processes of interaction which comprised this research.

Issues of reliability and validity in participant observation Issues of validity and reliability in participant observation have been addressed by Burgess (1984), Schatzman and Strauss (1973), Becker (1958), Lofland and Lofland (1984), and Denzin (1978, 1989). It is accepted that the researcher's understanding in part constitutes the meanings he grasps. The aim is to present understandings from within dynamic, emergent settings, which may not be 'replicated' by another person at another time. Nonetheless, rigour and openness about method and analysis enhance the credibility of fieldwork findings. Search for disconfirming cases and display of enough data so that the reader can form alternative interpretations are strategies for assuring warrantability of interpretations. Feeding back understandings to actors tests the 'adequacy' of the researcher's interpretations. These strategies were built into the method and analysis of this research.

Interviews and issues of reliability and validity in interviews in fieldwork Interviews in field work provide access to the understandings of participants. Becker and Geer (1957) outline the differences between participant observation and interviewing. In the present study data from interviewing was construed in the relation to other field work and account data. The issues related to reliability and validity of interview data are to some extent similar to those of fieldwork generally (see Whyte, 1960; and the comments on Burton, 1978, above). They relate to possible biases in respondents and interviewer, problems of recording and transcribing. In this research interviews were regarded as sources of data on respondents' views, not as 'objective' data. Interviews were also regarded as occasions for display of different 'accounting systems' (Potter and Mulkay, 1985).[7]

Accounts

Accounts were generated as a data base on tellers' resources for participation in interaction, and the resources they had for explaining it. In saying that accounts were generated I want to convey that they were grown through interaction, sometimes with great difficulty and in unlikely soil.

The sources on accounts cited in Chapter 3 indicated that 1) people can and do give accounts in the course or their everyday life; 2) these accounts serve to explain what a person is going to do, is doing or has done, in a way that might have been unclear without the giving of the account; 3) in giving accounts people may state, restate or change the meaning of what was done; 4) in telling, people might reveal that what they did was appropriate or inappropriate, proper or improper in that world, and in so doing illuminate aspects of what Harré (1979) and Shotter (1984) call the practical, moral and expressive orders in which they participate; 5) in giving accounts people demonstrate that they are able to give accounts, that is that they can and do monitor their doings and when necessary or appropriate can and will tell what they were doing, and are entitled to be recognised as having greater authority than others might have concerning their intentions, aims, plans and understandings (though others, including the researcher, might have access to those matters). These latter might be called the 'person implications' of the accounts methodology.

Many of the arguments that Burton (1978) made regarding the theoretical and methodological aspects of participant observation apply to an accounts methodology. Accounts are called for because theoretically it is assumed that social interaction is mediated by meanings, and that 'rough passages' in social life will require that meanings be negotiated. Accounts provide the occasions for that negotiation, repair and maintenance (see Chapter 3). However, the form of social life under investigation is only revealed through the process of account generation. Viewed theoretically, the form of social life is the organisation of accounting practices (Garfinkel, 1967). Methodologically, the form of social life is explored by locating or arranging occasions for accounting. The content of accounts provides the data for theoretical elaboration related to the substantive social issues in the area of interest, in this case the practices of patient-nurse interaction.

Previous studies using accounts include Brown and Sime (1981), Bunch (1982), Llewelyn (1985), Marsh et al (1978), Fielding (1982), Labov and Fanshel (1977), and Hughes (1980). Detailed comments on accounts methodology are available in Llewelyn (1985) and Brown and Sime (1981).

A trial of methods

Before the main study was undertaken, and prior to application for Ethical Committee approval, a 'trial' of the methods and analysis was carried out in an admission ward in a rural mental hospital. Access to the hospital was negotiated through informal contact with members of the local Ethics of Medical and Psychological Research Committee, subject to assurances that material was confidential and that I would not use the data for the study. The aims of the trial were to find out if patients and nurses could give accounts of conversations, and to see how the content of the accounts related to the wider context in which the conversations took place.

Among the relevant conclusions were the following: 1) patients diagnosed as 'neurotic' accounted for roughly 15% of admissions; thus, if diagnostic practices elsewhere were similar, data could be collected on a substantial proportion of patients in admission wards; 2) diagnosis of 'neurosis' often changed during admission, hence attention should be paid to how patients come to be diagnosed as neurotic, how that changes, and the implications of this for nursing research based on diagnosis; 3) nurses said that factors other than diagnosis, especially 'behaviour', mainly guided their practice with patients, hence it would be useful to enquire into the conceptual bases of nurses' practices; 4) as I felt awkward attempting to 'observe' interaction by sitting and watching nurses and patients, and observed few conversations, I decided not to 'watch' the patients and nurses; 5) a method of generating accounts, described below, worked; 6) field notes and account data were voluminous, hence a limit on number of sites and participants would be desirable; 7) the research was a social act, nurses and patients sometimes negotiating among themselves what sort of accounts I wanted and they should give; 8) 'non-diagnostic' use of the term 'neurotic' was denied by nurses but was observed, hence information on that use should be sought.

A note on the method of account elicitation will suffice to explain the later development of method. With few exceptions patients readily agreed to tell about their conversations with nurses, and nurses, asked to tell about the same conversation, agreed to do so. I took notes rather than tape record the accounts.[8] When asked what their aims were and what they thought the other's aims were in the interaction, some patients and nurses gave accounts in which, on analysis, intentions, actions and acts (Harré, 1978 and 1979) could be discerned. The importance of context in interpreting accounts was seen in two ways. When giving their accounts of conversations, participants often referred to much outside the conversation itself in order to explain it. This raised the theoretical and methodological question: what was an 'episode'?[9] Also, when I tried to tell colleagues about some accounts, I referred to what I had learned about the patient not only from her conversations but also from observation, ward rounds, and gossip.

Analysis of the data from this fieldwork trial yielded some themes that I carried from the trial and into the later fieldwork. One of the themes was nurses' concern with whether I thought I would get a 'true picture' through observation and account elicitation. Through analysis of various data I came to the conclusion that the question of the 'true picture' was a central concern of nurses, patients and medical staff. Much conversation was about whether what was said was really true; if not, how to discern the hidden truth; the problems and management of discrepant views; what was secret and who knew it; how to interpret action and talk. Belief and grounds for belief were vitally important. Such concerns were displayed in various arenas, private (bedrooms) and public (ward rounds, office). The 'true picture' was alternatively something to be discovered or to be produced. Appropriate management and strategic abilities were required. The relationship between the 'true picture' and diagnosis was complex.[10] Hence, it was clear that treating diagnosis as a given fact, and unproblematic, did not fit the observed practice.

On the basis of the fieldwork trial I concluded that the data were rich in potential for qualitative analysis.

A note on evolution of methods

Among the main themes of this monograph are the making of sense and the negotiation of realities. The methods used in the study were methods of making sense. In Burton's (1978) terms they were 'theories of data'. They were methods for elaborating theoretically salient aspects of empirical reality. In practice the methods were shaped to the emergent reality.[11] The forms of my questioning were shaped to the responses of the patients and nurses, shaped differently to different patients and nurses. The forms of my 'being around' the two sites of the main study were different: different stances and postures, literally, observable as me 'roving' from place to place or sitting in the sitting room in Site One; 'finding space' in the nurses' station in Site Two. Participation in the reality was the method for further participation in the reality. The stages in participant observation (socialisation into the actors' realities) were a theory of data (cf. Burton, 1978), in that what was 'found' was ongoingly interpreted as 'reality'. The theoretically salient implication is that 'realities' were continuously negotiated and constructed through practice of the methods of making sense.

The methods changed as I opened up and explored possibilities for making sense and constructing realities by allowing patients and nurses greater freedom to 'tell about' their conversations, without focusing on goals and intentions. One important evolution was that, whereas in the trial of methods I had specifically asked tellers about their goals and the goals of the other in conversation, in effect enrolling them in the analytic work; in the main study I only asked about goals when that seemed appropriate. Sometimes I heard and responded to the account as to a story or narrative, and did not respond to it as goal-orientated.

Methods in the main study

Participant observation

The data of participant observation were my developing understandings, based on observation, talk in the field and consultation of records. I recorded my understandings in field notes. I spent a few hours a day, four or five days a week over 3-4 months in each site. I recorded in field notes whatever I noticed.

Noticing and developing understandings Noticing was a practiced awareness that what I saw made sense or puzzled me, that it was new to me or that I was aware that it was routine. What I noticed were aspects of the sites as these stood out from the background of what I was engaged in or what was going on around me. I noticed talk in meetings and other formal and informal settings; aspects of the ward layout; my own understandings of events, moods, feelings; action, interaction; the passage of time; smells; and, as I will describe, others noticing me. I took notes at regular intervals during the day, usually in a quiet room if I could find one, or in the nursing station. I did not take notes when sitting with patients, or in meetings. The nurses or patients did not question my explanation that I took notes to help me keep track of how I was coming to see and know the sites as contexts for understanding the accounts of talk in them. However, nurses in both sites asked, as time went on, whether I was observing them or the patients. I explained that I paid attention to anything that I felt would enable me to understand the site and their interaction with patients.

Thus the persona I adopted was of someone wanting to understand the sites and the understandings of people in the sites. This was congruent with my stance in generating accounts. Nurses and patients knew that I was around the ward enough to know generally what the place was like and what was going on. That meant that in their accounts they could refer to features of the current reality in the site to explain something about the interaction which I had not observed. The data from field notes, accounts and interviews are interwoven in the main analysis chapters (Chapters 5, 6 and 7) because context and interaction were reflexively related through the processes of symbolic interaction.

In addition to field notes I wrote a series of theoretical notes, methodological notes and personal notes (Schatzman and Strauss, 1973; Glaser and Strauss, 1967; Strauss, 1987; Denzin, 1970). In theoretical notes I recorded emerging concepts or categories, or related field material to readings. Methodological notes concerned my understanding of how the methods worked to generate data. Personal notes recorded the times when events in the field touched me personally and called out personal understandings.

The second set of field work data were notes of interviews with doctors and nurses about diagnosis and its relevance for their practice (see below the section on 'Diagnosis').[12] I also interviewed nurses about other aspects of their practice as these raised questions for me.

I adopted new methods in response to developing questions and understandings. For example, when nurses said that diagnosis was not central to how they thought of patients, I used Canter et al's (1985) conceptual sorting system to find out the categories in terms of which they did construe patients. When I learned that nurses were concerned with the 'picture' they had of a patient, I compared Kardex notes with what they said about patients to see how the 'pictures' of them differed.

The method of gathering accounts

In explaining to patients and nurses why I wanted them to give me accounts of conversations I told them that I wanted to know more about interaction, specifically conversation or talk, between nurses and patients. I asked to see patients at times convenient to them. Typically, the setting for accounting was a room in which the account giver and I could talk uninterrupted. In initial interviews I explained the research and asked for the patients' written consent to being interviewed and to recording of the interviews. I explained that since I was not present at their talk, and in any case was interested in how they understood it, I wanted them to tell me about their conversations with nurses. Having got consent[13] I tape recorded the accounts using a portable audio tape recorder.

I explained to the patients that I was interested in understanding how both they and the nurse understood their talk together, and that this knowledge might be of use to future nurses and patients. I told the nurses that the patient had mentioned a conversation with them and asked that they tell me about it,[14] as I was interested in how both they and the patient understood the conversation.

I told them that the other participant would not know what they said, and that I was not after the 'right' view of what happened; but that nonetheless, I would hear the two accounts and my declared interest was in considering the two accounts together in order to understand how each understood their talk together. I thought at the time that this method implied (to them as well as to myself) the possibility of their speaking without fear of contradiction. However, it is clear with hindsight that through analysis I would be aware of contradictions which neither participant would be able to resolve. This ironically gave me greater power of interpretation than I intended; and reproduced a feature of the sites themselves, whereby staff members noted contradictions in patients' accounts to them but did not always discuss these with the patients.

First level accounts and second level accounts The definition of an 'account' emerged through the process of generating accounts, as did the definition of a 'conversation'.[15] An account was what was negotiated as an account by me and the nurse or patient. Understanding this enabled me to understand reflexively that nurses and patients were involved in negotiating understandings, not only of what what a conversation meant, but of what counted as a conversation, as just talk, as something trivial, as 'women's talk'[16]. In Chapter 5 I explore further the nurses' and patients' understandings of forms of accounts.

I gathered two kinds of accounts. 'First level accounts' were the patients' and nurses' replies to my request to tell about a conversation. 'Second level accounts' were what nurses (and in two cases, patients) who had given a first level account told me on a later occasion, when asked to read their own first level account and comment on it to help me understand better what was being done in the conversation. I suggested that the nurse or patient let me 'look over her shoulder' while she clarified what she and the other were doing in the interaction. The outcome was a new dialogue, now focussed through the text of the first account.

Second level accounts provided the opportunity to check out my interpretations of the first level accounts. With two exceptions[17], I did not ask the patients for second level accounts, on the grounds that asking patients to read their accounts and comment on them might have interfered with the ordinary process of interaction between nurses and patients more than asking for first level accounts had done; and that the patients might have suffered greater performance anxiety and inhibition in the interview setting.[18]

The term 'account' thus refers to two sorts of data: in 'first level accounts', the telling about an interaction, by a participant in the interaction; and in 'second level accounts', the elaboration of that ('first level') account, in response to me asking the teller to tell anything more that would help me understand the interaction, or in response to my telling how I understood it and asking for feedback from the nurse on my understanding. I told the nurse that I had read the account and had an understanding of it, but appreciated that my understanding might differ from his, and that I wanted to know further how he understood what he and the patient were doing in the interaction.

A second level account is thus more like Harré and Secord's (1972, p. 9) notion of an account as a device for telling:

> why he performed the acts in question, what social meanings he gave to the action of himself and others.

Second level accounts were thus more explicitly occasions for legitimation, for justification or explanation. It could be argued that in asking for elaboration on the first level account I implied a possible failure of understanding on my part, and a parallel failure, on the part of the teller, to make clear what he was doing. The second level accounts were highly unusual in nursing practice, in that they presented the nurses with text created from their talk, and thus raised new issues related to accountability (cf. Fielding, 1982, on nurses' accounts on their work with the elderly).

My way of asking for accounts varied, and the possibility that how I asked affected what I was told cannot be discounted.[19] The negotiation of understanding of what I wanted was part of the data and was heuristic, highlighting that my and the nurses' and patients' frameworks for understanding talk were at times different.[20] In each interview the nurse or patient and I did whatever interpretative work was necessary so that he or she could help me understand his or her interpretation of the conversation.[21]

Background understandings In hearing and understanding the accounts I had access to understandings of much beyond the accounts: what I knew of the site, of the patient, as a nurse, as a member of (broadly) the same community. In hearing the accounts I engaged with the tellers in an 'inner-temporal course of interpretive work' (Garfinkel, 1967, p. 25; cf. Schutz and Luckmann, 1974). I did not play the 'dope' who pretends not to know what he knows (Cicourel, 1976). I assumed that to have done so in a site in which I had spent some time (and where I could have been assumed to have developed some understanding as I went along) would have jeopardised my relationships with others, especially nurses.[22]

The important theoretical point is that I asked as I did and heard as I did because I came to know the setting, the people, and how to act and what to ask. My understandings developed through the interaction, through participation in construction of the reality(ies) of the sites. Theoretically, the implication is that nurses and patients in their interaction also knew in time, and that how they interacted was shaped by the situation and context their interaction reflexively realised. That my ways of making (common) sense with the patients and nurses varied implied that their (common) sense might vary (cf. Altschul, 1972).

With a few exceptions - times when my way of asking was clearly confusing to both me and the teller (see Appendix 15) - the various openings I used allowed the nurses and patients to tell about conversations, or to deny them; or to tell me that I did not make sense, and to work out a way whereby I did. If there were failures of understanding they and I brought into the foreground the background understandings which enabled us to negotiate a working understanding of what I wanted to do with them. This aspect of the method is of theoretical interest. I could negotiate understandings with these patients insofar as they were among the ones I could approach and engage in conversation. They were in 'my reality' (to use a phrase from a nurse in Site One, see Chapter 5) or a reality that could be negotiated. This, as I will explain later, was one of the ways in which nurses distinguished these patients from others who were considered more 'ill'.

Numbers and kinds of accounts: In Site One, six patients gave a total of twenty-five accounts of conversations. One gave seven, two gave five, two gave three and one gave two accounts. A few accounts told of conversations with more than one nurse, and some accounts told of no conversations or the nurse mentioned could not be contacted for their account or could not recall it. The total number of conversations mentioned was twenty-two. Nurses gave their accounts of eighteen of these twenty-two conversations. In addition one nurse gave one account of a conversation for which no patient account was collected. Nurses gave second-level accounts regarding five of the eighteen first level accounts.

In Site Two, seven patients gave forty one first level accounts, and two second level accounts; nurses gave twenty first level and two second level accounts; there were thus twenty matched pairs including two multiple accounts (two or more conversations with nurses mentioned by the patient in one account). In addition, in Site Two I asked nurses to give accounts about what the patient's stay had been 'about', from their points of view and from the patient's points of view. I collected five of these 'stay' accounts.[23]

There were thus eighteen pairs of accounts of conversations in Site One and twenty pairs in Site Two.[24] The first level accounts lasted from a few minutes to approximately twenty minutes, the second level accounts about fifteen to twenty minutes.

The accounts are regarded as resources for understanding how the individuals in interaction in the site constructed their interaction and understood it; with pairs of accounts allowing understanding of differences and similarities in understanding. The accounts were read as documents of the resources on which nurses and patients drew to interact and to tell about and explain their interaction.

Summary

In this section I have outlined the main methods used, and the evolution of methods in practice. The main method was the practice of developing understandings in several forms, based on observation and dialogue. In addition, the second level accounting sessions provided nurses, and in two cases patients, with occasions to 'tell more', to develop further my understanding of the interaction from their points of view.

In the next section I describe how I analysed the data produced through these methods, while in the third section I give a 'flavour' of the methods in use, by introducing the sites and the patients.

Notes

1 The reader is reminded that I have used the term 'neurotic patients', aware of the difficulty of interpreting its meaning in this and other research. Alternative and preferable constructions, for example, 'patients diagnosed as neurotic', or 'patients nominated as neurotic for the purpose of this study', are too clumsy; and those terms too would be subject to qualification.

2 The data were seen as created by these methods, products, things made rather than found (Shotter, 1984, p. 4), things 'cut out' from the flow of action (Silverman, 1985).

3 There is a sense in which the researcher sacrifices common sense and its function of binding perception with that of others, in order to show its workings.

4 'Analytic model' and 'source model' are Harré et al's (1985) terms for the elements of scientific theoretical imagination

5 Peplau (1952) conceived of nursing as a form of participant observation in which the nurse gains access to the patient's world; and Benner and Wrubel (1989, p. 88) argued that 'caring for a patient enables the expert nurse to be a participant in the subculture of being a patient'. During fieldwork as a relatively uninvolved participant observer I did not play the sort of role these writers had in mind, nor could I fully understand the site in the way a working nurse would have done. My degree of involvement with nurses and patients allowed me glimpses of the role I was not playing. Symbolic interactionism implies that the researcher is involved in the definition of the situation in which he participates. I wanted to be with both nurses and patients without playing the role of either, in order to negotiate a new sort of relationship based on their telling about their talk together.

6 Previous nursing researchers who used participant observation methods (Altschul, 1972; Cormack, 1976) already participated or later participated in the definition of nursing in academic or administrative settings.

7 This was especially relevant regarding the questions to psychiatrists on diagnostic practice. Interviews were occasions for distinguishing the 'official line' on diagnosis and the practical reality. This was theoretically salient to the concerns of this study, in that it enabled retrospective re-evaluation of nursing research based on diagnoses (see later in this chapter).

8 I decided to tape record accounts to free myself from the labour of note-taking during interview.

9 For example, a patient, upset, went for a walk and imagined conversations with the nurses. The walk and the 'conversations' formed part of the background to a brief 'episode' of interaction on the patient's return to the ward, and could be construed as part of a larger 'episode'.

10 It was possible for nurses to claim that the 'true picture' and diagnosis were incompatible, and to cite as evidence their

conversation or interpretation of conversation with the patient. Or, diagnosis could be held up to see if it matched the 'true picture' as that evolved; or offered in the hope it would be accepted as a clarification of an obscure 'picture'.

11 Eskimo carvers are said to 'find' the shape in the stone or the piece of wood. The carving is shaped to the form the wood 'really' presents. So it was with the methods of this research.

12 I wanted to know the 'local view' on the significance of diagnosis, and on its validity and reliability; whether diagnosis or formulation was a more important 'frame' for selecting patients; and whether both nurses and doctors knew of diagnoses or formulations (in light of MacIlwaine's, 1980, use of formulation as the basis for selecting patients in her study; and Altschul's, 1980, assumption that nurses knew diagnoses). It was important to know whether doctors and nurses thought that patients were identified in stable and meaningful ways through diagnosis, and what implications that was thought to have for structuring interaction and treatment. I wanted to know how much weight doctors put on diagnosis in understanding patients, and what, if anything, provided other bases for their treatment. My intention was to regard diagnosis as a basis for selection of patients for the study as potentially problematic. Altschul (1972) and MacIlwaine (1980) accepted diagnosis and formulation as the basis for selection of patients for study without considering how the patient came to be constructed as a 'neurotic' patient, and indeed, whether the patient continued to be so regarded during the period of their studies. Towell (1975) addressed the problem of changing and problematic diagnoses, and the dynamic interplay between interaction and diagnosis.

13 See Appendix 1 for letters to nurses and patients explaining the study, and the consent form completed by patients.

14 The account givers in this study were not regarded as 'reporters' of what happened; that is, what they said happened was not assumed to be an objective summary of what occurred. Rather, I regarded them as tellers (Shotter, 1984) about something in which they had taken part to someone interested in their understanding of their talk.

15 See Appendix 15 for a particularly clear example of a problematic process of elicitation.

16 See Chapter 5.

17 Two patients gave one second level account each.

18 Moreover, while one aim of the study was more fully to understand interaction from the points of view of both participants, the emphasis was on extending knowledge of nurses' (rather than of patients') ability to account for their interaction.

19 See Appendix 14 for an excerpt from an account in which a student nurse tells how a patient asked her what (not) to tell me.

20 For example, the meaning of 'conversation' had sometimes to be negotiated: was a comment at medication time a 'conversation'? My guideline was to say that I was interested in any conversation they wanted to tell me about, even if it seemed insignificant, since so little was known about the subject and because it was important to understand how they understood the talk.

21 In occasioning this interpretive work, I reproduced through use of this method some of the features of the nurses' and patients' work in interaction (see Chapter 6).

22 There are, as Garfinkel's (1967) studies showed, strong prohibitions against knowing too little. See also Altschul's (1972) and Fielding's (1982) discussions of the problems nurses face in claiming not to know what 'everybody knows'.

23 I asked more senior members of the nursing staff specifically to give me accounts of the patients' stays; even for patients who had mentioned no conversations with those nurses. I sometimes also asked other nurses in the course of accounts of conversations to tell be about patients' stays. I also asked several of the patients in Site Two to tell me what their stays had been about.

24 There are far more 'missing' nurse accounts in Site Two; that is, fewer matches. In one, the nurse denied that she was the nurse who had taken part in the conversation; in a number the patient did not remember the nurse's name; in some the nurse had moved to another ward before I could see her. I discerned no basis for thinking that the 'missing' nurse accounts differ from those for which matching accounts were found.

Section 2: Analysis

Introduction to analysis

In this section I will summarise the processes of analysis through which the understandings reported in Chapters 5, 6, and 7 were developed using the methods described in the previous section. Analysis involved trying out ways of understanding in interaction as well as of interaction. The analysis constituted a continuous dialectic between developing theoretical understandings and data.

The analysis was geared to the methods I had developed, which were based on letting nurses and patients go on to tell me about interaction, rather than directing them toward justification.[1] The methods were open, and analysis was intended to open the accounts for readings. The process of analysis after leaving the site was a form of 'deconstruction'. This process, in which the data were 'broken down' and reconstituted to develop further understandings, at times threatened to become a 'descent into the maelstrom' (Poe, 1967) of meaninglessness. I will outline how analysis of the accounts in terms of 'story' helped me to move through that 'descent' to the understandings developed in Chapters 5, 6 and 7.

Analysis was based on the main theoretical platform of this study: the proposition that reality is negotiated (constructed) by people on the basis of their interpretation of situations which they constitute through interaction based on their interpretations. Interaction was located first of all in the words of those involved in constructing it. The interaction reflected the subjectivities and the objectivity(ies) they negotiated. The order that analysis enabled me to impose was a second order based on the first order the actors imposed on the world (and each other) through their interaction.

Their 'first order' constructs are the basis of the 'second order constructs' elaborated in Chapters 5, 6 and 7. The complexities of analysis elaborated below reflect the complexity of trying to grasp a pre-interpreted 'reality' when the 'grasp' is itself an interpretation. What is rejected through this analysis is a view that the researcher has a privileged grasp on the reality, on the basis of which 'common sense' can be imputed or denied. My interpretations in this monograph are not more 'valid' than the actors', but are spoken from a different position and invested with different interests.

In the previous section I described the methods of this study as means of developing understandings, mainly through dialogue (interview and accounts and talk in field work). It was assumed that interaction and talk were everyday methods through which nurses and patients developed understandings (or misunderstandings) of each other. These methods enabled me to develop understandings and misunderstandings of the nurses and patients as sense makers making sense of sense makers. The process of analysis was the process through which I made sense of them in this way.

A note on some literature and the 'shape' of the analysis: a circle

The process of analysis was lengthy, multi-phased and recursive. These features of the analysis reflect the essential tension, indicated in the preceding section ('Method'), between a 'grounded', inductive approach tending toward theory (Glaser and Strauss, 1967), an ethogenic approach intended to discover the rules or generative mechanisms of interaction (Harré and Secord, 1972), and a hermeneutic phenomenological approach (Ricoeur, 1971; Denzin, 1989). Analysis was the process through which these distinct and in ways incommensurate approaches to understanding and explanation were 'tried out' to determine their usefulness in constituting and bringing out, through processes of interpretation, features of the data of this study relevant to understanding and exploring talk about interaction between these patients and nurses.

I reviewed discussions on analysis of participant observation, interview and account data in the work of researchers in the interpretive tradition. Among those whose work I reviewed were Blumer (1969), Douglas (1971), Cicourel (1964, 1976), Schatzman and Strauss (1973), Becker (1958), Clinton (1985), Ammon-Gaberson and Piantanida (1988) and Denzin (1989). These sources share an emphasis on the role of interpretation in the construction of first order and second order realities. Interpretation is construed, generally, in terms of the cycle of interpretation (the hermeneutic circle) in which one interprets what is happening in light of background understandings, the thus-interpreted forming part of new background understandings.

Sources of the method of analysis used in this study

The style of analysis can be construed as 'reading for social meanings' (Harré, 1982). The various analytic strategies can be understood by adopting the metaphor of talk and action as text, subject to hermeneutic analysis (cf. Ricoeur, 1971). This analysis was based on the 'documentary method' in which concepts are regarded as meaningful in relation to emergent themes (Glaser and Strauss, 1967; Wieder, 1974; Garfinkel, 1967). This accounts for the practice, outlined below, of reading parts of wholes in relation to the whole; for example, reading each transcript for a given patient in relation to all of the transcripts of her accounts; and reading each patient's accounts in relation to those of all patients in one site; and each site in relation to the other. This was the process of developing understandings (cf. Benner, 1985; Denzin, 1989).

Among the main guides I used in developing strategies for analysis were Glaser and Strauss (1967) and Strauss (1987). They describe in detail the analytic processes involved in generation of conceptual categories from data; and a theoretically guided process of analysis which involves making hypotheses about relationships between categories and properties, 'suggesting relationships into a theory'. I adopted some of the strategies used by interpretive and hermeneutic researchers. Giorgi (1975) outlined a process of analysis involving identification of meaning units and themes, 'interrogation' of the text in light of the purposes of the research, and writing of descriptive statements. These processes accord with those of Glaser and Strauss (1967). Gray-Snelgrove (1982) outlined methods of hermeneutic analysis, in which concepts which 'stood out' were regarded as uncovered meanings, initiating a process of questioning to illuminate other meanings and relationships.[2] Labov and Fanshel (1977) microanalysed psychotherapeutic interviews, 'expanding the text' with their understandings, documenting styles, identifying narratives and speech acts.

Account and story analysis

The main form of account analysis was that described by Harré and various others in several texts. Marsh et al (1978) outlined the ethogenic 'discovery procedure' involving: observation and description from the 'outside'; 'insiders'' commonsense construals of the episodes identified through observation; rule discovery and negotiation with the actors; and analysis of the 'realities' within which the analysed material made sense. Kreckel (1982) did a pragmatic analysis of accounts, based on the conditions for acceptance of statements. Harré (1982, p. 85) used a 'cognitive resources matrix' as a means of representing the social resources displayed in various documents.[3]

Bennett and Feldman (1981, p. 7) used analysis of stories (construed as ways of 'conveying selective interpretations of social behaviour to others') in their study of jury trials.[4] Denzin (1989) also notes the role of story in the creation of interpretive contexts, and gives analysis of story a central place in the 'biographical, interpretive method'. Mair (1987) is formulating a 'story-telling psychology' which emphasises the importance of story in development of self and person, and in therapy.

The key features of the analysis

The thread that ties together the analysis of the data of this study is a concern with language and with interpretation.[5] This is consistent with the understanding in the interpretive tradition that language, and participation in the social worlds language enables people to constitute, are the bases of personal and social being.[6]

I argue in this monograph that the concept of 'response' should be revised in relation to nurse-patient interaction.[7] Nurses' interaction with the patients makes sense if construed as responses to the implicit questions 'Why is she here now?' and 'What do I have to do for her?'. The difference is between a behaviourist conception of 'response', on the one hand, and a 'social-behaviourist' (Mead, 1934) or interpretive 'response' on the other. Interposed (in conceptual terms) between the patient and the nurse, in the latter case, is a symbolic process: a process between the patient and the nurse, but most importantly, within the nurse himself (through self-monitoring, Harré and Secord, 1972; or self-talk, Meichenbaum, 1977).[8]

The methods used in this study were ways of getting at those interpretive processes, by asking for accounts, and by observing interaction and taking part in interaction with the nurses and patients, on the basis of an assumption that interaction was mediated by meanings which I could come to share through participation, in the fieldwork and in accounting.

Analysis was the process of taking the data constructed through those methods and deconstructing them to 'read' for (interpret) the teller's interpretations. These interpretations were what constituted the interaction as meaningful, in the 'first order' of the interaction, and in the 'second order' of my understanding.

The main kinds of analysis

The main kinds of analysis I did were: 1) inductive derivation of concepts, categories and themes from field notes, interview notes and accounts (cf. Glaser and Strauss, 1967); 2) analysis of the meaning structure of accounts by analysis of behaviour, action, act and episode (Harré and Secord, 1972)[9]; 3) analysis of accounts using a Social Cognitive Matrix (Harré, 1978, 1979, 1982); 4) analysis of accounts as stories, using Burke's (1969a) 'dramatist' pentad of act, agent, agency, scene and motive; 5) analysis of the metaphors used in interaction and in accounts; 6) juxtaposition of various documents relating to a given patient, including medical notes, nursing Kardex entries, field notes and accounts; 7) simple quantitative analysis - counting and percentages - to determine the proportion of patients diagnosed as neurotic.

A few comments on each kind of analysis will suffice to give a picture of the aims and processes involved in each.

Analysis of field notes

Field notes were re-read as soon as possible after being written, and concepts which 'stood out' from them were noted on index cards. Examples of concepts were 'bad meeting' and 'what are we doing with (this patient)?'. The cards were sorted and the concepts were grouped into categories and themes; for example, 'varieties of interaction', 'nursing' and 'patient action', 'time', 'place', 'moral order' and 'working relationships'. The concepts were generally what Glaser and Strauss (1967) call 'in vivo' codes, that is, they were couched in the language of the people in the site. The categories and themes were second order concepts but related to 'in vivo' codes: for example, 'varieties of interaction' included 'the way I handled that'.

Analysis of accounts

Analysis of accounts began as I heard them. I paid attention and took part in the account interview by hearing and interpreting what the other was telling me, and asking for clarification when necessary. This part of the analysis only became available for further interpretation when I transcribed the audio-recorded account.

I transcribed the audio recorded accounts.[10] While transcribing I realised that I was understanding while hearing while transcribing, but the understandings were lost if not noted. I therefore inserted in the text notes to myself to indicate understandings which occurred during transcription.[11] I found that understandings which occurred during transcription, as the voices, recorded months earlier, one of them my own, were heard again, recalled understandings at the time of recording. In listening I understood again, from a new position, and noted my responses.

I listened more than once to transcripts that were particularly difficult to hear, and listened to difficult portions several times, until I felt confident that what was on the page was a faithful transcript. Those accounts which I heard less well I relied on less or not at all in the further analysis of the data.

Reading, interrogating and responding to the text: analysis of accounts from Site One Following the intention to produce theory grounded in the data, I analysed data during its collection/creation, and often guided collection of later data in order to further understanding based on ongoing analysis. The clearest instance of this is that each second level account depended on my having taken part in production of the first level account, listened to the audio tape of the account during the transcription, and in the course of doing so engaged on both occasions in an 'inner-temporal' process of understanding. My participation in the giving and hearing of the second level accounts was informed by this earlier process. Having heard, I understood or failed to understand, and asked or did not ask further accordingly. My understanding of the second level accounts, and my analysis of them, is built on understanding of the first level accounts.

I understood what I heard in the accounts in the light of what I knew about the nurses, patients and ward at the time. This fed into analysis, and was, of course, itself interaction. The 'inner-temporal work' was interaction with self and other (Mead, 1934).[12] My understanding was thus thoroughly grounded in participation in interaction. The important distinction is between interaction in which I took part, and interaction I was told about. The gathering of accounts is part of the former, but 'brackets' (see below) the latter.

The description of transcription applies to transcripts of accounts from both sites. Having transcribed the accounts and transferred them to a microcomputer, I read each transcript to recall understandings which had been noted during transcription. These were of different sorts, including identification of actions, acts and episodes; remarks on how the nurse or patient demonstrated her understanding of the interaction; and material from outside the body of the text which informed my understanding.

The method of analysis of transcripts from Sites One and Two differed in ways which I will now describe. Throughout the readings of transcripts from Site One, I asked the questions that underpinned the research: 'What does this tell me about interaction?' and 'What is happening here?'. These were the same questions that underlay the field work. During detailed re-reading of the transcripts I asked about each transcript in turn:

1. What is happening in the situation being told about here, and what is being done, according to the person telling me?
2. What is my understanding of what they are doing in the situation they are telling me about?
3. What does this account tell me about the patient?
4. What does this account tell me about the nurse?
5. What are the nursing actions in this account, according to the teller?
6. What are the nursing actions in this account, as I see them?
7. What are the patient's actions in this account, according to the teller?
8. What are the patient's actions in this account, as I see them?
9. What does this account tell me about interaction?
10. What does this account tell me about the method I am using?

I used the questions to identify in the accounts the episodes, acts and actions, which formed the basis for further analysis. The model of dialogue was preserved in this form of analysis, though now the dialogue was between myself and the text.

Analysis by patient and between patients in Site One I analysed the transcripts for one patient at a time, following the order in which the patients entered the study. My intention was to see all accounts for each patient as forming a meaningful whole. Previous British nursing research did not follow this idiographic approach (Allport, 1942).

Having noted common themes I decided to move beyond this analysis of the patients as single cases. Themes from the accounts related to themes from earlier analysis of field notes and interviews, enabling me to locate interaction with these patients in the context of the site.

The theoretical point brought out by this process of analysis was that the contexts within which I made sense emerged through the processes of interpretation in interaction in the Site and in the accounts sessions. The form of research shaped the content. Context and what was seen in relation to the context shifted as figure and ground shift in gestalts (cf. Ricoeur, 1971; Denzin, 1989). The process of analysis was one of developing understandings of accounts in relation to what else was known about that patient from other transcripts; in relation to what else was known about patients from other sources; in relation to what else was known about interaction with other patients.

Analysis of accounts from Site Two Because data collection and analysis proceeded together, both guided by developing understandings, analysis of accounts from Site Two differed from that for Site One. Each account in Site Two was summarised, preserving the main behaviours, actions, acts and episodes, but not simply cataloguing them. Instead, further analysis was directed toward asking what each account in Site Two 'said' about three broad themes which had emerged from Site One analysis: knowledge/communication, power, and moral order. Summaries related to these themes were written for each Site Two account. An additional analysis based on Harré's (1982) Social Cognitive Matrix was done on some accounts[13], but this strategy was discontinued when I began using a story analysis.

Analysis of stories I found, in early analysis of the accounts, that I missed important aspects if I construed them simply in terms of explanation, excuse and justification. The accounts were also narratives. They were narratives of conversations situated in the sites, and they were often re-narrations of the narratives given by the account giver or the other in the conversation. I analysed the accounts as stories because I came to see that interaction between the nurses and patients stemmed (explicitly or implicitly) from responses to the questions at the heart of work in admission wards: 'Why is she here now?' and 'What do we have to do for her?'. The form of response to these questions was often a story.

This analysis was thus partly based on empirical observation of the questioning and story telling in practice. It was based on recognising that story was a common form of response in interaction and in accounts. I could grasp key analytic concerns and important features of the empirical data more easily through analysis of story based on Burke's (1969a) pentad (act, agent, agency, motive and scene) than through other methods of analysis. For example, reading accounts as stories I could clearly understand the action that the nurse talked about from the point of view of the nurse. If a nurse said that a patient was lying on the ground and another patient was screaming, and that she noticed that a patient in the study was crying but could not do anything about it, I understood through the story analysis that aspects of the 'scene' were being emphasised to 'tell' that the nurse's 'agent' status in relation to the study patient was affected. The ratio of setting (ward with other demands) to agent (nurse/patient) to agency (patient/nurse) was highlighted in this way. The story thus told was a form of excuse: the nurse in telling it made the excuse. The analysis of story helped me grasp the relationship between agent and agency[14] in the nurses' and patients' stories, and to relate this to theories about nursing (see Chapter 8). In effect, story analysis contained the elements relevant to the problem of understanding what nurses and patients (agents and agencies) were doing (act, motive) in their interaction, taking account of the context (setting).

Story analysis also directed attention to metaphor and metonymy in nurses' and patients' accounts (See Chapter 6 below).

Analysis of form and content of accounts

I thought that accounts would somehow 'deliver' the content of psychiatric nursing. I thought that I would be able to find actions/acts/episodes, with meanings intact, and that this would provide the basis for saying what nurses and patients were doing. What I found was that I could catalogue these units of meaning, but that my perception of them as actions or acts depended on my interpretation of what the teller of the account told me. That interpretation was the product of 'inner temporal work' that I did shaped by the form of the account: how the teller told the story (cf. Garfinkel, 1967). Thus an analysis of the methods of understanding, based on consideration of form-as-content, followed identification of the content.

The importance of form Earlier nursing research in this area has emphasised the content of interaction, generally by some form of content analysis of qualitative data (Altschul, 1972; MacIlwaine, 1980; Cormack, 1976). The content of accounts has been privileged. This accords with attempts to find the content of psychiatric nursing, and this in turn accords with the attempt to hold up that content for comparison with some other content. In these analyses I brought out the 'submerged pole' of the form/content binary opposition. I focused on form. Form was brought out by attending to how content was established. In this analysis, form was considered prior to content, and content construed as contingent on form. The nurses stressed this priority in their emphasis on style and on forms of interaction (see Chapter 5).

Closer attention to the form of the data is justified on two grounds. Firstly, it is generally the case in interaction that how something is said in part determines what is said (Garfinkel, 1967; Harré, 1979, 1981). Secondly, as the method of this research was flexible and somewhat variable, and was deliberately so in order to be responsive to what was found, so the form of interaction between myself and the respondents intertwined indissolubly with the content of the accounts which were the basis for further analysis. The accounts were themselves forms of interaction. As such they were both resources for understanding what they told about (resources for content analysis like that done by other researchers) and forms of interaction which told something about the resources of nurses and patients as tellers, reporters and narrators, and thus about their powers and liabilities at the times when their interaction occurred in the sites. Silences and pauses structured some accounts (see Appendix 2).[15]

Aspects of the form of accounts: framing and bracketing All of the devices available to the dramatist or narrator were available to the account givers. Thus nurses sometimes spoke in the patient's voice, from the patient's position. The nurses thus re-presented the patient dramatically. What the teller and the other said and how they said it were mediated by the teller in the account. The teller and the other thus became characters in the teller's narrative (cf. Brown and Canter, 1985). Accounts were occasions for dramaturgical production.

The account was a set of brackets which framed the conversation. 'Bracketing' refers to the fact that nurses and patients told about conversations. 'The conversation' was never heard or witnessed. The theoretical stance of this monograph is that while 'the conversation' as something objectively there - the words, the pauses - could have been captured by some technical means, the conversation as a social event existed only in the interpretations of the participants and in the accounts given thereafter.

Accounts expressed formally an aspect of the work of the nurses. Speaking in the voice of the other was one device for asserting strongly that what the nurses said had been said could be taken as what was said, whether or not the nurse explicitly claimed to be giving a verbatim report. Formal devices could be used to accomplish a claim that the nurse was speaking the exact word when this was important for understanding (cf. Raffel, 1979).

The nurses' power to speak demonstrably in the voice of the patient and, where precision was important, to relate the patient's actual words, was part of their claim to be able to represent the patient and what was said and done. This was part of their work in the ward. They could only do this if they had spoken to, attended closely to and remembered what the patient said. In addition they needed the power and facility to employ dramatic devices - demonstrably precise recall, mimicry - in order to show that what they said was to be heard as what the patient said. The nurses in doing so were not using extraordinary methods: abilities to recall and relate effectively are part of the stock of ordinary powers. Nonetheless, the patients in giving accounts did not 'speak in' nurses' voices (see analysis of an account from Site Two below for an exception) or pointedly use their exact words. It was part of the nurses' work, not the patients', to use ordinary methods to assure that assessment of the real case was shown to be done. This was accomplished through forms of talk.

As the reality of what happened was established through forms of talk which established the basis for interpretation, so forms of talk established what was not really the case. Thus speaking ironically, joking and speaking dismissively all established reality. A nurse recounted that an old woman had told him that she was too old to go to the geriatric day centre. The nurse laughed and repeated 'too old for the geriatric day centre'. In joking he established the 'reality' that one could not be 'too old' to be considered geriatric.

This discussion foreshadows discussion of the main themes of this monograph, discussed in Chapters 5, 6 and 7. The powers of nurses and patients were conveyed in their forms of talk as well as in what they said: their forms of talk were forms of power. Their forms of assertion of reality were forms of knowledge. Their forms of claiming the right to speak for others or to speak over (monologise) others' voices were forms of participation in moral orders.

The analysis of forms of talk is thus a main pillar of the claim of this monograph that through their talk these nurses and patients negotiated social reality. I will establish through the next three chapters that the nurses and patients were engaged in a form of 'therapy' (Berger and Luckmann, 1967) involving determining what was 'wrong' with the patient, what had to be done for her and the 'rightness' of what was done. I will argue that stories were among the devices through which they accomplished the work of restoring the patient to the main reality, the world of everyday life in the community. The use of the everyday communication device, the story, enabled them to do that work. The concept of story and analysis of stories enabled me to 'handle' the accounts they gave of how they 'handled' their interaction.

Analysis of stories as methods of constructing realities: stories as forms of rationality Being asked to tell me about what happened gave nurses and patients scope for use of the formal possibilities of narrative to construct stories whose beginnings could reach beyond the interaction into past and future. The reasons for their parts in interaction could be established by tying what was done at the time to what had gone before and what would come after. This was the process of constructing the sense of what was done in relation to the 'stay'. Stories conveyed the temporality of stay, and compelled the listener to honour the morality of everyday life, the ontological conditions of which determine the need to wait to know what will happen (Garfinkel, 1967; Schutz and Luckmann, 1974).

Analysis of documents

For each patient, a 'file self' (Harré, 1983) existed, consisting of medical, nursing and administrative records. The records were examined as data on interpretations of the patient from different points of view and for different administrative purposes. They were treated as documents created for specific institutional purposes (Garfinkel, 1968; and Cicourel, 1976). In particular, in light of Altschul's (1972) and MacIlwaine's (1980) contentions that nurses' accounts did not reflect awareness of diagnosis, I read nurses' records to discover how they accounted for interaction in records which could form the basis of professional accountability.

The role of theoretical concepts in the analysis

The mode of analysis of this study was consistent with the theoretical perspective. The theoretical perspective is that theoretical concepts are second order, and depend for their adequacy on the degree to which they are explanatory of first order constructs. In studies of practical life, including nurse-patient interaction, the first order constructs have ontological and hence epistemological priority. In this section I will outline how second order constructs emerged from the data and how they were related to other theoretical constructs and to the developing understanding of the empirical reality being studied.

I have indicated that my understandings throughout the field work were informed by 'sensitising concepts' (Blumer, 1969). At different points in the process of analysis, key theoretical understandings led me to undertake extensive analyses. These understandings were grounded in the empirical reality of the sites. For example, the emergence of the main themes of communication/knowledge, power and moral order derived from a process of inductive analysis of field work concepts, and sensitivity to the relationship between these grounded concepts and key features of Harré's (1979, 1983) theoretical position.

Examples of analysis and theoretical elaboration: cycling to a double hermeneutic

To give an example of the 'play' between data and theory, I will quote from two 'method' notes made a month apart, in which I recorded thoughts I had while cycling to Site One. In the first (11-2-87) I wrote:

> Cycling to Site One yesterday I wanted to 'be more human' - to see and respond to and reflect to the patients - and learn thereby. Today I felt I wanted to let patients see I respected them and their position in being in hospital...

In the second (17-3-87) I wrote:

> Thinks on cycle ride out 'I'll have to remind myself to think "what's going on here?"'

These data reflect understandings that had developed after a few months in the field. The first reflects a feeling that the site somehow called for a show of respect. The second reflects that by that stage the process of developing understandings had to be deliberate and conscious. I knew enough to know that I had to 'keep knowing going'. These notes can be read as signs of a stage in field work, steps on the road to 'going native'. In addition, the first especially reflects something about the empirical focus of this research (cf. Burton, 1978): I had come to see Site One in terms of nurses working to accord respect to 'individuals'; I saw their work as nursing with a 'human' face. These notes formed part of the data base that on analysis yielded three core concepts from Site One: communication/knowledge; power; and moral order. These second order themes of 'knowledge, power and moral order' emerged through a lengthy process of analysis. One day at the end of this process I had an insight that shaped subsequent analysis and the development of this monograph. I saw these terms in relation to the central terms in Giddens' (1976) analysis of interaction: 'communication', 'power' and 'morality'.

A note on Giddens' concept of the reciprocal production and reproduction of interaction and structure

Giddens (1976) elaborated the dialectical relationship between interaction and institution. He argued that social reality is structured and structuring, and that the processes are reflexively related. The microprocesses of interaction and the macroprocesses of institutions are related through intervening 'modalities', thus (p. 122):

INTERACTION	↑	Communication	Power	Morality
(MODALITY)		Interpretative scheme	Facility	Norm
STRUCTURE	↓	Signification	Domination	Legitimation
		(*Weltanshauung*)		

Giddens (1976) argues that in any interaction including talk people draw on 'interpretive schemes' within 'frameworks of mutual knowledge' drawn from a 'cognitive order' and in doing so reproduce the cognitive order. Giddens (1976, pp. 122-3) claims that this is also the case for facilities of power and structures of domination; and for norms drawn from a legitimate order and structures of legitimation.

In later theoretical analyses I realised that Giddens' analysis is part of the interpretive tradition which sees interaction as production of social reality. This understanding led to incorporation of some of Giddens' arguments into the developing theoretical perspective of this monograph. Thus I wrote in theoretical notes:

> **The double hermeneutic: forms of reality and ordinary and technical language**
>
> Because language is construed not as a lens through which to see reality but as a mode of action, it follows that different languages or usages will be found in areas of social life organised for different purposes and interpreting the language is essential to apprehending the reality. Giddens (1972, p. 158) writes: '(S)ociology, unlike natural science, deals with a pre-interpreted world, where the creation and reproduction of meaning-frames is a very condition of that which it seeks to analyse, namely human social conduct: this is...why there is a double hermeneutic in the social sciences..' .

Return full circle to the data

The circle from empirical data to emergent theoretical insight to connection to the literature led to another circle, this time of return to the data. From reading Giddens I returned to reanalyse the data from the first site in terms of 'interpretive schemes' and 'facilities of power', and more generally to consider the institution as interaction. That analysis in turn fed into the analysis of empirical data from the Second Site. It was through this hermeneutic process of analysis - interpretation of what arose in light of background understandings - that the understandings of this monograph were generated.

Conceptual development and 'working words'

In the next Section, 'Sites', I discuss diagnosis in this study, noting that a consultant said that 'neurotic' was not 'a working word'. The concept of 'working word' is apt for capturing a key feature of this analysis, one directly related to issues of reliability and validity. The aim in generating concepts and categories from the data was, as with grounded theory (Glaser and Strauss, 1967), to ensure that the emergent understandings remained tied to the empirical phenomena. The phenomenon was the interaction of the nurses and patients. I will outline in Chapters 5, 6 and 7 that the key themes or categories that organised the data centred on the concept of 'work': knowing 'the main thing' (knowledge related to assessment: the answer to the question 'Why is she here now?'); the 'working relationship' (facilities of power: the answer to the question: 'What do I have to do for her?'); and taking the 'right attitude' toward 'the kind of person' the patient is (norms, rules for according respect and observing rights and obligations: the answer to the question: 'What kind of person is she?'). The categories are expressed both in the actors' 'first order' words ('in vivo codes': Strauss, 1987) - working words, closely tied to the questions that directed work - and in 'second order' codes.

The conceptual development that followed from 'finding' that these working words related to theoretical concepts (see above) was always accompanied by tying the developing concepts back to the language of the site, in field notes or transcripts. This was true even where language seemed least connected to the empirical phenomena. For example, as will be elaborated in Chapter 6, nurses and patients used metaphors in telling about their conversations. Conceptual development through analysis led to understanding that metaphors 'bridged' or 'bound' actions meaningful on different levels: the metaphor of 'weaning' was used to convey what was done in face to face interaction (action), to what that interaction meant as a step in a staff plan (act), and to the overall understanding of the stay (episode). The metaphor was a 'working word' on all levels; the work being clarified through the process of analysis. This argument can be extended: conceptual development was part of the work of the actors in the site. The nurses developed the range of application of common-sense concepts, for example, 'weaning', in doing the work of the site. They used terms from common language as 'working words'. The 'working words' I picked up were the first order constructs they used in the work of restoring unproblematic reality (see Chapters 5, 6 and 7). My understanding of the nurses' working words was tested when I saw if they 'worked' in getting the nurses to confirm or disconfirm my understandings. The issue of validity was addressed by keeping the developing theoretical understandings rooted in the language of the nurses and patients themselves.

The 'play' of empirical and theoretical concepts was part of the ongoing interpretive process. Thus, for example, analysis of 'in vivo' concepts of 'readiness', 'coping' and 'responsibility' generated the category of 'power', which in turn led me to consider Harré's concept of 'powers' and its relationship to concepts 'agent' and 'patient'. This led me in turn to revision of how these concepts functioned in mainstream nursing theory (Henderson, 1966). Again, for example, analysis of the grounded concepts 'knowledge' and 'moral order' led me to review literature on deviance, and occasioned a further analysis in which I 'tried out', by return to the data, a reconceptualisation of the accounts as accounts of deviant patients. This in turn led me to review recent work in medical sociology on the sick role (Turner, 1987). A third example: the theme of 'problems' emerged from the data, originally featured in analysis of the categories, 'knowledge' and 'power', and at a later stage became central to understanding the patients' accounts as narratives of problems, through which they established their character as patients. This then led to consideration of Baruch's (1981) 'moral tales', and to consideration of 'normal problems' (cf. Cicourel, 1976, on 'normal troubles'). Again, this led back to consideration of the nurses' commonsense basis for understanding these patients.

The cycle of interpretation, potentially endless, was brought to closure through an act of commitment (Ricoeur, 1971) sealed through feeding back to the nurses the understandings formed through my participation with them in the process of this research. Developing understandings were thus checked out or confirmed by my continually working out how my interpretations allowed me to understand the world. This process operated when I was checking out the data for disconfirming evidence and to see if my concepts and categories enabled me to make sense. It operated during the field work when I checked to see if my interpretations 'worked' to enable me to get by in the admission wards (or sites of the study) (cf. Burton, 1978). Finally, it operated in the feedback and checking out with the nurses in the sites.[16]

A note on differences and contradictions

The reader will recall that I noted a tension that ran through the analysis. This tension can now be elaborated. I have noted that analysis had a circular form: parts were read in relation to wholes and through the hermeneutic process new understandings developed. This is the model of 'dialogue', the growth of understandings. The metaphor might be the circles of growth marked by rings in a tree. The tension in this monograph lies in the other sort of analysis I did: that which focused on differences. Thus I noted differences between accounts given by a single nurse or patient, and differences between different patients' and different nurses' accounts, and between accounts in one site and those in another. I focused too on differences in concepts drawn from field notes.

The tension lay in contradictions. An analysis of differences consisted of noting, for each pair of accounts, what the main episode/act/actions were according to the nurse and the patient. Then a note was made of similarities and differences. For example, a patient said that she had panicked on a visit to a day centre, accompanied by a nurse. The nurse had calmed her. The nurse said that the patient panicked on the visit, but that walking around, not what the nurse had done, had helped her. Analysis of the corresponding accounts given by patients and nurses (the 'matched pairs') revealed that differences were common. Nurses and patients claimed, in general, to have talked about the same topic. They talked about the same episodes (visit to the Day Hospital), but sometimes different 'acts'[17] ('she comforted me'; 'I didn't do anything'). The ratios often differed: agent to agency, motive to setting. Thus their stories differed. These differences will be explored in Chapters 5, 6 and 7. I will discuss further in Chapter 8 the 'tensions' of contradictions.

Some further comments on reliability and validity

In the Section on 'Methods' I discussed some of the issues of reliability and validity related to the methods used. The process of analysis raised issues of reliability and validity, exploration of which may help the reader appraise the interpretations in the next three chapters. I will summarise the main issues. The reader will find these issues more fully dealt with in Appendix 3.

The main issues with regard to validity in the qualitative interpretive analysis were whether the actor's interpretations and understandings were elicited fully; whether they were interpreted in such a way as to preserve the actors' meanings; and whether they are presented in such a way that the reader can understand the phenomenon from the actor's point of view. I made every attempt to give nurses and patients opportunities to give as full accounts as they wished. There were problems in eliciting accounts from patients who had problems of hearing or speech (see also later chapters). However, these problems reflected issues related to interaction and formed part of the data. There is also a question as to whether, in some cases, accounts from patients were brief or curtailed due to their 'mental state'. It is possible that patients were selective in what they chose to tell about, and this study makes no claim to represent the range or 'quantity' of patients' conversations with the nurses.

Regarding the second point, it is clear that my understanding and interpretation was involved in all stages of analysis, and that, broadly, interpretation was guided by my interests in doing the study. I tried to be sensitive to my biases, and searched for disconfirming as well as confirming material during analysis. I also tried as much as possible to feed back my understanding of what the actor was saying in the interview to clarify that I had 'got it'. That actors could and sometimes did contradict me meant that the 'lead' in understanding lay with them (at least sometimes).

One reply to the threats to validity was that I returned to the nurses in two sites, and in some cases to individual nurses, to check out my whether they 'recognised' themselves in my interpretations. They recognised, not their own, daily, working view of themselves, but a view from a different perspective that captured important aspects of their work.[18] The feedback was not universal nor was it complete. In one site, because most of the nursing staff had changed by the time I gave feedback, I discussed with nurses who had worked in the site at the time, some of whom were working in different wards, what form of feedback would be most helpful. We agreed that I would feed back to as many of the nurses who had taken part in the study as possible, rather than to the whole team working in the ward at the time feedback was given. This meant that some understandings which related to conditions and staff at the time of the study could not be confirmed by all staff. I did not give the patients the same sort of later feedback as I gave the nurses. This was due partly to pragmatic considerations - they had all been discharged by the time I returned to give feedback. Moreover, the main intention of the study was to develop further understandings of use to nurses in their practice. I did not feed back details on differences between patients' and nurses' accounts, as to have done so would have violated the agreement on confidentiality. Nor did I feed back to staff members details of differences in accounts or in interviews given by different nurses.

Another bolster to validity was that I constantly related data of various sorts and from various sources to each other: fieldwork observations to accounts to interviews. This meant that I had a basis to 'check out' understandings at various points .[19]

The issues of reliability are closely related to those of validity. The usual questions - whether another researcher would produce the same 'results' using the same methods and whether the study could be replicated later producing the same results - are not relevant to this research. The study was intended to interpret the actors' interpretations of the interaction they took part in producing. The understandings were of there and then. The theoretical stance was that new interpretations constitute new acts, not 'truer versions' of old acts.

I could have asked other researchers to analyse a portion of the data. However, since the thread that ran through all of the data was my developing understanding of the data, and since that understanding was informed by background understandings and what had 'percolated' through from various sources during the fieldwork (for example, as a result of learning all I knew about Site Two after I had been in Site One), it would have been impossible to ascertain the meaning of agreement or disagreement between my interpretation and that of someone who had not been involved in the same process of understanding.

I have raised the question of differences in understanding and will return to the question in Chapter 8. Here, it is important to conclude that while the aim was to develop understandings that took account of those of the actors, it was not the intention simply to report the actors' understandings. I have developed a set of understandings rooted in the data, but also informed by the interplay of insights gained from the two sites of the study, from the literature and from reinterpretation of the range of background understandings I brought to the study. The main understandings generated through the process of this study are reported in Chapters 5, 6 and 7.

Summary

In this section I have outlined the ways the data were analysed, emphasising that data collection/creation and analysis proceeded together. I highlighted issues related to interpretation of the data as accounts and stories, and stressed the importance of form in analysis of data on nurse-neurotic patient interaction. In the following section I will introduce a 'taste' of how data collection and analysis were done, in presenting the background to the sites and the patients in the study.

Note on the presentation of data

Because I gave assurances that data would be presented in such a way that those who took part in the study could not be identified, I have had to change various details of data presented in the text. Unavoidably, this has in some cases altered meanings. Performing this excision and revision of text, I realised that the process of analysis and presentation in some instances 'cut out'[20] or distorted the meanings the nurses and patients had 'worked' to bring into their talk or shape in conversation.[21]

In some transcripts I excised the minor grunts and rejoinders with which I peppered the flow of nurses' and patients' talk. This lends to some accounts the appearance of 'paragraphical' speech, when the process was much more interactive.

I have tried to retain the usages of the nurses and patients, but recognise that my command of their dialects is imprecise.[22] Likewise I have tried to portray hesitancies and other characteristics of individuals' talk, but have not done so where that seemed to portray the person so obviously that confidentiality was threatened.

I have referred to patients throughout as 'Pn' (e.g. P1) or in transcripts, simply as 'P'. In some places the site is indicated as well, e.g. 'S1P4' is 'Site One, Patient 4'. Nurses are referred to by level of training or experience where relevant. In some instances, when a nurse is referred to over several pages, pseudonyms are used. Nurses are referred to as 'N' in transcripts. I am referred to as 'R' in transcripts.

Notes

1 In asking patients and nurses to give accounts I drew on the work of Harré and Secord (1972) and Shotter (1984) among others. The seminal work of Lyman and Scott (1970) identified the key role played by accounts in the maintenance of social order. One strand of research following their work focuses on accounts given in the 'context of justification', when things go

wrong (Garfinkel, 1967) or when moral standing is called into question (Baruch, 1981). Fielding (1982) used the situation of accounting to create a context of justification in which nurses were asked 'Why did you do that?'. A second strand of accounts literature sees accounts as forms of explanation, not necessarily given in a context of justification (e.g. Becker, 1967; Diers, 1979; Fay, 1975; Bunch, 1982; Hammersley and Atkinson, 1983; Melia, 1981; Nisbett and Wilson, 1977; Smail, 1984; Benner, 1984; Potter and Mulkay, 1985; Askham, 1982.)

The accounts as I gathered them in the main study were not as clearly focused on explicitly asking for the actor's motives and reasons as was the case in Fielding (1982). They were freer forms of 'telling'.

2 She moved from what stood out to connections in wider contexts, continually asking 'so what?' until she reached 'the most fundamental level of meaning - the root of significance for me' (Gray-Snelgrove, 1982, p. 80). She presented the fruits of this analysis in terms of concepts, themes and penetrating features.

3 In the matrix (Harré, 1982, p. 85) are displayed the social situation as perceived by the researcher, the rule system the researcher presumes to be operative, the personality displayed by the participants, and the arbiter of propriety of action in the situation. The main elements of behaviour-action-act-episode analysis are subsumed in the 'cognitive matrix' analysis.

4 Their analysis of story draws on Burke's 'dramatist pentad' (see Chapter 3).

5 Chapman (1987) focuses attention on language in nursing.

6 See the section on subjectivity in Chapter 3.

7 Compare the use of the concept 'response' in Altschul (1972), reviewed in Chapter 2.

8 Compare Peplau (1952), see Chapter 2.

9 See Harré and Secord (1972) and Harré (1979) on behaviour-action-act-episode analysis.

10 The quality of tapes was variable, some being less audible or in parts unintelligible. My goal was to transcribe only what I took to be a warrantable hearing of what was said. Where material was not intelligible it was not transcribed, its place in the transcript being indicated by a question mark in brackets, thus: '(?)'. Where I felt I understood what was said but could not fully warrant the hearing, I transcribed the possible words in brackets with a question mark, [thus: ('the words'?)]. My intention was to

produce as full a transcript as possible, but to indicate ambiguous or uninterpretable portions.

I made sense of how the nurses and patients made sense by being an active participant in the construction of accounts. In transcribing the accounts I transcribed my participation as fully as possible, complete with prompts, 'Mnhmn's, 'OK'. Where sighs and laughs were clearly noted, they are included, but tone of voice, while definitely important in understanding what is said throughout, is only noted where it seems particularly important to indicate how I understood what was being said [thus: '(Note:...)'].

I have omitted many of the 'Mnhhns' and other annotations in presenting data in the text, for the sake of brevity and ease of reading; but only where I considered that this did not substantially alter the sense of the text.

11 These are likewise indicated thus: '(Note:...)'. They can be distinguished only by their content from the notes on tone of voice.

12 One of the themes of this monograph is the constant exchange between self and world. This applied to me as well: my self was involved in the process of this study, and part of the method was paying attention to my feelings, understandings, misunderstandings. In Chapter 8 I return to consider the implications of these methods and modes of analysis for nursing research. Hunt (1989) has explored 'psychoanalytic aspects of fieldwork' and the rich potential for understanding unconscious processes in research (through dream analysis, for example; and analysis of transference).

13 An example of a situation was an old woman talking to a student nurse about her home town, the 'rule system' being the norms of social conversation, the 'personality' a friendly person from the same locale, and the 'arbiter' (imagined) another local person.

14 'Agent' and 'agency' are two of Burke's (1969a) pentad terms, the others being 'act', 'scene' and 'motive'. By 'agent' is meant the actor whose intention is the central concern of the story, while by 'agency' is meant the means through which the agent acts. For example, in the board game 'Cluedo', the stories are based on someone (the agent; e.g. Professor Plum) killing another (the act; e.g. the murder of Colonel Mustard) with an implement (the agency; e.g. the candlestick), somewhere in the house (the scene). The motive is never an issue in 'Cluedo'.

I will argue that nurses and patients are both agents and agencies in relation to each other. The nurse is an instrument (agency) of the patient's (agent's) action, sometimes and in some ways. The patient is an instrument (agency) of the the nurse's (agent's) action, sometimes, in some ways. The 'ratio' changes with changes in relationship and as 'work' is advanced.

15 The subject of silences, gaps, and how to understand them has been addressed by Faulkner (1979) and Clark (1981), in discussions of 'opportunities' missed by nurses.

16 I will elaborate in later chapters that this process of analysis represents reflexively what nurses and patients had to do to operate in the sites.

17 See Burke (1969a); and Harré and Secord (1972).

18 See also Chapter 8.

19 See Denzin (1970) on 'triangulation'.

20 See Silverman (1985) on 'cutting out'.

21 In Chapter 8 I consider how these methods could be used in practice. There, indexical and personal material could become the explicit focus of attention.

22 During work as a therapist I was alerted to the possibility that some emotions might only exist in the culture in which a word could name them (cf. Harré, 1983). Retention of the local meanings is vital in psychiatric nursing practice.

Section 3: Description of the sites

Introduction

In the previous two sections I described the method and forms of analysis used in this study. In this section I will first describe how I gained access to two sites. Then I will describe the process of entry to the sites, the beginning of the process of data collection and analysis. Next, I give 'thumbnail sketches' of the two sites, giving information on situation, layout and other features relevant to understanding the sites as the contexts for the interaction reported in this monograph. I then outline the practice of diagnosis in the two sites; review the significance of diagnosis in this study; and describe the patients who participated in the study. This section thus sets the scene for the three chapters which follow, in which the understandings developed through this study are presented.

Through the process of gaining entry to and early days in the two sites, I began to realise that the sites were the processes of interaction in the sites. The objective worlds of the sites were known first of all subjectively through participation in the interpretation of intersubjective reality. The knowledge of social life reported in this monograph was gained through participation in the construction of social reality. The understandings developed here were context-related, developed through the temporal course of the fieldwork and accounts. What I knew later I knew in light of what I had known earlier, and what I had known earlier was reinterpreted in light of constant comparison with what I knew later.

In the section on 'Diagnosis', I indicate that understanding the processes by which patients were nominated as suitable for the study opened the door to understanding more general features of the construction of social reality in the sites. In indicating the complex issues related to how patients came to be in the study I highlight more general issues regarding the difficulty of drawing inferences and making explanations about nurse-patient interaction.

The two sites are not being evaluated in relation to each other. Theoretically, interaction is assumed to make sense in the sites it reflexively realises. The aim of the study is to develop understanding of the interaction in each site, to enter the worlds of the sites. Nonetheless, movement from one 'world' to another involved realisation that each 'world' was part of the larger macrocosm of nurse-patient interaction, some of the more general features of which are noted in Chapters 5, 6 and 7.[1]

Gaining access

The Ethics of Medical Research Committee

Permission to conduct the research was granted by the local Ethics of Medical Research Committee following correspondence on the potential value of the research and the possible risk of intrusion into the normal therapeutic practice of the wards. The Committee approved the study subject to satisfactory early feedback from the consultant and nurses in the first site. This was given and the Committee granted full approval.[2]

Selection of sites

Following the trial of methods (see 'Methods' section), two sites were chosen from among the psychiatric admission wards in the area. The decision to study two sites was based on the rationale that comparison would enable better understanding of how interaction related to context. Within the limits of my resources, I wanted to get access to as many 'worlds' of interaction as possible, to see variations in 'local' social resources.

The first site was chosen partly because informal contacts indicated that it might be open to the prospect of research. The second site was chosen from among several admission wards in a nearby hospital. I approached one of these wards first, on the grounds that it had in the past specialised in treatment of neuroses. The new consultant, an academic psychiatrist, offered me access but declared that I would find no patients diagnosed as neurotic on his ward, and that moreover the concept of neurosis was no longer commonly used in diagnosis, having been supplanted by the concept of 'personality disorder'.[3]

Having no reason to think that any one ward would be preferable as a second site, I chose as Site Two the ward whose consultants first responded to my letter requesting access.[4]

A flavour of methods: negotiation of entry involved negotiation of understandings

Site One The first days in each site were especially important sources of data. My notes on the process of entry into the sites contain seeds of the themes of knowledge, power and moral order, which emerged through analysis of all the data and which will be analysed in depth in following chapters.

Entry to Site One began with informal contact with a nurse who indicated that nursing administration and staff on an admission ward might be receptive to involvement in research. Following approval by managers I contacted the ward's consultant, who said that the charge nurse could handle negotiation of entry. This negotiation involved meeting with, discussing the research with and getting the collective agreement of all ward staff and patients.

In my first meeting with the staff, the consultant suggested that my research was somewhat anthropological and that I might offer them beads; whereupon I, an American (albeit long resident in Scotland), felt suddenly and acutely under the scrutiny of a strange tribe.

The power of scrutiny was brought home to me many months after the research ended. I met a nurse who had started in Site One on the day I began my research. I had felt we were 'new boys' starting together, and used him as a valuable source of impressions. Only when I met him later, in neutral territory, did he tell me that his anxiety at starting in a new ward was magnified by the thought that I was going to be observing not only the ward but him.

The staff in Site One negotiated first with me and then among themselves what role I should claim in telling the patients about the research. They and I agreed that the patients might not understand my interest in 'neurotic' patients[5], and that I could explain that I was interested in the sort of 'problems' that had brought some people to the hospital. They concluded that I would be better saying I was a student at the University (true) rather than a nurse (also true), on the grounds that if the patients thought I was a nurse they might not feel free to tell me as much about their talk with nurses.

I duly claimed the student role in a meeting with all staff and patients, during which the staff encouraged the patients to consider what implications my being around and asking them about conversations might have for their sense of privacy and for confidentiality.

During this meeting I realised something of the importance of interpretations and the potential for confusion of meanings. After my explanation a patient asked about my religious convictions. The group watched and waited for my reply, and I understood again that observation and knowing in this place would be not one-way but a continuous hermeneutic process. I knew that I had to find a way of replying that recognised that the question should not be answered there and then - that I did not have to give an account of my beliefs in this setting - but that did not display that I knew the question to be inappropriate. I came to know the site in part by feeling how the people in it came to know me and let me come to know them.

The staff and patients agreed to let me come into their place. In early days I was aware I had continually to negotiate my role, as patients in meetings asked if I was a nurse (I hedged until saying that I used to work as a nurse but was now a full time student); as I had to find someplace and some one to have coffee with; as I had to 'read' when to stay or leave rooms as others came and went; as patients asked me to do things for them and I declined. A patient who had been in the site for months acted as a sort of 'guide'. When I tried to wash dishes with the patients, she took the towel from me and directed me to the day room, saying that my 'job' was to sit there.

I was acutely self-conscious during early days in the sites, and felt strong urges to find a role the playing of which would reduce my discomfort. At the same time, staff and patients tried to identify or define a role for me. I found that I could not be in the site without a role, and that others would define me in ways meaningful to them but sometimes discordant with my own claims.

I finally adopted a kind of 'roving' role. This roving was a method for knowing the site and a product of knowing the site. I 'responded' to what felt like expectations and demands to be in one place and not another, to leave a room when some things were said and not others. I sat with the patients in the sitting room when this felt right; I sat in 'community meetings'[6] with staff and patients; after these meetings I usually joined staff to hear their review, but sometimes stayed out with patients to see if they had an alternative review; I went to staff meetings and staff hand-overs (when nurses changing shifts told the new team what had been happening). If it seemed that a nurse and patient wanted privacy to talk I left them alone; if it seemed my presence was not intrusive I stayed. If in doubt I asked if it was all right to be where I was, doing what I was doing.

Site Two The 'rules' according to which 'strangers' were 'incorporated' (Harré, 1979, pp. 214-220) were different in Site Two. There, entry was controlled by senior nurses and consultants. I did not have to negotiate directly with or get the permission of all nurses or the patients. Instead, the consultants gave permission, on behalf of the patients, for me to spend time in the site as a participant observer; junior nursing staff met me separately from senior staff; and I was not asked to seek student nurses' agreement to participation. It was left to my discretion how to present myself to patients. There was, in effect, no patient group to which I was accountable. The attitude of the nurses was summed up when I asked a nurse whether I should tell the patients at the morning meeting who I was and what I was doing. He said that the patients were used to people coming into groups and that I did not need to tell them, but could 'if the spirit moves you'. The nurse said that patients here were so used to being asked questions that they did not ask 'Why?'. Had I said I was doing research, the nurse said, patients would have asked 'Into what? Soap?'.

Being subject to the gaze I found through the fieldwork experience that being in the sites was being subject to gaze and to interpretation. I want to highlight this: I want to convey by 'being subject to' not the relatively passive gerund, but the fact that I was a kind of being (subjective and objective) that/who was subject(ed) to the gaze of others who likewise were subject(ed) to my gaze (cf. Goffman, 1963; Foucault, 1979). The period of entry to the sites was the period of most obviously intense interaction through gaze and talk. Threads of what emerged as main themes through the course of ongoing fieldwork and analysis could be seen in early days. For example, in Site Two, access to patients and to nurses - to the public arena which observation implies - was controlled from the top down through professional hierarchies, and I never had to negotiate my rights and obligations with the patients as a group. Conversely, I found it much more difficult in Site Two to sit among the patients; and none of them 'guided' me as had happened in Site One. I often felt that no one in Site Two wanted me to be there. A consultant suggested at the first meeting that I would be better doing the study in a Day Hospital attended by more patients diagnosed as neurotic. I felt that a senior member of the nursing staff similarly steered me away from other nurses during early days. A consultant suggested that the nurses were somewhat unsure how they would be seen in a study of this sort, since the focus of their work was with psychotic rather than neurotic patients, and they therefore might be judged inappropriately. Thus in entering the sites I began to form impressions about structures of knowledge and control of access to knowledge; guidance, control and power; and management of moral orders; themes to be explored more fully in Chapters 5, 6 and 7.

The flavour of the sites

The theoretical significance of these comments on entry to the sites is that understandings developed through processes of interaction and negotiation of meanings. These processes were structured in the ways that the knowledge, power and moral orders were structured. Thus participation in the sites necessitated entry into the belief systems in the sites, and interaction based on the systems. I have mentioned the 'persona' I adopted in the sites. It is important to emphasise that this does not imply that I wore a 'mask' during fieldwork. I played a role and tried to negotiate that role to enable me to do the work of understanding that I wanted to do. However, the way I felt, what I could do, who I understood myself to be on an ongoing basis reflected the responses of others to me. My entry into the knowledge of the sites was through entry to a form of self-knowledge earned through interaction.

Site One: a description

One of the main themes of this research is that situations are defined through interaction. An implication of this is that the problem of saying what psychiatric nursing is can be reconceived as a problem of describing where psychiatric nursing occurs. This problem is 'glossed over' (Garfinkel, 1967) if the site in which psychiatric nursing takes place is tacitly assumed to be stable, accomplished, somehow already 'there'. My argument is that the site, the 'where' of interaction, must take into account the four-dimensional character of the location of practice.

Site is a 'when' and a 'whom' or 'with whom' as well as a 'where'. The first site of this research was different at different times and when different people were working. One aspect of the complexity of what the nurses did was the complexity of the physical and social contexts in which they worked and which they sustained through their work. In attempting to illuminate a context for understanding of interaction, I had to take account of this complexity. My aim as researcher was congruent with that of the nurses; namely, to tell what the place was like. The nurses constituted the site for their practical purposes through telling what it was like.

Site One: the place

Site One was the main admission ward in a small hospital in the country. The hospital was seen by the staff working there as closely linked to the community and reflecting it. The nursing staff mostly lived locally and knew the local towns and, not infrequently, the patients or their families. Ward based nurses liaised with day centres and general practitioners and often knew a patient's psychiatric history or reputation before seeing the patient. People coming from the community were not wholly getting away from it when they came to the hospital. The ward was geographically isolated from the centres of population yet was a distinct part of the community, or a distinct location of part of the community.

The admission ward had twenty beds to which one consultant admitted adult patients including patients over the age of sixty-five. The staff working there comprised: one consultant and two junior doctors, two charge nurse/sisters, one staff nurse (these latter three trained as Registered Mental Nurses), two state enrolled nurses, student nurses, an occupational therapist, two variably attending social workers, and sundry domestics and porters.

The ward was arranged on two floors, with dormitories and women's toilets on the upper floor, and all other facilities - sitting room, nurses' station, offices, kitchen, interview rooms and men's toilets - on the ground floor.

Privacy and gaze A pervasive feature of the ward was lack of privacy. I was acutely aware from the moment of entry into the ward of the difficulty of avoiding the gaze or presence of others. The glass walls of the nurses' station allowed the nurses to look out at the patients and the patients to look in on the nurses. The walls of this glass room were not wholly soundproof so that any dramas (and any ordinary interaction) not removed from the sitting room/nurses' station area were available to any who did not deliberately disattend. The mutual availability to gaze was echoed in the sitting room where a tank of gold fish provided an alternative focus of attention. The gold fish had a 'drug sheet' on which was prescribed 'fish food', fed by the patients. Availability to gaze and the management of conduct in conditions of close contact in a confined space were central features of the ward. I felt under the gaze of the others and, initially with acute self-consciousness, avoided meeting their eyes.

Goffman (1963), Foucault (1979) and Bloor and McIntosh (1987) have described the relationship between observation and control, especially the power involved in subjecting others to gaze. Asquith (personal communication) has noted that location of site may relate to power of gaze. Hospitals located in rural settings stand out more than do urban ones, and they and the folk in them may be more readily the focus of gaze. Thus the focus of gaze inside 'reflects' the focus of gaze of those outside, through the eyes of the nurses, other staff and patients who move from the outside to the inside and see those within the institution. The gaze in urban hospitals may be more anonymous. This 'reflection' of the outside world may be a feature of the 'common sense' linking nurses inside with the community outside. In Chapters 5, 6 and 7 I will examine public-private exchange as a key feature in the construction of knowledge, power and relationships in the moral orders of the sites.

I have described the layout of the ward to highlight how ward architecture affected use of space and time (cf. Altschul, 1972). Lack of space presented many problems. During busy periods in the ward one could have no certainty of getting a chair in the main sitting area. Twice daily the sitting areas had to be transformed into settings for group meetings by importing chairs from the kitchen. In the cramped quarters peoples' bodies and bodily functions were available to others' attention. In group morning exercises in the sitting room all fit patients and nursing and occupational therapy staff were expected to jump and stretch in unison; other displays were unintended - gut sounds in quiet spells in the sitting room, treks across the room to the toilets.

The ward was arranged on two floors. Because nurses could not routinely be deployed during the day to 'observe' on the upper floor, access to the upper floor, to beds and to lockers with personal possessions, was restricted from breakfast time till evening. If patients wanted to get something from the dormitories, they had to get a key from the nurses. Thus during the day patients generally carried what they needed, bundles of knitting or reading, handbags. The dining room was usually a throughfare, and at times was locked off for use as an occupational therapy area. Small interview rooms were sometimes claimed by patients, on one occasion for small prayer meetings, but such use could be interrupted by other patients or staff.

The lack of space and privacy extended into the night. The male and female patients slept in two adjacent dormitories, separated by a door usually locked at night. If a patient got up in the night, to go to the toilet or to talk to a nurse, she risked disturbing others. A recurrent theme in meetings was disrupted sleep. When patients were tearful, angry or disorientated and wandering in the night, nurses and patients had to try to suppress or tolerate the disturbance. A bad night for one patient meant bags under the eyes of many.

The ability of staff and patients to accommodate all that occurred in the public areas of the ward, especially the sitting area, was remarkable. During the period of observation a patient stripped in the sitting room, two had fits, one was fed from a drip, fire alarms were set off, furniture was smashed, and a number of people wailed, shouted or behaved oddly. Whether these unusual displays could be removed from view depended on the 'situation in the ward', that is, on the number and grade of staff and the state of other patients. Most of the time most of what went on in the sitting room was utterly normal: sitting, knitting, gossip, television viewing, games, and so on. It was, though, observable and hence remarkable normality.[7] Such normality could be seen as 'deviant', as will be elaborated below: if patients pleasantly pursued ordinary activities, the ward could be likened to a hotel or a holiday camp, rather than what it was 'really', a psychiatric ward. The problems of construction of 'the reality' of the ward as a psychiatric ward will be discussed in Chapter 5.

Site Two

Site Two was one of several admission wards in a large teaching hospital in the city. In this site there seemed to be none of the close-knit links between staff and patients that I had found in Site One. Each of the admission wards in the hospital in which Site Two was situated was said to have a different character, with Site Two said (by its own nurses) to be the quietest. It was a modern ward with side rooms accommodating from one to several beds. There were two main day or television rooms, and patients ate at a cafeteria off the ward. There was a sense of more space, more separate spaces and less crowding than in Site One. There was a corresponding sense of less intimacy. Site Two felt less homely, more clinical, though it is difficult to explain in what way.

The Second Site was arranged on a single floor, with side rooms and dormitories, two sitting rooms, and offices. From the nurses' station the patients' main sitting room and the main dormitory could be observed through windows. Blinds were adjusted in the station so that the effect was like that of a one-way mirror, enabling observation of patients by nurses but not vice versa. The nurses in the office could thus be more cut off from patients, a point noted by one nurse who commented that the nurses spent a good deal of time in the office while patients sat in the day room. The nurse thought that this was due to the ward architecture, saying that in other wards nurses had to make a point of sitting outside the office to be with patients. It is noteworthy that the use of space and time in the two sites differed markedly in part due to the requirement that sites of quite different architecture were used for purposes of observation. The quality of life of all patients was to an extent affected by the administrative and clinical purposes of the sites. The patients in this study, who generally were not 'under' 'close observation'[8], nonetheless had to live in spaces organised to allow observation of others. Hence, they too were 'observed'.

Site Two had 21 beds, for both male and female patients. Nursing staff comprised two charge nurse/sisters, three to four staff nurses, and at times several student nurses. Two consultants admitted patients to the ward, and a senior registrar and two junior doctors completed the psychiatric staff. The ward was serviced by a number of other professionals: an occupational therapist, a social worker and sometimes a social work student, sometimes a psychologist. There were lines of communication and referral between the Site and other specialist units in the hospital.

Diagnosis and selection of patients

A note on the concept of diagnosis in this research

I noted that a consultant in Site Two claimed that the concept of 'neurosis' was no longer current in his or others' practice. His claim led me to consider whether I should abandon conducting the research on the basis of the concept of 'neurosis', and substitute a concept more likely to be used, for example, 'non-psychotic' (see below)[9]. However, I decided to continue using the concept on the grounds that the problem posed through previous nursing research related specifically to this concept, it was still in use in other research and training programmes relevant to nursing (Marks, 1977, 1985), and it was still used for psychiatric 'administrative' purposes (see below). Indeed the consultant's response raised the theoretically salient point that the existence of a group of people might be in doubt in one place and not in another, or for one set of purposes and not another. In addition it highlighted that previous nursing researchers' reliance on the concept for explanation, in particular their reliance on ironic juxtaposition of diagnosis with commonsense meaning, might have led them to conclusions the validity of which is difficult to assess retrospectively.

Diagnosis and the selection of patients

In the proposal for the study submitted to the Ethnics Committee I indicated that patients would be selected on the basis of diagnosis of neurosis, comprising International Classification of Disease (ICD9) diagnoses 300.1-300.9 inclusive and 306.2 (World Health Organization, 1978).[10] These diagnoses were chosen to correspond to the formulations used by MacIlwaine (1980)[11]. The definition of which patients were suitable for inclusion in the study under these terms was negotiated with the medical staff in the two Sites. I will describe that process and then note the diagnoses of the patients in this study. I made no a priori assumptions about the validity or reliability of diagnosis, nor about the relevance of diagnosis to medical or nursing practice.[12]

Site One

The consultant in Site One noted that there would be few patients with the relevant diagnoses at any given time, and that diagnosis might change during admission. We agreed that the patients suitable for the study would be those nominated by the consultant on the basis that, had they been given a discharge diagnosis[13] on the day on which selection of patients started (after the first month of field work), they would have been given a main diagnosis of neurosis; and patients admitted subsequently with such a diagnosis as an admission diagnosis. I had to negotiate with the consultant which diagnoses in ICD 9 would fall within the term 'neurotic'.

Selection of patients and routine practice in Site One Asking the consultant in Site One to select patients on the basis of diagnosis highlighted features of the routine working practices of doctors in Site One. He explained that diagnosis was not at the front of the doctors' minds when they considered patients on a day to day basis. Diagnosis was done routinely five days after admission, in part to satisfy administrative regulations. The doctors' practice was guided more by formulation than diagnosis, with 'personality' as well as 'illness' factors being taken into account in diagnosis. The concept of 'neurosis' was little used; instead the main working distinction was between 'psychotic' and 'non-psychotic' patients.

Thus in asking the consultant to select patients in this way I was asking him to make extraordinary judgements; to diagnose patients at an unusual point in their stay, for reasons other than those that guided his routine practice. This diagnosis, in particular for the patients chosen when selection began - selected on the basis of what diagnosis they would have received had they been diagnosed that day - was an artefact of the research.

The routine practice of diagnosis in Site One In light of the weight previous nursing researchers had placed on diagnosis as an explanatory variable, without enquiring into the social construction of diagnosis, I wanted to know what the concept 'neurotic' meant in the Sites. I interviewed medical and nursing staff about diagnosis, asking when it was done, who did it, who knew of it, what changed as a result of it, whether the terms 'neurotic' and 'neurosis' were used and what they meant, number of patients thus diagnosed, whether they knew of it, and whether staff used the terms in a lay sense.

The consultant distinguished between diagnosis - 'a shorthand label to tell us something about the patient' - and formulation, a summary of 'why the patient is presenting this way', including a description of the patient's stresses and supports. He considered formulation the better guide to treatment, helping him in 'trying to arrive at the right attitude' to the patient. Diagnosis referred to the patient at one point in time, while formulation was dynamic, a hypothesis or set of hypotheses tested in the practice of treatment (Sladden, personal communication). A junior doctor who had worked in both sites said that more weight would be given to diagnosis in Site Two than in Site One. The doctor emphasised that in Site One the consultant's view on the patient was the last word: 'what the consultant thinks would determine what would happen for the patient'.

Diagnosis as label in Site One The charge nurse in Site One, like the consultant, referred to diagnosis as a label. He indicated that regarding patients in terms of diagnosis was reductionistic: the diagnosis was only 'part of the individual', and it was with each patient as an individual that the nurses were concerned.[14] Other nurses confirmed this anti-reductionist stance.

Diagnosis and guidance Thus asking about patients in terms of diagnosis brought out important features of the work of medical and nursing staff. Thinking about patients in terms of diagnosis was not, at least explicitly, the basis of routine practice. Indeed, it violated some aspects of the ethos of the place. This view was the dominant one, but not shared by all. A student who had worked in Site Two complained that patients in Site One:

> never have a diagnosis. They remain in assessment until they're discharged... (The consultant) is uncompromisingly against labelling people (hence the nurses) never know what (the patients) are being treated for.

What was at issue was whether diagnosis was necessary to work as nurses were meant to work in the site. A newly qualified nurse said that knowing a diagnosis:

> gives me a starting point instead of saying 'this is a person' and you just have to flounder about...I'm just in the job and looking for a certain amount of guidance.

An experienced nurse said that he had to know diagnoses to meet the students' need for 'security', 'to put patients in a box', but 'nursing wise' the trained nurses were 'not strong on labels'. Raising the question of diagnosis thus brought out understandings of what the work of the site was, who could define the work, and the basis of competent practice.

Diagnosis of neurosis in Site One

The consultant, who said that his orientation was 'psychotherapeutic', said that diagnosis of neurosis was a matter of distinguishing 'levels' of illness. In saying that a patient was neurotic he was saying also that they were not psychotic or organically ill. It meant that the patient was suffering from a disorder in which 'anxiety is a feature', and where the patient's 'way of handling bad feelings' was 'maladaptive'. Neurosis was 'maladaptive processing of bad affect'. He considered that 'neurosis' and 'personality disorder' were matters of degree: if 'more of the personality were involved' the person would be diagnosed as a 'personality disorder'. The junior doctors claimed that neurosis was a 'diagnosis of exclusion'[15], based on excluding psychoses and organic conditions. Some nurses said that the term 'neurotic' might be used in a 'lay' sense in 'privacy', to mean 'a patient full of complaints at their life situation', or to mean 'she's neurotic - meaning, she's driving me crazy'. Another said such a 'lay' use would be a 'misuse of the term for people getting anxious for valid or invalid reasons or for acting out or childish behaviour'.

The consultant said that instead of using diagnostic terms in speaking to a patient he might use the terms 'ill' or 'problems'. He said that by 'ill' he meant 'not responsible at this time'; illness 'excused them a lot of behaviour'. He meant to convey a different 'message' regarding responsibility in telling a patient 'you've got problems'.[16]

Diagnosis in Site Two

In Site Two I interviewed the two consultants, junior doctors and several nurses, using the same interview schedules as in Site One. Both consultants emphasised, as had the consultant in Site One, that formulation was more important than diagnosis in organisation of their work. The formulation was meant to say something about why the patient was 'presenting in this way now'. As in Site One both consultants referred to the administrative requirement that diagnoses be done within a given time. The diagnosis had to be approved by the consultant, and in this sense the diagnosis was what the consultant said it was. One consultant usually told patients their diagnoses, the other said diagnoses were mainly useful as a shorthand in interprofessional communication, avoiding the necessity of repeated description, and were not routinely told to patients.

One of the consultants said that the ward nurses' role in diagnosis was to provide observations which informed the doctors' decisions. Some nurses in the Site said that they sometimes disagreed with diagnoses, in which case they provided the doctors with information intended to change the diagnosis, rather than challenging the view directly.[17] A trained nurse said that his disagreements, when they occurred, were over 'management issues' rather than diagnosis, and that he had no skill in diagnosis.

Something of the character of Site Two can be gleaned from these comments on diagnosis. In one respect, Site Two was like Site One: in both sites the consultants emphasised the importance, for practical management of the patients, of the view conveyed by formulation. However, in Site Two the nurses emphasised the doctors' responsibility for diagnosis and management, and the etiquette involved in managing discrepant views.

Diagnosis of neurosis in Site Two The consultants in Site Two noted, as had the consultant in Site One, that the diagnosis of neurosis was less reliable than that of psychosis (cf. Kendell, 1975). The more meaningful distinction from the point of view of practical management was between psychotic and non-psychotic patients. The nurses shared these views, saying that they would 'approach' psychotic and non-psychotic patients differently, this term conveying features of the nurses' work involving close proximity and need to communicate with patients some of whom were considered out of touch with one's reality.

One consultant said that the ward was 'geared up to' the treatment of psychotic patients. He and a senior nurse referred to another ward in the hospital which had specialised in treatment of neurotic patients. Both said that in comparison the nurses in Site Two felt unsure of their abilities in nursing these patients. They also referred to a day hospital to which most neurotic patients would go, the implication again being that other nurses elsewhere were more competent in management of patients diagnosed as neurotic.

Site Two was thus characterised by clinical and administrative division, including specialist units, which effectively rendered other units less competent by comparison. The senior nurse likened Site Two to a 'casualty department', with various sorts of patients coming in and being channeled to more specialist services.[18]

Issues of communication and power in relation to the patients diagnosed as neurotic In Site Two both nurses and doctors said that talking to the patients would be a more important aspect of treatment with patients diagnosed as neurotic than with those diagnosed as psychotic. However, the difficulty of talking with these patients was stressed by several nurses. One said that neurotic patients were 'palmed off' on students because senior staff had little time. Another said that the patients had one-to-one 'formal interviews' with the doctors, the content of which the nurses did not share, and that this enabled the patients to avoid talking to the nurses by saying that they had already discussed things with the doctor. Some nurses noted that their role involved 'observing' the patients, not being involved with them, and that what they observed at times conflicted with what the patient told a doctor. From the nurses' point of view it appeared that the doctors, lacking the evidence of observation, often took the patient's view against the nurses'. This situation created problems in attributing responsibility to the patient. (The issue of responsibility will emerge as important in Chapter 6.) The nurses also felt frustrated in their effort to 'offer a service' to the patient when the patient denied that she had problems (cf. May and Kelly, 1982). If the patient offered discrepant stories the nurses could not help her. The frustration was directed toward the doctors, the nurses wondering why the patient was kept in hospital when she denied her problem.

Issues of communication and power were closely related. A number of nurses mentioned that the neurotic patients were more 'equal' to or more like the nurses than were psychotic patients. The neurotic patients could challenge what the nurses said.[19] They were thought to dislike talking to trained staff (compared to students) because trained staff were always looking for 'meaning' in what the patient said whereas students were 'innocent'. Psychotic patients were thought to see the nurses as there to do a job and manage the ward, whereas it was difficult to know what the neurotic patients thought the nurses were there for. The nurses experienced the frustration of feeling that nothing they said to these patients made any difference. They felt like saying to the patient, but could not say, 'if you could just sort it out...'.

'Neurotic' not a working word The doctors said that 'neurotic' was not used in its lay sense. That sense was thought to be pejorative, meaning:

screwed up, having emotional difficulties and relationship problems.

The nurses said that the term was not often used in its technical, diagnostic sense: it was 'not a working word'. However, the nurses said that when the term 'neurotic' was used it was used by doctors to refer to patients who were 'difficult, not rewarding', taking up much time, 'not fulfilling their contractual obligation', 'someone who wants you to do something you regard as unimportant'; or to refer to patients' relatives they considered 'overconcerned', 'dissatisfied, infringing on medical territory and decisions' ('we have our own ideas and don't want them to be questioned'). One nurse said that the term 'neurotic' when used by the nurses meant that the patient should not be in hospital. The nurses also said that nurses more often used the term to refer in a derogatory way to other staff than to refer to patients: 'to stop you (the nurse) in your tracks and devalue what (you) said'. The student who said this also said that in order to understand the site, it was important to pay attention to how the medical staff valued what the nurses said.

The nurses' 'working words' were explored by asking them to 'sort' patients on the basis of the concepts they used in their day-to-day work (Canter et al., 1985). The nurses' sorts can be found in Appendix 10.

These data suggest that the concept 'neurotic' was meaningful in a number of ways in Site Two. Examination of its uses always pointed to issues of conflict, between patient and nurse or doctor, and between nurses and doctors. The conflict centred on communication, on discrepancies between what was said and what was seen, or between what was said to one person and what to another. That conflict was inseparable from the process of diagnosis, part of which involved the nurses feeding observations to the doctors who decided what was wrong with the patient and whether she should be in hospital. The image of the nurses was of a group of people constrained in what they could say and low (sometimes lower than the patients) in the 'hierarchy of credibility'. Nor, apparently, was the superficial similarity between such an image and the commonsense image of the 'neurotic' meaningless, for the nurses used the term 'neurotic' in its lay sense to demean each other. The power to mark another as abnormal in her response to ordinary events of life was evident not only in the professional discourse of diagnosis and interprofessional communication. It was likewise evident in the informal discourse of the nurses and doctors, when the fear was that the power would be wielded on them. One nurse in conversation with other nurses and a doctor said that she would hate and avoid being admitted to the site, more so if she had a 'nervous breakdown' than if psychotic, because she and they knew what got known about the patients, what got asked and what got talked about.

The question of diagnosis of neurosis thus raised issues of power, of making claims about claims and making the claims stick. It intersected the myriad other questions of power in Site Two. The implications of this feature, whereby the 'official' use of the concept was infrequent, and the 'unofficial' use was considered improper but was clearly functional in the site, have not been noted by previous British nursing researchers (John, 1961; Altschul, 1972; MacIlwaine, 1980).

A retrospective conclusion on the value of using diagnosis as the basis for patient selection

The above discussion highlights some important issues related to selection of patients on the basis of diagnosis. If research is conducted on the basis of a logic that seeks to explain findings as effects of or as correlated with variables, then diagnosis raises certain issues. The reliability and validity of diagnosis are central concerns, and it is important to stipulate the conceptual basis on which diagnosis is claimed to be responsible for effects, and whether it mediates the effects of other variables. Some claim must be made about whether a diagnosis considered as a variable is thought to have explanatory power because as 'label' it mediates social processes or whether it is thought to indicate something about the nature, character or powers of the person diagnosed; which in turn are responsible, through some processes, for differences in what is observed.

Those were not the concerns of this study. Diagnosis of 'neurosis' as a basis of selection was chosen, not because I considered it a variable to be used in explanation, but because a number of explanations in the nursing literature were based on it. What I wanted to find out was whether people in the two sites considered diagnosis meaningful in structuring their work with patients, and to elucidate better than had previous nursing researchers the relationship between the meaning conveyed by diagnosis and the common-sense meaning, from the point of view of the staff in the sites. This recalls the arguments in Chapter 2 regarding the relationship of common sense to 'special' meanings. The nursing researcher 'policing' the boundaries of common sense and special meanings is obliged to consider that the language he takes as his topic is the product of nurses and other staff themselves policing the meanings.

What I found was that in highlighting the term 'neurotic' I discovered aspects of the working practices of nurses and patients that were relevant to my understandings of nurse-neurotic patient interaction. These understandings will be elaborated in Chapters 5, 6 and 7. However, the value of those understandings was not dependent on any assumption about what 'neurotic' patients were 'really' like, or whether nurses or doctors had 'got it right' or 'wrong'. What was of theoretical interest in this study was the social construction of reality. I could 'read' aspects of that construction by paying attention to how others negotiated with me and with each other the meaning(s) of 'neurotic' in the course of interviews and processes of patient selection.

A description of the patients selected for the study

Site One

Six patients in Site One agreed to take part in the study by giving accounts of their conversations with nurses. Five were females, one male. Two were young, two middle aged and two elderly. I took no written note of their other demographic data, though this information might have been relevant to analysis (cf. Altschul, 1972). Three had been in the site for periods of several months when they became available for selection, while the other three were nominated by the consultant early after admission or when the formulation changed to one occasioning the consultant's diagnosis (for the purposes of the study) of neurosis.

The consultant diagnosed them on the basis that at the time of nomination the main problem for which they were being treated was anxiety and/or depression. The discharge diagnoses (main and secondary) of the six patients[20] were as follows, with ICD 9 classification in brackets: acute confusional state (293.0) and neurotic depression (300.4); reactive depressive illness (309.0); schizoaffective disorder (295.7), inadequate personality and hysterical personality traits (301.6); neurotic depression (300.4); schizophrenia (295.3 or 4); endogenous depression (296.1) and dependent personality (301.5 or 6).

Only two of the six patients had discharge diagnoses that matched the original selection criteria. The consultant said of the others at the time of selection that 'diagnosis' would have been of an anxiety state or depression in the context of personality disorder or schizophrenia. The point must be made that at different points in their stays in hospital these patients would not have been considered suitable for the study, since in three cases the main focus of intervention was psychotic or organic conditions. On the other hand, the consultant's formulation for one patient selected as suitable (who declined to take part) later shifted toward 'psychosis'.

Staff in Site One spoke of some patients as 'moving targets'. The 'picture' of these patients changed, and with it formulation and diagnosis. It is clear from the above data that some of the study patients in Site One were or had been 'moving targets', and that all that is said about interaction with them is said of people who can be called 'neurotic' or said to be 'diagnosed as neurotic' only provisionally and with qualifications. This finding raises retrospective questions about the meaning of 'neurotic' in the work of John (1961), Altschul (1972) and MacIlwaine (1980). Whether the patients in their studies were 'neurotic' during the periods of their studies in the same sense as were the patients in this study is indeterminable.

Site Two

The discharge diagnoses of the seven patients in Site Two[21] were: 300.4 and 300.3; 300.4; 309.1; 300.0 and 303.9; 309.0; 300.4; 300.4.

A note on the proportion of patients diagnosed as neurotic

Information from the data office indicated that, of patients admitted in the year prior to the study, 29 of 162 (18%) of patients in Site One and 21 of 253 (8%) of patients in Site Two had discharge diagnoses of neurosis (ICD 9 300.0 through 300.9, and 306.2). These figures compare with 15% in the site of the field work trial.[22]

A note on issues of selection, participation and non-participation

Two patients in Site One and two in Site Two declined to give accounts. One patient in Site Two was transferred before I could ask her to take part. Two patients declined to take part because they felt too anxious; one declined on the grounds that she was 'dying' (see below); and one declined giving no reason, during a period when staff were reformulating their view of her, toward a diagnosis of psychosis. Thus the reasons for non-participation in the study were related to the patients' moods or clinical features.

It may be that the most distressed patients self-selected out of the study. In addition, I suspended interviewing one patient who became very disturbed (possibly psychotic) during the period of the study. My decision was guided in part by reluctance to risk increasing her distress. It is a reasonable assumption that some of the patients who declined to take part would have been critical of the nurses, since they were in open conflict with them during the periods in question. Thus, the processes of patient selection themselves brought out the problems of talking to some of the patients, highlighting issues related to knowledge (I 'knew' the patient was not 'really' dying, but could not say so to excuse what she regarded as my offence in asking her to take part, or to justify perseverence), power, and rights and obligations in a moral order. I tried to give nurses and patients maximum power to say 'no' to participation, at what cost to the value of the data I cannot say.

Summary

I have introduced the sites and the patients, and indicated that data collection/creation and analysis proceeded together. In the following three chapters I will present the products of analysis of the data. The main themes which emerged from the analysis of nurse-neurotic patient interaction as interpreted in the sites were: knowledge, power, and moral order.

Notes

1 These 'worlds' in turn are parts of larger 'worlds' of interaction. I read this interaction as nurse-patient interaction, but the actors could be and were 'read' by themselves and each other, and were read by me at times, in other ways, or other ways as well: as women, as old people, as people talking.

2 With a colleague I had earlier conducted a study (Pollock and Tilley, 1988) of our own and other novice nurse researchers' experiences with Ethical Committees, and found that others using qualitative methods had also been required to justify their research to Committees more used to appraising the value of quantitative research.

3 See the section below on diagnosis.

4 It could be argued that this method of selection of Site Two was biased, in the sense that I cannot account for the non-response of the other wards, and ruled out as unsuitable the ward first approached, on the grounds that patients with the relevant diagnoses would probably not be found. However, the intention of this study was not to generalise to a larger population of sites, and the main purpose of exploring situated interaction was fulfilled by this method of selection.

5 There is an unresolved conceptual and, it may be argued, political issue involved in research based on a word that cannot be used with some of the participants. The problem relates to the double mediation of the word: its use in this research is related in undetermined ways to both its lay use and to its psychiatric use. The necessity of negotiating alternative ways of indicating why I was doing what I was doing (using the term 'problems') heightened my awareness that I was involved in a socially constructed (and constraining) reality and had to construct my participation in it accordingly.

6 I will explain more fully the function of community meetings in the two sites in Chapter 5.

7 See Sacks (1984) on 'being ordinary' as an accomplishment.

8 The meaning of 'observation' is explained below, Chapter 6.

9 The local Data Officer said that doctors wanting to do research generally asked for breakdowns of patients on the basis of 'psychotic' and 'non-psychotic'.

10 The neurotic disorders in ICD 9 comprise: anxiety states (300.0), hysteria (300.1), phobic states (300.2), obsessive-compulsive disorders (300.3), neurotic depression (300.4), neuraesthenia (300.5), depersonalisation syndrome (300.6), hypochondriasis (300.7), other neurotic disorders (300.8), and 'unspecified' (300.9). MacIlwaine (1980) also used cardiac neurosis, (306.2) (World Health Organization, 1978).

11 MacIlwaine (1980) selected her patients on the basis of formulation, without indicating how the definition of 'neurotic' was derived from formulation.

12 Kendell (1975) reviewed general issues related to reliability and validity of psychiatric diagnosis.

13 Discharge diagnoses were considered by medical staff and Data Office staff to be more reliable than admission diagnoses.

14 See Pollock (1989) on the 'ideology' of individual care. See Chapter 8, below for further discussion of the relevance of

Foucault's (1979, 1982) analyses of power and practices of 'individualisation'.

15 See Kendell's (1975) notion of neurosis as a 'ragbag' diagnosis. These comments should be read in light of the discussions, elsewhere in this monograph, of 'residual categories'.

16 See Towell (1975) for a similar distinction in a 'therapeutic community'.

17 See Hughes (1988a) on the role of nurses' 'stories' in informing diagnosis in casualty wards.

18 See Hughes' (1988a) suggestion that it is in casualty departments that one might look for evidence of the current relationship of nursing power to medical power.

19 See May and Kelly (1982) and Chapman (1987) on the fragility of nurses' authority.

20 Note: the order of patients has been changed from that indicated by the notation used in the text, to help preserve confidentiality.

21 Note: the diagnoses do not correspond to the order of numeration of patients in the text, to help preserve confidentiality.

22 These proportions may not represent the proportions of patients in the sites during the period of the study. The consultants 'guesstimated' that 10-20% of the patients they admitted would have principal diagnoses of neurosis. Despite the best efforts of the local Data Officer, I was unable to arrive at a proportion of patients with these diagnoses during the period of the study.

5 Knowledge, or 'the main thing'

Introduction

In this chapter I will discuss the interaction between the patients and nurses as forms of knowledge. 'Knowledge' emerged from the data as one of the main categories in terms of which the nurses and patients made sense to me of their conversations together. The knowledge was what they needed to know to take part in interaction in the sites. I have used Berger and Luckmann's (1967) concepts of 'therapy' and 'reality maintenance and repair' to interpret the interaction of the nurses and patients as a form of 'therapy' involving maintenance and repair of the 'paramount reality', and recovery of patients 'strayed' from its bounds. The aim of the 'therapy' was to establish a common sense.

The nurses' and patients' accounts and interaction made sense when they were regarded as if they were forms of response to the questions 'Why is she here now (Why am I here now)?' and 'What do I have to do for her (What do I have to do)?'. These were the commonsense questions responses to which constituted assessment and treatment. The focus in this study is not on whether nurses and patients got the answers to these questions 'right', but rather on how they negotiated their parts in interaction to make sense with each other.

The knowledge outlined in this chapter was the knowledge needed to make sense in interaction as a patient or nurse in the two sites I studied; the knowledge needed to do the 'work' of the sites. The knowledge of the sites was knowledge of what the work was, what people were there for and what to do with them. That knowledge was ongoingly articulated in the negotiated interaction of nurses, patients and others. In negotiating the work of the place, including work on illness and problems, nurses and patients relied on background understandings, on common sense.

Sense makers making sense of sense makers

Through interpretation of the data, the nurses and patients are revealed as sense makers making sense of sense makers. The work of the sites was, from the point of view of the nurses, making sense of (assessing) patients and then doing something on the basis of the sense that was made. From the point of view of the patients it was making sense of what had happened to them and what to do about it.

Talk was a main vehicle through which the work of the site was accomplished. It allowed the patient's subjective reality to be interpreted in terms shared by the staff, and it allowed responses to be articulated. Through participation in talk the patient came to see how she was seen by the nurses and other staff and what she needed to do to get back to the community. Through talk the nurses and patients located and explained disruptions to ordinary intersubjective reality and sought ways of restoring it.

Everything that counts as knowledge: accounts, maxims, frames of meaning, and stories

I understood what was going on in interaction between the nurses and patients because their accounts enabled me to 'place' people in settings and follow the action. The answers to the question 'Why is she here now?' and 'What do I have to do for her?' took the form of accounts which shared the features of Burke's (1969a) pentad: act, agent, agency, setting, motive.[1] Accounts were the common-sense vehicles for assessment and treatment, devices for following the development of the social action of being a patient in the admission ward. In their accounts nurses and patients drew on common knowledge of character and scene to structure the way they acted. They used metaphors, for example that of a patient being 'weaned', which allowed the actors to draw on and explore implications of the parent-child relationship (including implications about the nurse knowing best, having to curb demand, transferring the source of satisfaction). Accounts 'bridged' symbolic orders of illness and ordinary reality. For example, an account of 'weaning' was familiar from common sense, but also had elements relevant to understanding 'dependence' on the institution as a consequence of a long illness.

In this Chapter I present the forms of knowledge used by the nurses and patients to make sense to each other and to me. They sometimes drew on 'special' or 'technical' knowledge; for example, knowledge of diagnosis. Often, though, the knowledge was in the form of accounts, maxims, frames of meaning, stories and metaphors. These constituted the 'cookery book knowledge' and the 'recipes' (Schutz and Luckmann, 1974), used to do the practical work of the sites. Recipe knowledge was replete with the dilemmatic characteristics of common sense (cf. Billig et al, 1988).

Different kinds of knowledge and different realities: the patients as sense makers

Understanding of the interaction is based on the distinctions the nurses and patients made in their accounts. The logic of this section is based on an assumption that the terms they used conveyed distinctions in the social reality meaningful to them. Their accounts formed discourses the meaning of which was constituted by systems of differences and binary oppositions. They made these distinctions in order to tell about their talk and the subjective and objective realities created in the talk. The distinctions conveyed knowledge of differences in reality.

In coming into the sites, and into conversation in the sites, the patients entered a new reality, one sustained through the discourse in the sites. The relationship of this reality to the reality outside was determined through interaction and talk. The patients learned the reality through participation in it, especially in talk. In participating in interaction, they learned the terms in which everything, including themselves, made sense. The patients drew on knowledge they had when entering the site to realise differences between it and the reality outside.

The data indicate that nurses and patients drew on different knowledge in making sense in episodes of interaction. Their talk was sometimes explicitly about the differences in knowledge: a patient knew that she was ill, the nurses that she was not. In other cases, the differences were noted by one or other participant or were apparent when pairs of accounts were analysed.

Throughout this monograph I adopt the stance that differences in knowledge constituted differences in reality. Thus, I interpreted disagreement between a patient and a nurse over whether the patient was ill as indicating two realities, in one of which the patient was ill. I found that empirically the nurses' 'reality' was 'paramount'. It was 'the' reality ('my reality' in the words of an experienced nurse) in relation to which other (others') realities - delusional, confusional, etc. - were ordered. This ordering was one of the main kinds of work in the site. Nurses were able to claim, explicitly or implicitly, that their reality was the primary reality; the sense that ultimately was made was the sense that was made in their reality; and patients' understandings were required to move into accord with the claims of the primary reality.

The patients ordered their own knowledge in what I will refer to as two 'frames of meaning'. I will describe these and then describe how the nurses' frame of meaning, that of 'work', ordered the patients' frames of meaning and thus constituted the paramount reality. The argument that I am advancing is that it was through this ordering of knowledge and the practices through which it was accomplished that the work of assessment and treatment was done. Thus the ordering of realities in face to face interaction reflexively constituted the sites as psychiatric admission wards.

The first of patients' two main frames of meaning: ordinary talk

By 'frames of meaning' I mean the 'interpretive schemes by means of which sense is made by participants of what each says and does' (Giddens, 1976, p.122). Such frames allow the 'tokens' of speech to be seen as 'types' related to other terms in the frame. (See Chapter 3, especially notes on meaning in Harre and Secord, 1972). In such frames are sedimented the experiences which constitute knowledge (Schutz and Luckmann, 1974). The frames of meaning described here were derived inductively through analysis of the fieldwork and accounts data. Not only do frames of meaning structure communication; they structure action and the processes of legitimation. They are thus central to the question of what nurses and patients do in their interaction. The simple answer, with regard to knowledge, is: psychiatric patients and nurses negotiate understandings and act through processes of interpretation mediated by frames of meaning. In this section I outline the two main frames of meaning derived from analysis of patients' observed interaction and accounts.

'Ordinary talk' - also called 'social talk' - was one of the two main frames of meaning in terms of which the patients made sense of their talk with nurses. The second was 'illness or problem talk' (see below). The distinction between 'social talk' and 'problem talk' or 'illness talk' was made by a patient in Site Two. I had asked her to tell me about talk with the nurses:

> P: I think, um, in this hospital, mostly it's really, um the conversation starts, em, on a **social**, sort of, basis, **unless**, unless you're upset about something and, a nurse'll come and talk to you.

In both sites the main feature of the patients' talk was that it was primarily social and unremarkable. Ordinary talk, mediated through a frame of meaning shared with the nurses, constituted a common and primary social reality. It was the mode of realisation of the primary reality in the sites. Its very ordinariness kept it 'submerged': it was an ideology, a system of knowledge not subjected to question or comment.

Ordinary talk ranged from 'talk in the passing' to longer talks, and was often communal. The topics of ordinary talk were those of ordinary day-to-day conversation: television, holidays, sport, make up, cars and so on. In talking about the ordinary things of ordinary life[2] the patients and nurses realised a shared reality. Thus S2P10:

> P: Eh, well, for conversations today, I usually just speak about **general** things, like, if a nurse asks, 'How are you feeling?'.. I'll say if I'm feeling fine, or, if I'm feeling tired, or, maybe other conversations come in, like, eh, my husband phoned, and, told me that the washing (laughs) got stolen off the back green. And, so, I was telling the nurses about that, and, talk about things like, make up and, eh, if you go for a walk, they ask you, what shops you went intae, what you bought. Usually just ordinary things.

In ordinary talk the patients brought into the ward the reality of social life outside the hospital. They brought themselves into the shared social world. They realised in ordinary talk the 'common ground' of shared social reality. The paramount social reality (Schuetz, 1943; Berger and Luckmann, 1967) was sustained in ordinary talk. Through it patients and nurses reproduced in the sites features of the wider social world. The sites were away from the rest of society, but in ordinary talk society penetrated the sites. If it was Christmas outside, it was Christmas inside. The nurses decorated trees at home and talked about this with the patients in the ward. The patients decorated the ward tree and an old woman told young nurses about decorations that she used to make.

What was shared in the frame of meaning 'ordinary reality' was a set of distinctions. Ordinary talk was the means of realising the distinctions in everyday social life, and the means of 'placing' others in relation to oneself in the reality. Though the symbols of everyday life were shared in ordinary talk, their meanings for the patients and the nurses were often different. The nurses' trees were at home, the patients' tree was in the ward (cf. Banton et al, 1985, pp. 21-28). The patients were away from home. The old woman declined to help make decorations, talking instead of what she used to do elsewhere. The patients realised through their ordinary talk distinctions between their place in the social world and the nurses' place. They realised something of what was shared and what was unshared, common and uncommon.

In their ordinary talk the patients and nurses in this study realised distinctions between people at home and people in hospital; people in work and people out of work; people caring for children at home and people whose children are cared for by social agencies; 'women's talk' and 'men's talk' and, correspondingly, women's world and work and men's world and work. They reproduced the binary oppositions in the common discourses of social life, the privileged and submerged terms. The patients in their ordinary talk with the nurses participated in the construction of themselves and the nurses in a shared and unshared social world, with its attendant tensions and contradictions.

Through the 'social' frame of meaning the nurses appeared in the patients' accounts as the 'types' (Schutz and Luckmann, 1974) of characters they might appear 'outside'. A conversation between an old woman and a young female student was, for the old woman, 'a young girl's talk'. In ordinary talk the patients 'saw' the nurses outside the hospital. Conversely, in ordinary talk the patients saw themselves 'in here'. Thus when patients and nurses were talking about work - an ordinary, day-to-day aspect of ordinary talk - a glaring fact was that the nurses were in work, the patients not. Thus P5 in Site Two:

> P: Because o-, obviously we can't talk on the same level, because, um, (?) on the same level I mean as, we've done a different job from, nursing, we don't know anything about nursing. So, maybe they talk about nursing, and I talk about what I did (laughs) before I came in here...

Patients knew that some nurses could understand ordinary talk depending on their sharing or not sharing the patients' social experiences. A man could 'communicate quite good' with a male nurse because he liked sports too. A patient and a nurse, mothers, talked about children; two others about the town they knew. Social knowledge yielded the power to discourse and to claim a place in the conversation. However, the places were structured by the distinctions in the wider society.

A second frame of meaning: talk of illness and problems[3]

Patients in both sites drew on and referred to a second main frame of meaning drawn on to make sense of and in their accounts of talk with the nurses. This frame was 'talk about my illness (my problems)', 'medical talk', or 'personal talk', talk about 'why I (the patient) am here'. All these terms distinguished this kind of talk from ordinary talk.

The distinction between 'ordinary' and 'illness' discourses, made through participation in them, marked a distinction in reality. The distinction was between the (broadly) intersubjective reality of ordinary life, and the patients' subjective reality revealed in 'talk of illness/problems/personal things'.

Distinctions between the terms 'illness talk', 'problem talk' and 'personal talk' will be discussed below. Here the distinction to be made is between, on the one hand, 'talk of illness', 'problem talk' or 'personal talk'; and, on the other hand, 'ordinary talk'.

Characteristics of talk of illness/problems/personal things Talk of illness was talk of the subjectively experienced world of the person who was ill. The world of illness was described by S1P2[4]:

> P:...medication, feeling groggy, feeling depressed, not being able to cope, feeling..to cry, wanting to get out of hospital. These are the symptoms when you first come in to hospital.

Illness talk objectivated this subjective world: the patient experienced 'symptoms' of an illness. Talk was about 'my condition'. The subjective world intersected an objective world: time passes, and things become different from 'when you first come in to hospital'.

The distinction between 'ordinary talk' and 'illness and problem talk' marked a distinction between realities An example of talk of illness or problems is found in S1P3:

> P: It (Note: the conversation with the nurse) was about deciding if I could go home or not. Eh, I found it very hard to make a decision...Things if I say that eh, something I'm gonna do, it doesn't work that way, it goes the opposite way, and I find that if I was making any decisions at my work I was making too many, too many mistakes.

Another example is S1P7:

> P: Well, they don't speak to me...They don't eh...Oh there was one this morning, n-, nursing officer. I'm sure, I think that's what he was, very nice too, very nice. He was speaking, talking about my own condition of course.

Or (S2P6):

> P: Eh, well, one girl, I was giving her a bit of, I was a bit upset. And we were sitting along at the seats at the telephone, and I was just sort of telling her about my family and, you know, my sister's been on holiday and, things like, like that, you know, she was just back on holiday...and I was asking her, about her holiday and, I (?), got carried away with myself, telling her a wee bit of my worries, you know.

Getting 'carried away' from ordinary talk into talk about illness and problems was part of being ill and having problems.

Through illness talk the patients realised that - made sense of how - in mood and situation they were different from the nurses. Subjectivity was negotiated through objectivation and commentary on the patient's objectivated experience, generating a discourse:

> P: ...(W)hen I told her, just general things that I worry about, she said that **she** actually worries about the same things...Well, I didnae really **believe** her, at the time, but I've s-, I suppose it **must** be true because, nurses **are** just the same, really, they **do** suffer frae tension, and, it's just the way that, if you're the kind of person that's used to being tense, then, it, it sort of gets **exaggerated**.

In this discourse the patient constructed oppositions and tensions through which the reality of illness or problems was negotiated. Among the oppositions were 'general things'/specific things; what is 'true'/what is not 'true'; what is believed/what is not believed; nurses 'the same'/nurses different; 'the kind of person that's used to being tense'/the kind of person who is not; normal tension/'exaggerated' tension. This discourse may be read as the negotiation in talk and in reflection on talk of a common understanding of the patient's illness or problem.[5] The distinction between the patient's experience and that of the nurse was made by negotiating the binary oppositions in a shared discourse, and subjecting the discourse to judgements of validity ('true', 'believed'). In discourse which structured the tensions of common sense the patient disputed the nurse's claim to 'worry about the same things'. The common remained subject to dispute: the tensions shifted to the meaning of 'exaggerated'.

What was structured through the patient's discourse was a set of claims about reality. In another example a patient (S2P6) talked about taking part with nurses in an occupational therapy session:

> P: And, eh, Millie (Note: a nurse) was with us, as I say, yesterday and, we were to do these cards, you know, and we all (?) cards, and she got hers, compl-, her, writing on the card was a bit trivial to, **our** problems, which is only natural, because she's, **well,** and we're not well.

Through examination of their own and nurses' discourse the patients constructed accounts which ordered reality. The oppositions were: 'nurses' problems'/'patients' problems'; 'trivial'/'non trivial'; 'well'/'ill'. The discourse structured a hierarchy of knowledge. The patient (S2P6) used the frame of 'illness/problem' to make sense of her interaction with the nurse, and through the interaction reconstituted the frame. Use of the frame enabled the patient to order reality so that it appeared commonsensical, 'only natural'. Command of the discourse was claimed (as in the previous example) by the ill person, on the basis of her objectivated subjectivity as someone who was ill and who from the position of one who was ill knew the triviality of the not-ill. The patient's claim was based on the privilege of someone with 'illness sense' to recognise the triviality of the 'well''s problems. However, the nonprivileged term can be seen as potentially dominant. The patient was taking part in an occupational therapy group designed (by the well) to get the ill to talk about their problems in order to get better. That is, the aim was to re-establish a different 'natural order', the goal of which was 'well sense' and 'well talk'. Occupational therapy was akin to 'carnival', in which values and roles are inverted, and from which order re-emerges (Bakhtin, 1984).

The distinctions in common sense were called on to make common sense, to distinguish illness sense and 'well' sense in relation to common sense. The distinction was made in the realm of common sense. Knowledge of illness had to be objectivated in a shared reality (cf. Simm, 1978, on 'insight').

In such talk the patients constituted knowledge of their experiences and understandings, their subjectivity as patients. Patients as well as nurses 'policed' the boundaries of social talk and talk of illness (Berger and Luckmann, 1967; Robinson, 1985; Chapman, 1987). They thus sustained the distinction 'ill' and 'not ill' (cf. Billig et al, 1988), and the reality of illness. I will argue later that this negotiation was complex. A nurse's account claimed that the above patient (S2P6), by claiming illness, avoided 'work on problems'.

The relationship between 'ordinary talk' and 'talk of illness' for patients diagnosed as neurotic

Some patients considered that ordinary talk was potentially meaningful in relation to talk of illness. Even in social conversation 'you might be giving them (the nurses) information without really realising it' (S2P6). The patients constructed the nurses as people who knew, perhaps knew better than the patients, what was wrong with them (the patients). They correspondingly constructed themselves, in the sites, as people to be known.

The nurses and patients played different roles in articulating the distinction between 'ordinary talk' and 'illness talk'. These patients construed the nurses as translators, mediators of frames of meaning. The patients understood that what they said in ordinary talk could mean something else in another frame of meaning. They thus realised their participation in a process of interpretation, the product of which was the reality of their illness.

The data support three further observations. Firstly, patients referred to the ordinary things of everyday life to tell me, as they told the nurses, that they could not do these things as they once had done. They defined their illness or problem against the backdrop of ordinary life: for example, an inability to make decisions; exaggerated anxiety. Secondly, the patients knew that in listening to ordinary talk the nurses might notice, understand and act on something concerning their illness or problems (S2P4):

> P: ...You think it's just an ordinary conversation you're having about the weather or your family, and they possibly relate that to the doctor... And, it gives the doctor a, more understanding of where you're feeling at the time, (?if they're) having to

come to you every time, the doctors, well like everybody else they're very busy.

Or S2P6 said that the nurses did not help with problems, but qualified her claim:

> P: The nurses talk about your **social** life, and, what **they've** been doing and what you've been doing, and, what you **intend** to do... (They) watch you closely. And, I think in here, all, your movements, and your reaction, are taken into account, when they maybe go into their meeting, in the office, I think probably you're discussed, if you're a bit uptight, cos they know by your face if you're, sorta clenching your teeth or if you're sitting fidgeting with your hands. And, I think, probably, (? they're or ? their) training as well, to, (? they'd) be able to notice things like this.

The patients construed the nurses as interpreting them through participation in ordinary talk. Thirdly, some patients understood that the nurses construed ordinary talk itself as a form of help, not only diagnostic but therapeutic. Thus S2P2 said that the nurses pushed her to 'socialise' because they knew that 'socialising' was better than lying in bed if you were depressed. In talking ordinarily, patients construed themselves as being construed from the point of view of the aims of the sites: assessment and treatment.

The patients thus construed themselves as taking part with the nurses in an interpretive process the explicitness of which varied, as did the role of the nurses. The patients in negotiating their interaction with the nurses may be understood as using a 'code' (Wieder, 1974) the existence and operation of which they picked up as they went along. The code translated terms meaningful (or meaningless) in the 'ordinary talk' frame of meaning into terms meaningful in the frame of 'illness or problems talk'. The implication is that patients understood that even ordinary talk had potential value for interpretation of why there were in the sites. That the patients imputed mediation of frames of meaning to the nurses suggests a similar mediation on the part of the patients. They talked on the assumption that sense might be made of them. From their point of view, the patients thus participated in the realisation of their illnesses and problems through their participation in both 'talk of illness' and 'ordinary talk' (and facial expression) interpretable as 'talk of illness'.

Other features of patients' knowledge: location and distribution of knowledge

The patients knew - it was knowledge shared in meetings - where knowledge was located. Knowledge of illness was located in the sites. They knew that people 'outside' did not understand their illness (S2P6):

> P: Oh well, it's, em, you come in, you're all confused and, jus-, you just don't know what's **hit** you. But once you come in here you feel safe...you feel that people really **care** for you, you know? Whereas sometimes your family are a bit distant, because they just dinnae understand what, a problem you've got. Cos they dinnae understand it about mental, problems, you know.

They talked differently with the nurses than with people outside, casting them in different roles (S2P5):

> P: talking to somebody else, about, things that you probably wouldn't talk to friends about, or even close family, really, you know?

The patients thus knew that different constructions of reality, including the reality of their own subjectivity (as 'someone with mental problems'), were located in different places in the wider community.

They also knew that the work of interpreting them, constructing the objectivity of their subjective reality, took place at different places and with different people in the sites. Talk of problems or illness was institutionalised in group meetings, or on what the nurses called a 'one to one' basis. In Site One, problems and illnesses were often talked about in the community meeting attended by all patients; while in Site Two, the community meeting was used to discuss administrative matters, and discussion of patients' illnesses or problems was discouraged. In Site Two, talk of illness and problems was shared in a 'small group meeting'. This meeting was 'closed' to some patients on the grounds that they might not have been able to benefit from it. It was also closed to student nurses, and I was told that it was the one meeting it would not be appropriate for me to attend. The rationale for closing the meeting was that 'observers' would inhibit patients' and staff members' sharing of feelings and experience. I assume that forms of subjectivity not elsewhere realised in Site Two were realised in the small groups. Thus forms of discourse and knowledge were differently institutionalised, defined and protected in the two sites.

Patients knew what sort of knowledge nurses, doctors and others had. In Site Two, most patients knew that the main work on their problems or illness was done by the doctor, psychologist, social worker. They knew that nurses knew about their moods and interests. They knew that nurses, possibly due to their training, knew better than they themselves did how they were. The nurses saw how they looked and told them, they saw improvements and told them. Some patients knew what helped them and what the nurses, doctors and others were doing for them in hospital (S1P2, S1P3). Some knew that they were not being helped (S1P7). Some knew what was unhelpful: for example (S2P10), a nurse dismissing the patient's claim to be distressed.

The patients knew that the nurses knew by looking and listening: 'he's watching you all the time', 'he misses nothing', they said of the charge nurse in Site One. In Site Two P6 said 'I think they're, watching you, and, **in a nice way**' (cf. Altschul, 1972). They knew that the nurses remembered. These observations suggest that the patients knew how the nurses knew because, by implication, they watched the nurses and saw the nurses watching them; they remembered that the nurses remembered. In knowing the patients the nurses were themselves known.

Patients knew who among the patients was more ill and which patients were responsible for what they were doing. They knew that people who were more 'ill' needed more help and that it was right - it made sense as well as being morally right - that the nurses helped those most in need, even if that meant they helped patients other than oneself.

The patients made sense of the site in terms of knowledge of the site, of illness and ordinary reality, of patients and people in the site, and of the stay (period of admission) in the site. Patients knew that greater severity of illness meant that the nurses spent more time with the more ill patients:

> P: And, em, but wh-, the, I mean, what they do is very good, but, you feel that they're, if **you're** taking up their attention, they're taking (? a-), you're taking them away from somebody else, you know?

They knew that if you were really ill or really upset or disturbed then the nurses would talk with you.

That the nurses had helped meant that they could help; there was a potential for help (cf. Altschul, 1972). What the patients knew was that the nurses would try to comfort, try to console, try to reassure. The patients also knew, especially in Site One, that what the nurses did was limited: in the end, 'you've got to do it yourself'.

Summary of patients' knowledge

Patients commonly understood and constituted the meaning of their interaction with nurses by drawing on two frames of meaning: talk as 'ordinary talk' and as 'talk of illness'. The patients' knowledge was of their subjective experience being realised objectively in the sites, in part through talk in which the distinction between 'ordinary life' and 'illness' was realised.

'Ordinary talk' as a frame of meaning was not only 'about' ordinary social life. It was social life in the sites. The patients, in saying that they were talking ordinary talk, identified themselves as members of the society in which washing hung out to dry, holidays could be taken if affordable, and so on. Thus S2P10:

> P: And then, we spoke about, eh, he suggested that I should get a holiday. And I told him I can't afford it. And he was telling me that he had been away on holiday, to Skegness. But, that it was quite expensive. (Sighs 'Eh'). That was really all...(He made) good suggestions, which I had, I, I thought of myself, like, I need to, I need to get a job, and I could **do** with a holiday, but that means, eh, saving up money and I cannae do that till I get a job...But it was a good conversation...It just sort of seemed that he was i-, he seemed interested in me as a person, no just a, patient, if you see what I mean...He just seemed to be interested in, why I was there and, eh, he seemed to want to know, what kind of family I had...And, I don't know, it was just as if he wanted to understand maybe why I drank, or why I was anxious. I I, I quite like the conversations, cos, it lets you know, eh, what the nurses are like, **away** frae here...Knowing what he (?), his wife does, and knowing that he's got two girls. And that they go to Skegness. Just, things like that.
>
> R: It may sound a stupid question, but why is that good?
>
> P: I don't know (sighs). You can, sortae relate to them. Like, for me it would be different if, if he wasnae married, and, didnae

have a family. I dinnae think I could relate to him so much, then...Where uh, I could relate, to him.

R: Because he wouldn't have..

P: The pressures o', like say, bills, or saving for a holiday, or,

R: Right, I've got you. Right...Some of the things that **you**, can understand.

P: Mnhmn.

Ordinary talk was a device for establishing membership in the society (Hughes, 1988) in which such features were features of reality.

Similarly, talk of illness was a device for establishing membership. To talk about your illness was a mark of illness. Illness showed (or was seen, interpreted) in what was talked about in illness. Talk of illness was talk that had been placed in the bit of the wider community that was the site (cf. Bott, 1976). Illness was a part of the wider social reality set apart from it, a reality experienced by the patients. Forms of talk-as-reality-construction took place in different places in the reality. Reflexively, the sites were constituted as places for definition of reality through talk and other signs.

Talk of illness occurred most when the person was most ill, usually when she came to the site, and dwindled as the person got better (S1P2):

> P: ...I've been doing things on my own, because once you're better, you, like I said the nurses are very nice you just have general conversations with them.

The ratio of talk of illness to ordinary talk located them in their stay (less talk as you got better), in their illness.

In talk the patients constituted themselves as subjects in the discourses of illness and ordinary reality. In talk the patients located themselves and were located in the realms of ordinary life and illness. Through their talk they could be located by nurses. Interpreting and being interpreted by the nurses through the 'illness' frame of meaning, some patients were able to make sense of what happened to them as 'illness' or 'problems'. For example, S2P4 understood that she had been wrong when she thought that she was physically ill and the nurses had said that she was anxious.

The negotiated character of the reality: points of articulation and dispute

Here I am setting out the frames of meaning in terms the patients used to make sense in and of their talk with the nurses. These frames of meaning were drawn on to account for interaction. That is, they were drawn on to make intelligible what had happened - to explain, justify or excuse it - by indicating in what frame the action was meaningful. To say that something had happened due to one's illness, for example, was to appeal to be heard and interpreted in relation to a frame in which it was understood that one as an ill person could not help oneself, was not responsible.[6] In ordinary life, one was responsible for one's actions. To frame action as illness meant also that whatever rights and obligations attended recognition of oneself as ill were potentially called into play. For that reason, a patient's ability to recognise and articulate the frames of meaning, 'ordinary life' and 'illness', was vitally important. That ability was the basis for a patient's participation in communication about her subjectivity, indeed, in the establishment of its objectivity.

Knowledge of illness and ordinary life may be thought of, not as a corpus already established to which patients referred, but as a set of claims advanced, subject to acceptance or challenge. What counted as 'everyday' and 'illness' depended on face to face negotiation in interaction between patients and nurses. Common sense was always subject to negotiation. In their talk the patients and nurses negotiated the meaning of the patients' experiences in one discourse or the other, negotiating whether the claims they made were valid claims in the discourse of 'ordinary life' or 'illness'. In further analysis I will argue that the talk of the patients and nurses was often negotiation of or dispute about whether something 'counted' as illness or not. The objectivity of the patients' subjective reality had to be negotiated: 'it's the pills' versus 'no, it's you' (S1P4). In talk the patients negotiated whether they ought to have 'placed' themselves or been 'placed' in the place in the wider society where ill people were: they negotiated why there were 'here'. They negotiated whether their personal states made sense (were best interpreted) in the frames of meaning, 'ordinary talk' or 'illness talk', and what they were meant to do about their personal states in these public places.[7] The negotiated character of the reality of their illness or problems is emphasised below.

The nurses as sense makers: the frame of meaning 'work'

I have presented the knowledge the patients needed to manage their interaction with nurses in the sites by presenting the two frames of meaning within which they had to be able to make sense (and to make sense of the sense that was made of them). I now turn to the main frame of meaning within which the nurses had to make sense (to make sense of the sense made of them): the frame of 'work'. The 'work' of the nurses comprised, to a varying extent, negotiation, with the patients, of the reality of ordinary life and illness/problems. That was the work of the sites: in their interaction the nurses and the patients shared the work of the sites, constituting them as psychiatric admission wards in which people with private troubled states were accounted for as patients.

Analysis of interviews, card sorts, field notes, and patients' and nurses' accounts highlighted six elements of the accounts and stories nurses told in telling about their interaction with these patients. The elements were: site, stay, illness/problems, remedy, patient/nurse, person. These elements featured in stories meaningful within the frame of meaning used in doing the work of the site.

Knowledge of these elements was the knowledge needed to answer the questions which informed the practical work of the site: 'Why is she here now?' and 'What do we have to do for her?'. The elements featured in accounts of the work of the sites and reflexively constituted it as work in the sites. As patients' ability to give accounts and maintain claims about what happened in interaction depended on their capacity to articulate the frames of meaning of 'ordinary social life' and 'illness', so the nurses' ability to give accounts and sustain claims depended on their capacity to articulate the frame of meaning 'work'. Although the meaning of 'work' differed in the two sites, in ways which I will elaborate, the six elements featured in accounts in both sites.

I am not arguing that any single nurse knew all that is detailed here, though often I have drawn on accounts given by experienced nurses[8] because in them are represented the common themes.[9] Nor was this knowledge monologic: different nurses knew different things and disagreed. The claim here is that the nurses' accounts taken together constituted a discourse with both common and contradictory themes, drawn on in their work and accounts of their work (Billig et al, 1988). These nurses' knowledge was mainly practical and not theoretical, mediated through accounts and practices rather than theories (Shotter, 1984); pragmatic, expressed in terms of knowing how and knowing what (or who) rather than knowing that (Shotter, 1984). It was not usually a topic, but became one when a problem or a new situation arose; when new people came to work, or when a stranger (cf. Schutz, 1944) appeared and asked what was being done, as I did during field work.

I present the six elements separately in order to explain them. However, they are inter-related in the same way that the elements of a story are (Burke, 1969a; Bennett and Feldman, 1981). The argument of this section is that the work of the site was accomplished through managing interaction and accounts of it so that the elements cohered into a story of work: on the macro level, the story of the site at the time, including the stories of all patients in the site; and on the micro level, the story which guided the nurse in interaction.

Features of knowledge in the frame 'work': knowledge of site

The practical meaning of interaction with the patients was always meaning in the context of the ward at the time and as the place it was. There were institutional features of the site, regular meetings, the structure of the buildings, quiet days, and so on. Nurses drew on knowledge of the institution to understand and direct interaction. However, the meaning of any feature of the site was its meaning at the time. 'The time' was the 'real time' of the ward in which all that was going on in it had to be accounted for. This was highlighted in an account in which a nurse emphasised that she needed to respond to the patient ('she was there, you know') despite being unable to do so at the time:

> N: I felt that, (?) during the Kardex I was running after Mary most of the time, and Elsa was lying on the floor, but P4 was there too, you know, she was there, but like I didn't have any time at all with her, and she was sitting crying, so I said that, basically to let her know that I, I was still speaking to her...And, eh, let her know that I was, I was noticing her.

'You know...to let her know...to let her know...'. The nurse acted so that her action would be correctly interpreted for its meaning at the time. Her action was a form of account, the meaning of which referred to the site at the time. Reference to the time and to the place as it was were essential to understanding this as action based on knowledge, as knowledge in action. Decontextualised, the action would have lost its meaning. Its meaning was indexical (cf. Garfinkel, 1967).

The main form of indexical, contextualised knowledge was 'noticing'. To 'notice' was to reflexively constitute the site as the place within which what was noticed appeared as the focus of accountable action. 'The site' was the site as the location of noticing as accountable action (cf. Garfinkel, 1967).

Knowledge that the site was a psychiatric hospital: the knowledge in maxims needed to 'keep the work going' The main responsibility for defining, constructing, maintaining and repairing social reality in the sites lay with the nurses. The nurses shared the responsibility with the patients. The 'floor' account (see above) was given during a period when Site One was, in the nurses' words, 'like a madhouse'. I shared a view that everything felt chaotic, everyone had trouble keeping up with what had to be done, nurses were stretched with too few on duty, patients were sometimes abusive or bizarre. The nurse with her look called on the patient to acknowledge that this was the reality and to count what the nurse did as accountable work. Patients in both sites indicated in their accounts that they recognised that the nurses had to respond to others in greater need - the equivalents of the woman on the floor, the woman screaming - who formed part of the shared reality.

At other times the ward was somnolent, lazy, 'like a hotel' or 'like a holiday camp'. It was part of nurses' knowledge at these times that they had to assert the definition of the place as a psychiatric hospital. The knowledge of the site as a psychiatric hospital was the knowledge the nurses needed to work in the place. That knowledge was expressed in a number of maxims. The maxims can be understood as responses to the questions 'Why is she here now?' and 'What do I have to do for her?', implicit in the nurses' work.

The main nurses' maxim was: 'keep the work going', also expressed as 'keep the programme going'. The 'programme' was not only the organised work but its meaning: 'healing' (Site One) or the 'solution of problems' (Site Two). 'Keep the programme going' meant make sure that the main priority was met: in Site One, 'keep the place anxiety free'; in Site Two, 'keep the patients safe, fed, then happy'. To do this the nurse needed to 'keep to my (Note: the charge nurse's) agenda', if possible. The 'programme' was the order of the site - literally, its temporal order of meetings, groups, admission, treatment, discharge - as well as the content.

'Savvy', the essential nursing knowledge (see below) was knowledge of the order and priorities and how to maintain them. To keep the work going it was necessary to 'know the patients' stories' or 'know the current picture of the patient', implying 'talk to the patients regularly', and (in Site One) 'pay attention to the patients, because they know what's really going on'. Maxims related to illness or problems and to remedies included: 'be sound in your clinical knowledge' (implying that the nurse should know typical illnesses and problems in order to be able to interpret for a patient what was illness and what a problem – an additional part of 'savvy' was knowing how to recognise 'cons' and distinguish between 'normal problems' and problems which constituted 'the main thing'). A maxim related to 'keep the work going' and 'keep to the agenda' was: 'handle the main thing at the time'.

The knowledge in the nurses' maxims was drawn on to 'keep the work going'. The reality of the site was never fully accomplished. It was always vulnerable to re-definition. Work always needed to be done to maintain the definition of the site as a place for assessment and treatment. Use of the 'code' (Wieder, 1974) contained in the maxims enabled the nurses to define the site as a hospital where the work was 'going'.

Knowledge of site was also institutionalised in routines and common occurrences, ordered through following the maxims. One learned the institutional knowledge by being in and working in the site. For example, definition of Site One took place regularly in community meetings, while written knowledge of both sites was sparse. In Site One, for example, a document entitled 'Ward Objectives' was required reading for all nurses new to the ward. The objectives were:

> Primarily to assess patient's condition, taking into account, reasons for admission, background, presenting features, etc.; diagnosis by medical staff, assess patient's needs, discuss/finalise treatment plan and initiate same with emphasis on treating the patient as a 'whole' rather than just the illness itself.

The knowledge in the library The knowledge really needed to manage the ward was located not in the 'Ward Objectives' but in what an experienced nurse in Site One called 'the library'. The library was not merely the notes, records, orders, contact sheets and other systems of data relating to the patients. It was the ongoing knowledge of who and what was going on in the ward at the time. Much of the library was not written, but 'catalogued' in the nurses' own minds.

'Savvy': knowing the main thing Knowledge in interaction constituted knowledge of site. Knowledge of site 'appeared in' the accounts of interaction. The sense that was made of and in interaction had to make sense in terms of the site if the work of the site was to be kept going. The 'floor' account (see above) can be read as revealing that the 'main thing' in interaction with P4 at that time was that her distress was not, could not be, 'the main thing' in the site at the time. Keeping the work of the site going then meant getting someone off the floor, quieting another, all while other nurses and doctors in another room reviewed cases and discussed how to keep the work of the site going.

There were two aspects of knowledge of site: knowledge of the site and knowledge in the site. One got knowledge of the site by finding what counted as knowledge in the site. One found out what counted as knowledge in the site through interaction and accounts of interaction. This was the way I learned about the sites, and the way nurses and patients learned. Knowing 'the ward at the time' was part of what may be called 'knowledge of site'. 'Knowledge of site' was what was needed to work in the ward, knowledge that when a patient was on the floor when you were the only nurse in the ward meant that you could only show another patient that you noticed her. This was knowledge of 'the main thing' at the time, of the main threat to the reality of the site as a work place.

The most important aspect of knowledge of site was knowledge of what it was most important to know: knowledge of the hierarchy of knowledge. When resources were stretched (when nurses were stretched, knowledge was thin, it threatened to break), an experienced nurse in Site One said that what they needed was not just any nurse - a nurse who did not know the ward would have been 'as much use as a cold' - but a nurse with 'savvy'.

'Savvy' meant, among other things, knowledge that the charge nurse liked to spend time with the patients, not be stuck in the office doing paper work. Other nurses with 'savvy' took care of the ward administration so that the charge nurse was free to be with the patients. The charge nurse knew the site by knowing the patients; he knew the patients in order to know the site. The nurses' knowledge was practical knowledge and the hierarchy of knowledge related to the hierarchy of aims in the work. The charge nurse's aims in Site One were to 'keep the clients happy and keep the place anxiety free'. He could ensure that this was being done if he was able to be out in the ward with the patients. His style in working was to use humour to keep anxiety down. Thus 'savvy' in organisation of work was knowledge needed to keep the site the way it was meant to be. An experienced nurse in Site Two said that the aims were to keep the patients 'safe, fed and happy, in that order'. Knowledge of this knowledge was vital. This nurse said that if a patient were missing and a nurse said 'We were being psychotherapeutic with another patient' the nurse manager would say 'You could do that any time'.

'Savvy' was knowledge of how to maintain the reality of the site so that the realities within the site were ordered to sustain 'my (Note: the charge nurse's) reality' - the paramount reality recognised by the nurses, and especially the charge nurses[10] - as the paramount reality. Knowledge of site was the knowledge needed to reflexively constitute the site. It was the knowledge needed by nurses to conduct themselves accountably.

Knowledge of knowledge of site (reflexively claimed here) was thus knowledge of valid accounts, acquired through hearing and giving accounts and seeing the consequences of different practices of accounting. This was the knowledge I checked out in giving and getting feedback in the sites. The sites were constituted by the nurses as the places they were meant to be, as the nurses, their managers and the consultants knew they were meant to be, at least insofar as public accounts (and especially documents) were concerned. Garfinkel (1967, p. 24) noted that in any organisation there are always some things that are 'none of somebody-else-in-that-organization's business'. These were the sorts of things that would have been considered invalid knowledge and were omitted or expunged from public accounts.

In the nurses' accounts, the sites were the sites as rendered accountable through the nurses' practices. Because knowledge of site informed action and action was intended to be accountable in the site, and by virtue of the indexicality of talk about interaction in the site, the site appeared through nurses' and patients' accounts. It was realised in the accounts:

> N: Ella had a shower this morning. I can't really, remember much about the conversation. I had said to the other nurse that was in the bath, 'I'll go and get P7 for a shower', and she says 'No, P7's no wanting one'. And P7 shouted frae the toilet 'Yes I am', and I says 'It's a good job I wasna talking about you,

P7'. Em, but that was really a-, about all. I can't remember anything, significant.

This ordinary talk about ordinary talk constituted the ward as a place where humour compensated for lack of privacy. Unremarkable to the nurse, it displayed her capacity to moderate with wit the immodesties of interaction in the ward. The texture of 'being with the patient twenty four hours a day' was revealed in accounts of conversations in bathrooms, kitchens, occupational therapy, dormitories, offices. When a patient in Site Two said that the nurses knew the patients, their moods and interests, because they were with them all the time, she conveyed something of the meaning of this intimate and prolonged contact.

Government of statements about the main thing A corollary of knowledge of site and 'savvy' was that 'the main thing' in any account had to be appropriately placed in relation to the main thing in the site at the time. Thus in the 'floor' account (above), S1P4 appeared on the periphery of the main action in the site at the time. From the nurse's point of view, the site (including P4 in the site) was constituted, as a set of relevances, in relation to the 'main thing' she was 'handling' at the time.

This was typical of action with the patients in this study. It was often 'talk in passing', at 'quiet points', talk with students when senior nurses were engaged in more demanding reality maintenance. Only rarely was it 'the main thing' in the site at the time.

Knowledge of stay

The second meaning of interaction was the meaning it had in the context of the patient's stay. This was the context provided by the ongoing developing sense of what was being done in relation to a patient, including the intentions the nurse had with regard to her. Knowledge of the stay located the patient in relation to admission from and return to the community (cf. the concept of 'trajectory' in the work of Glaser and Strauss, 1965).

As knowledge of the site shaped the story about interaction (P4 at the periphery), so knowledge of stay was conveyed in the sense of development of the story about the patient during her time in the site. The basic fact of knowledge of stay was that patients came in, stayed and were discharged. Some would come back and this would be one of multiple stays. Part of knowledge of stay was that there were typical features of a stay. For example, patients generally did not go home during the first few weeks of their stay. A student nurse in Site Two was surprised when S2P2 suggested going home during the first twenty four hours. 'The patient's stay' was the point of reference for the current understanding among the staff of 'What is she doing here?' and 'What are we doing for her?'. As with knowledge of site, knowledge of stay was pragmatic: it provided the context for knowing what 'our job' was.

The meaning of a stay could be clear or unclear. This related to whether nurses thought they were 'getting anywhere (or nowhere) with her'. A student nurse said[11]:

> N: (Sighs) Mn, maybe I'm showing my ignorance here. I havenae really read, P7's **notes** or anything. Em, I just know that she is very lonely. She used to have a purpose in life..She moved into a flat, it's her own property. And, eh, didnae see anybody, day in and day out, and she had, seemed to have lost, this purpose for living...and, eh, **she** deteriorated as **well**, (? put) depressed. So she was **in** here. I I don't feel we've done an awful **lot** for her...P7's just, dittering away and enjoying the company, but she's to go back to her own house. Though they're going to try and get her into Phinnie House (Note: day centre)...

Knowledge of stay implied a sense of time and direction of action, essential to 'keeping the work going'. Interpretation of this element in accounts with neurotic patients 'brings out' the knowledge needed to work with these patients in the site in order to keep them moving through it. To maintain the site it was necessary to keep the flow going.

Knowledge of patients

The third meaning of the interaction was the meaning it had in the context of the nurse's knowledge of this person as a patient. There were two aspects to patient knowledge. One was knowledge of what typical patients typically did or were like. This was related to both knowledge of site and knowledge of stay, as can be seen in an explanation by a trained nurse in Site Two:

> N: Um, when patients come in initially, they either adhere straightaway to, the limits that are set upon them, or they deliberately flaunt (sic) them...Um, it's, unusual, but often people that are in quite high powered jobs or, or who aren't

used to having limits set on them, they quite **enjoy** it, to sit back and relax, and have someone, say, 'You can do this' or 'You can't do that'. And, it takes the responsibility, **off**, them...

Knowledge of site, knowledge of stay and knowledge of patients were all referred to in making the point. The patient was known as typical through her response to having 'responsibility taken off'.[12] The patients were interpreted and constructed in terms relevant to the nurses' responsibility to 'set limits' to manage the site. The objectivity of a given patient was established in part through perception of her as (a token of) a general 'type' ('patients who have high powered jobs and like responsibility taken off them'); and in part through construction of her as an 'individual type' (Simm, 1978), that is the 'type' of the individual herself constructed on the basis of documentary interpretation of interaction with her over time. For example, an experienced nurse in Site One knew that patients did not ask if they were ready to go home, and it was up to the doctor or nurse to tell them. That 'general typification' was accompanied by perception of the patient as the type of person who looked glum but never 'demanded' time. Part of knowledge of typical patients was knowledge of typical accounts given by patients, whereby they were reflexively known as the types of patients they were. Thus a nurse in Site One:

> N: It was more the, type of person he was, because of the type of person he was, you know, maybe, if it had been (?someone else) I might have said something like, 'Go home and say to, your son, how you feel' and that..and most, not most, but some folk would have, coped with that. But he was the type of guy who needed a lot, of eh, support..
>
> R:...where did the, where did the, notion that, eh, he needed a lot of support come from, (?)
>
> N: Eh, (sighs) just because a lot of the times he s-, you know, he said he couldn't do things...

Typification distilled what happened 'a lot of times'. It helped the nurses cope with interaction by providing a set of expectations matched by standard responses. One typification of particular interest was that of the patient as 'actor'. This typification was seen one day when nurses, crowded into the nurses' station after a meeting, saw a patient fall to the floor. They looked onto the scene and carried on talking. One student nurse looked concerned. After a pause another student nurse went from the office to the day room, bent down and told the patient 'You can get up now'. The patient did not respond. The nurse returned to the office, exclaiming that the patient deserved an 'Oscar' for his 'performance'. The nurses' review of the meeting resumed. More generally, patients were typified as capable of strategic action and 'conning'. Knowledge of reality, and the ability to distinguish between and to order (the paramount) 'reality' and appearance (illusion, delusion, hallucination, fantasy, act), were essential to the nurses' work.[13]

Illness or problem knowledge

The fourth meaning was of interaction as indicating a problem or illness. Typically, talk of problems or illness occurred in the context of common-sense, ordinary understandings of typical life. For example, a patient's 'anxiety' was accounted for by noting that 'old people dinnae take changes very great'. The latter understanding was drawn from a stock of knowledge which could broadly be called, in one nurse's words, 'worldly knowledge'. The nurses' more specialist 'explanatory schemes' (Berger and Luckmann, 1967) articulated with ordinary understandings. In another account, a nurse greeted a patient returning from a weekend home:

> N: And then he volunteered a wee bit more information saying that he had had a nightmare, um, or, he said 'a dream'. Said he dreamt about his, his father...um, and then he volunteered that he's known other people who, you know, have dreamt about somebody that has died quite recently, or, feel that they're...about, you know, somewhere round them, who knows what's going on, and...I agreed with him, you know, this often does happen. And, em, asked him if he could remember anything specific about this particular dream, and, he just said that his father was talking to him in his dream so I was asking, you know, 'What did your father say, can you remember anything about the dream?', and he said he couldn't. Um, so I really just said that it's, it is quite normal for people, you know, when somebody has died to, to dream about them or feel that they're about.
>
> R: You, you said that..
>
> N: I said that, yes, and, em, in his case it was possibly just a delayed reaction since he hadn't sort of come to terms with it

until very recently, that his father had died, actually accepting it, he was having all these feelings coming, you know, a much later date, but very similar to somebody who's, maybe just died recently.

R: Mnhmn.

N: So I was just trying to tell him that this is all quite normal, (?not) not to...be frightened.

The nurse drew on knowledge of dreams, death, the return of the dead: all to negotiate an understanding of the 'normality' of what the man had experienced. In doing so she also drew on what may be regarded as 'specialist' knowledge: first, that what he had told her was a sign of 'delayed' grief; and second, that the staff understood that the delay in grief partly accounted for the man's depression and his admission. Another nurse on another occasion responded to the patient's worry about his father by telling of his regret at not having talked more to his own grandfather before his death. Again, the nurse told the man it was a 'common' experience. The distinction I marked in patients' understandings, between 'ordinary life' and 'illness or problem talk', appears here as the negotiation of an intersubjective reality, shared by nurses and patients, in which the dead may appear in dreams and regret may be common. The nurses surveyed the talk and acknowledged what was common. In surveillance they also 'picked up' what was not common. The second nurse, above, heard the man's despair at a return of 'bad days' as a sign of a stage in depression, and told the man that this was typical of the illness. 'Being sound in clinical knowledge', the nurse was able to distinguish the commonly painful from what he counted as illness.

The aim here is not to parse the nurse's understanding into common sense and specialist sense. Only through further interpretation and dialogue would it be possible to negotiate a claim that his action made sense in either frame or both frames.

Emotions, ordinary reality and the reality of illness and problems: 'what's everyday for us is not for her' In nurses' accounts, the basis for patients' action (patients' knowledge) was always 'bracketed' from its context in the patient's account and interpreted in terms of the nurse's knowledge. By 'bracketing' I mean that what the patient said was relayed in the nurse's voice (even when a verbatim quote was intended) and was therefore interpreted in the nurse's frame of meaning. Thus a student nurse accompanied P6 to a day centre. When P6 found that she was meant to attend the day centre as part of continuing treatment, she panicked and wept. In her account, the student nurse said that she (the student) had not realised that 'what was everyday for us was not for P6'. Knowledge of P6's illness or problem - the 'not everyday' - emerged from the background of the 'everyday' through the nurse's bracketing of P6's knowledge.[14]

These examples illustrate an important point regarding description and explanation of nurse-patient interaction construed in terms of personal states in public places specialising in the treatment of mental illness. Nurses (generally, discounting the times when the display was discounted as a 'con') knew that patients' displays of emotion showed where a problem lay. The work associated with this knowledge will be explored more fully in the next chapter. The point to emphasise, with regard to knowledge, is that the shows of emotion were read for their meaning as signs of an 'underlying' illness or problem.

Understanding what 'it' was The nurses' understanding of illness and problems had two aspects. Emotion was seen as meaning that there was some illness or problem to be interpreted further. And there were understandings of what that 'something' might be.

Understanding that 'it' was responsible and understanding of what 'it' was were distributed unevenly in both sites. In both sites, there were sometimes competing claims about 'it'. For example, in Site One, the staff were puzzled by P6. At times the consultant and nurses thought that her bizarre and offensive behaviour was due to some mental illness, for which she could not be held responsible. At other times, some thought that she was 'putting it on', 'acting'. The nurses finally appealed publicly to the other patients and to P6 herself to tell them whether she was ill and not responsible, or not ill and responsible. The patients' discomfort at playing this role indicated the violation of a tacit assumption: 'the nurses and not the patients have the right to know and should know what is really wrong with a patient'.

In Site Two, there were often conflicting accounts of what 'it' was. Those nurses who had vestigial knowledge derived from earlier work in a unit treating neurotic patients on the principles of psychodynamic theory gave accounts of 'it' as an intrapsychic process: for example, 'anxiety about marital problems put off onto things around the patient'. Questions of knowledge of whether there was an 'it' and what 'it' was have been construed in the nursing literature in terms of professional and lay judgement (John, 1961; Altschul, 1972; Sladden, 1979). It is not the intention here to allocate the knowledge in this way, but rather to claim that some knowledge of some 'it' formed one element in the nurses' accounts. What 'it' was, and whether what the nurses saw as 'it' was what 'it' really was, cannot be determined through the methodology of this study. The claim will be advanced below that the nurses acted to get 'it' out of the way in order to move the patient on. This claim does not depend on the 'validity' of their interpretation of 'it'. I will explore in Chapter 6 negotiations and disputes between nurses and patients and among staff about what 'it' was, and in Chapter 7 I will explore the implications of certain understandings of 'it' for action in the moral orders of the sites.[15]

Knowledge of remedies

Typically, accounting for a problem or illness was accompanied by accounting for a remedy. This could range from the look toward S1P4 to let her know that she was noticed, to reassurance that S1P3's dream was normal, to 'the usual five minutes talk' given when patients were upset, to getting a doctor to prescribe a laxative for the patient's constipation. Remedies mainly appeared to be 'recipes' (Schutz and Luckmann, 1974): 'the usual five minutes', 'reassurance', 'getting the family together'. Remedies were contrived when unexpected or new situations were encountered. For example, a student who had 'never been prepared for anything like this' had to devise a means of quieting a distressed woman (see Appendix 9). A new staff nurse had to work out a personal response to a patient. When staff in Site One had to take over an occupational therapy group, they worked out how to use a game to let a particularly difficult patient know how they felt about the way she treated them.[16]

Personal knowledge: the interpreting nurse

Lastly, the meaning of interaction was the meaning it had for the nurse as the person in the interaction. The nurses claimed that each nurse would understand and handle situations differently. They took it for granted that their impressions were based on what patients were expressing (Goffman, 1969), but also that 'hearing' involved interpretation. An experienced nurse in Site One used the metaphors 'reading into' and 'picking up' to claim that some nurses 'picked up' more than others. She claimed that one could 'read into' something more than was there. It was one of the strongest claims made by nurses, in particular in Site One, that what happened in interaction depended on the nurse involved. I will explore in Chapter 7 the relationship between this finding and the constitution of the sites as different moral orders.

Nurses thus acknowledged the possibility that they might 'know' more than there was to know. However, the nurses were not typically plagued by doubt. The reason for this might be that, through participation in a discourse in which action was typified, they typically encountered non-problematic reality. A nurse in Site One saw P7 looking fed up and went to see what she needed reassured about. The remedy of 'reassurance' was already 'to hand'.[17] The availability of 'reassurance'[18] as a remedy structured what the nurse saw as needing done. The indexicality of action itself militated against doubt. A default account was: 'that's what I think'.

Some nurses, especially learners, admitted to doubt when giving some of their accounts of conversations and of understandings about patients, and collectively the nurses could be unsure of what they were doing with some of the patients. Common sense became a topic for nurses when common sense as a resource was called into doubt (a trained nurse in Site Two). Different nurses could also disagree about what a patient was doing or expressing. In the latter case the nurses acted to resolve the disagreement, for example, questioning a patient said by some nurses to be 'hiding'.

Features of knowledge: location of knowledge and points of view

When patients and nurses gave their accounts of occasions of talk with the patients, they did what story tellers do. They set characters in some scene and told what happened. They established 'the point', 'the main thing'. However, the main thing only emerged from the background through the frame provided by the story teller. In the case of the patients, the frame was sometimes that of their subjectivity, their illness or problem. The nurses generally interpreted the patients in terms of what I have called the frame of 'work', the background of site/stay/patient/illness-problem/remedy/personal knowledge. Sense was made from the point of view and through the frame of meaning of the teller.

By focusing on the narrative, indexical and reflexive features of nurses' accounts I am highlighting an important feature of nursing knowledge, hitherto not noted in nursing researchers' interpretations of nurse-patient interaction. The implication of the above analysis is that in telling their stories and giving their accounts, the nurses reflexively constituted the site as the site in which the accounts, and they as accountable subjects, made sense. The ability to give the accounts testified to the nurses' role in maintaining and ongoingly producing the reality of the sites of interaction through interaction in the site. The sites as sites of nursing practice were sustained through that practice. Any attempt to account for the interaction without taking into account the background, taken for granted reality of the sites implied in the frame of 'work' would be incomplete. The nurses legitimated their part in interaction by calling into play knowledge of the knowledge needed to keep the work going and to maintain the site as the paramount reality within which their action made sense.

The background knowledge included knowing where things happened, with whom, when. When nurses in Site One said 'Saturday morning', they knew but did not have to tell that Saturday mornings were quiet, that this was when nurses' own projects could be undertaken, that people could be seen before leaving for weekends. In turn, 'leaving for weekends' had to be placed in the context of the patient's stay, 'quiet' had to be contrasted with the busy-ness of other parts of the week. Nurses, the patients and I came to know these things through participating in the daily life of the sites.

In any account, the explicitness of these understandings was always incomplete. Hearers in the site 'repaired' indexical particulars in hearing them (Garfinkel, 1967). When a nurse said 'Saturday morning' and acted in accordance with the tacit understanding that 'Saturday morning' entailed all that it entailed, Saturday morning was constituted as what it was through the action. Similarly, 'here', 'we', 'you' were constituted as what they were through the action. The nurse, the patient, the site, were constituted. A nurse's account in which 'Saturday morning' occurred was part of the site in which Saturday morning occurred.

Nurses' knowledge focused on the patient located in patients' accounts Nurses depended on the indexicality and reflexivity of their own and patients' accounts to do the work of the place, to act accountably. Patients' accounts were used by nurses to locate the patients in their world, knowledge of that world being drawn on in doing the work of location. If a patient said 'I couldn't help it' the person located by the indexical 'I' could be pinned down and challenged if the nurse thought that 'I's generally or this 'I' now was responsible for 'helping it'. Use of the indexical features of patients' accounts enabled nurses to locate the patient as a subject and to challenge the objectivation of the patient's subjectivity. The patient could be subjected to the 'gaze' (Foucault, 1979) that works through examination of indexical particulars. Thus in a nurse's account:

> N: Just information, really, and eh well she also felt that she told me how her weekend had gone and she felt that the drugs had a lot to do with it and let her know that the drugs really didn't have much to do with how she had been at home, eh, it was mainly up to her, a lot of it was up to her. And she says well, you know, 'Do you think that's, you know, do you not think it is the drugs?', I said 'No, I think I think a lot's something to do with you and you've got to try maybe to get on with Phil (Note: husband)...'

Regardless of what 'it' was, responsibility for 'it' was pinned to the 'I' of the patient's account. Nurses depended on the indexicality and reflexivity of talk to know and to speak of an interpretable 'it' which meaningfully explained and made sense of their interaction with the patient. Interaction was organised through 'work' on 'it' whatever 'it' was.[19]

Indexicality and looking: telling and interpretation The indexicality and reflexivity of the nurses' and patients' talk meant that in giving accounts to each other and to me they were always 'telling' more than they were saying. The debate about whether one can know more than one can tell or tell more than one can know (Polanyi, 1967; Shotter, 1984; Harre and Secord, 1972; Nisbett and Wilson, 1977; Mair, 1987) will not be addressed here. It is sufficient to establish that nurses and patients acted on the understanding that they were telling more than they were saying and that the other was involved in 'mutual work' (Giddens, 1976) to realise what was being said. I have already argued that the patients knew that the nurses might know more than 'ordinary talk' revealed.

The nurses' knowledge that they could tell more is explicated through analysis of the uses of the term 'telling' in nurses' accounts.[20] The nurse could 'tell' about the patient on the basis of what the first order interaction 'told' him. The patient could be speaking but 'it', the first order conversation including what was said and how it was said, was 'telling' the nurse about 'second order' matters, for example the patient's concentration. The nurse could be taking what the patient said (first order) with 'a pinch of salt' but that she was saying it was 'telling' that the patient was keen to leave the hospital. The patient's first order 'telling' could be interpreted by the nurse as deliberate 'signalling' of a meaning that the patient could not express directly. The patient was then seen as 'presenting'; that is, first order talk was seen as directly translatable into second order meaning ('well', 'ready to go').

'Telling' was an essential aspect of nurse-patient interaction. Interpretation was the work. Thus, an experienced nurse in Site One said:

> N: ...she's telling me things and I'll uh, you know I've got to kind of see them, I've got to kind of see her..(laughs) through her words uh uh what she's doing, where she's at, uh, what she wants..and similarly I've got to try and convey things.

Nurses thus had common-sense understandings of the features of language and interaction adequate to their practical purposes of 'telling' what was meant, what was being done as well as what was being said in interaction with the patients.

The 'main thing' was a product of interpretation. In 'telling', the nurses saw from within a reality reflexively realised through the interpretive processes of the sites. They saw a 'second order' reality related through hermeneutic processes to the first order reality shared with the patient. The objectivity of that second order reality was taken for granted but it could not be fully explicated. Nonetheless, the objectivity of important features of the second order reality were established through 'telling'. For example, nurses could 'tell' patients' motives, and their willingness to 'work' on problems.

The above account of telling, and of 'seeing through', indicates an assumption, on the nurses' part, of intersubjectivity. The site was established as a place where much went without saying and mutual resources for understanding were assumed. The patient said, but 'it' told. Understanding 'it' was a mutual accomplishment. The nurses needed to do 'documentary work' and to refer to features of the interaction, including the patient's understanding, to accomplish the rationality of their work with the patients.

Situating interaction: nurses' first and second order understandings

In second level accounts nurses interpreted in second level terms actions and acts already interpreted in first level constructs. I asked a nurse to clarify a point from a first level account:

R: Um, yeah, and you were saying at the beginning it just s-, sorta started off insignificantly, um, that, you'd seen her sitting, and, she looked bored. Um, so that you thought you'd have a general chat with her. So the sense I got from that is, em, that, these conversations just **arise**, in some way, through, in, just in the course of the day, through, you know, you could be walking by and see somebody looking bored, and take the opportunity...

N: Yeah, uh, depending on the circumstance. Like, I knew P2, to be in quite a good state of mind then. So I wasn't going to take the opportunity to, sort of, have a therapeutic chat, or anything. That time it was just, 'Ah there's P2 looking bored'.

Second level accounts provided occasions for nurses to display knowledge different from or additional to that displayed in first level accounts. They used concepts like 'observation', 'assessment', 'therapeutic chat', 'clinical', which constituted a second level discourse not used in telling about conversation. They also referred to important explanatory concepts (for example 'at that time': indexicality itself) which were key background features to the accountability of their knowledge. These further legitimations may have been occasioned by my wanting to know 'more', to understand better.

The important implication of this is that nurses had more than one accounting system (cf. Potter and Mulkay, 1985). Which one was drawn on may have depended on their interpretation of the requirements of the research setting (cf. Harre and Secord, 1972). The same actions were re-interpreted as different acts. The reinterpretation displayed a different sort of competence: in the example above, competence in distinguishing situations in which 'therapeutic talk' was called for.

Form of knowledge: accounts as stories as 'capsule versions of reality'

I have argued that patients made sense through 'ordinary' and 'illness' frames of meaning, and that in their accounts they referred to the work of the nurses and other staff. I have outlined the frame of meaning 'work' in terms of which nurses made sense of their interaction with these patients. I noted that through their accounts nurses articulated understandings of illness and problems, established against the background of common sense. In this way I have introduced a key claim of this monograph. The claim is that nurses and patients used the concepts 'illness', 'problem' and 'work' to make sense of each other and their interaction together. Each of the concepts articulated with an unspecified background common-sense knowledge. That articulation allowed nurses and patients who met as strangers to use these 'working words' to do the 'main thing' and sustain the work of the site - treatment of illness and problems related to personal states in public places - so that the patient could be returned to the community. These concepts were articulated in different discourses in the two sites. They constituted 'living ideologies' (Billig et al, 1988).

The nurses' and patients' accounts were forms of knowledge in the way that stories are. The key to understanding this claim can be found in Bennett and Feldman's (1981, p. 4) analysis of the function of stories in the administration of justice in American jury trials:

> (F)ormal justice procedures...must engage some parallel form of social judgment that anchors legal questions in everyday understandings...(A) particular everyday judgment and communication device, the story, fits into a formal scheme of legal judgment...The story is an everyday form of communication that enables a diverse cast of courtroom characters to follow the development of a case and reason about the issues in it.

In the following two chapters I will argue that the nurses and patients judged patients' and staff's responsibility for the patients' personal states. Here I argue that the story form of accounts enabled nurses to play their role(s) in this work. Accounts as stories defined the 'dramatist' elements of 'cases' and thus enabled nurses to play their parts in assessment and treatment or care of patients diagnosed as neurotic.

The processes of judgement of responsibility were processes of reality definition. This claim rests on an argument that knowing what really happened depended on knowing what was responsible for what happened (cf. Goffman, 1972). This argument is based in the empirical data of this study, as will be elaborated more fully in Chapters 6 and 7. It also accords with the theoretical perspective of this monograph, according to which social reality is constructed through grasping the meanings of social action, meaning implying motivation (Goffman, 1972; Schutz and Luckmann, 1974). Responsibility for what happened was established through establishing motive: was the patient responsible for an outburst, or was it just 'a state'? Did the patient do it, or did it happen to her? Was she an agent, or a patient (an agency of some state or illness)? Stories were the vehicles for these processes of reality definition, maintenance and repair. If the reality was disputed, if a shared reality was threatened, with two accounts conflicting - agent, patient; 'up to you', 'a state' - accounts were the devices by means of which reality could be repaired. The appearance of responsibility could be accounted for in another way; the existence of a 'state' and recognition of it as a cause of an outburst could be agreed. In an ongoing way, the work of reality maintenance and repair constituted the work of the sites. In this process, accounts were the vehicles for 'therapy'. They conveyed (usually implicitly) that a deviation from ordinary reality had occurred and what sort it was (illness, problem); indicated how the patient was thus deviant (made sense of the problem or the illness); and provided the basis for remedy, for the means by which the patient could be returned to the paramount reality (Berger and Luckmann, 1967). The paramount reality was the backdrop in relation to which the nurses' accounts made sense.

The significance of the structure of nursing knowledge and the structure of story: the construction of the main thing

The first five elements of nurses' knowledge are akin to Burke's (1969a) pentad of elements of story. 'Site', 'stay', 'patient', 'illness or problem' and 'remedy' can be compared to 'scene', 'act', 'agent', 'agency', 'motive'. The sixth element, 'personal knowledge', corresponds to the narrative 'voice'.

The similarity is meaningful. Burke (1969a) proposes that understanding of motivated action is accomplished through narration in which the 'dramatist pentad' (the above five elements) are arranged in 'ratios' which convey the meaning of the story, its 'point'. The work of the sites centred on understanding of motivated action (cf. Burke, 1969a): 'Why is she here now?' can be read as 'What is responsible for her being here now?'; and 'What do I have to do for her?' can be read as 'What is my responsibility to and for her?' Nurses and patients worked to understand action, and understand its motivation, for the practical purposes of 'getting or feeling better' (from the point of view of the patients) or of 'assessing and treating patients' (from the point of view of the nurses).

Accounts in the form of stories were the means by which the main things in the day to day interaction between the nurses and patients were articulated with the account in the form of story of the main thing, the return of the patient to the community. Nurses acted so that a story could be told to the effect that the main thing related to the patient had been grasped and handled.

Stories, assessment and treatment: the development of a case and judgement of what is 'wrong' with story and person

In this section I explore the knowledge embedded in the nurses' and patients' practices of 'reading' and telling accounts, construing the accounts as stories. Practice, from this perspective, is an interpretive process.

The analytical concept 'account', the analytical concept 'story', the analytical concepts 'maxim' and 'frame of meaning', all have this in common as used in this monograph: they refer to forms and devices of knowledge drawn on and reconstituted in structuring the world, including the subjective worlds of the patients, for practical understanding and action. They provided common forms for interpreting and ordering worlds and realities in relation to the paramount reality. These forms and devices of knowledge were used by nurses and patients to define, interpret, maintain and repair the intersubjective worlds of the sites.

Empirically, the interaction between these patients and nurses could not be understood as context-independent knowledge. The nurses and patients had to elaborate the context of interaction in order to make sense of how they and the other made sense in the interaction. In second level accounts I had to elaborate with them and refer to contextual features of their first level accounts in order to understand further what they were doing. These empirical conclusions accord with theoretical understandings of practical knowledge (Wieder, 1974; Dreyfus, 1983; Benner, 1984, 1985; Shotter, 1984). The meanings of interaction as practical knowledge can only be conveyed by elaborating its context. The meaningful context can be documented, but never exhaustively (Garfinkel, 1967). Interaction and accounts of interaction constitute as meaningful the features which form the ground for interpreting it. That context is, in the course of interaction, still open to further interpretation (Ricoeur, 1971).

Story was one of the main forms used to accomplish the practical work of the sites. The practical work of the sites was interpretation, but interpretation of a sort that yielded social facts: diagnoses, treatments. The patient's action and interpretations of her action - her subjectivity, her 'story' as the document of her subjectivity, her account of what had happened to her, and claims of excuse or justification - were subjected to observation and interpretation, the sense of which was conveyed in further accounts and stories. Story was the medium for interpretation. Accounts were among the varieties of stories told in the site. They were specifically the stories told to clarify ambiguous action, or to provide the grounds for justification or excuse.

Getting stories from patients was part of the work of assessment. Assessment was the set of methods for answering the question 'Why is she here now?'. Stories told by the nurses about the patients created the interpretive context for social action in the site. The relationship of story to site was reflexive.

The value of patients' stories lay in the possibilities they afforded nurses for interpreting what was 'wrong' with the story: a grief that had gone on too long, a helplessness that was unrelated to physical illness. What was wrong could only be determined by reference to 'normal' stories and to common sense (see Hughes, 1980, 1988a). Stories that were 'wrong' indicated what was subjectively problematic for the patient, 'the main thing' from the patient's point of view. This formed the basis for further interpretation of what 'the main thing' was from the nurses' point of view. What was wrong with patients' stories was often precisely that they did not tell stories about problems.

These observations are rooted in the empirical data. Readings of the data in the sections on 'frames of meaning' have indicated how nurses 'read' and interpreted the patients' stories. For example, the nurse heard the patient's story of the dream and 'ordered' it as normal, thereby ordering the dream world in relation to paramount reality, and normal odd experiences in relation to the 'non-normal'. The site was thus established as a site of knowledge about these aspects of reality. In the next section I will stress the role of story in establishing the continuity of sense across episodes of interaction, the basis of work with the patient, to establish 'the main thing' and work on it to move him through his stay. Story was the medium for defining the unit of analysis, the 'case', meaning the patient as the focus of knowledge and power during his or her stay.

An example of the development of a case through story

The story of the patient's stay developed through interaction, as exemplified in this account of how an experienced nurse in Site One - referred to in the following section as 'Nurse Val', a pseudonym - understood what was wrong with P3:

> N: And...just really introduced myself cos I didn't know his wife, and..just asked how things were at home and how P3 had been and, she said that they didn't really have have many problems, em, P3 was saying though that he felt that it was bit of a strain because of the son, he'd been hard on the son and em felt that he hadn't really been a proper father... so, we (?) talked about that a wee bit and decided that it might be a good idea to see the son with P3 and his wife and, maybe it would be better if they came up to the ward prior to him going home overnight on Sunday, so that it would all be over and done with before they went home...

In her second level account, with me 'looking over her shoulder', Nurse Val elaborated:

> N: Right. Well, first of all, I just really, as I said, (Note: in original transcript) I'm just introducing myself, to the wife, really, right, because it was the first time I'd seen the wife. I had, in previous Kardexes it had been said there was something underlying between the wife, and, P3, right? Em, so I just thought, Well, I'll see if there's anything I can pick up, (?), eh, seeing if they have any, (?), (?) having problems. Em.. That was the marriage, right? and I felt that, it was true, because like they both denied that there was any real problems, just the basic, sort of everyday, husband and wife, problems, right? Eh, and then it came out that, the main problem was, em, P3's relationship with his son. Eh, his wife (?agreed) with that, she was quite tearful at that point, right? Eh, so, having picked up on that, I decided that, it might be quite a good idea, to have the son up, because P3 was going home on on pass, he didn't particularly want to go home, because the son would be there and he felt pretty rotten about how he'd treated him, right? I felt that it would be a good idea, to have the boy up, then, P3 could confront him..and I would be there, as a spectator, sort of neutral body, right? Em, and that's (?), P3 thought it was really good, because it was giving him support, and the wife thought it was a good idea, because finally, it had

> all come out in the open, (?) their feelings and how they felt, and, em, because although she, she obviously loved P3, she felt a great deal for the son, she didn't like them not getting on.

'The main thing' develops through this account as it did for the nurse in interaction, in time, through an intersubjective process of interpretation and response. The account accomplishes the 'getting into the open' which is the main thing. In the second level account can be seen the form of assessment. Through the story and interpretation of it several developments take place: the development of the story about P3, on the basis of what he told Nurse Val and his wife, in the course of which 'the main thing' to do not only with his weekend pass but also with his stay becomes clearer; the development of P3's character through the story he tells - a father unable to express his feelings; the development of P3's stay, in that he went on pass; and the development in the interaction itself - the tears, the new knowledge - which P3's story accomplishes. A fourth development is important. Through dialogue recounted in the second level account Nurse Val developed the background understandings - of 'normal problems', for example - which informed her understanding and hence her accountability. She used what she called her 'worldly knowledge', implicitly acknowledging her dependence on common sense as well as special understandings to do the work of assessment. Nurse Val needed common sense to do the work of the site.

P3's story developed in, and in turn played a part in the development of, his interaction with Nurse Val; and the story about P3, as a patient during his stay in hospital, developed through this development. The nurse developed knowledge of P3's problems through the interaction, by bringing up from a background of 'normal troubles' 'the main thing', the 'real problem' (cf. Cicourel, 1976; Garfinkel, 1967). What developed through the interaction, through Nurse Val, P3 and the wife making sense with each other, was knowledge of reality previously hidden, brought into the open and into intersubjective reality through the story.

Nurse Val explained later how that knowledge articulated with other knowledge about P3:

> N: That was the major problem at the time. (?Right.) It didn't actually relate to his illness, or why he was here, but it was a ma-, well, in a way it did, because he was worried about it, right? Uh, it was one of his major worries.

The signification of action could be elaborated, but did not need to be elaborated for practical purposes. Knowledge of 'the main thing' was pragmatic, confirmed in its consequences. Knowledge of reality - the 'real problem' and how to deal with it - was a product of conversation. The reality negotiated by the nurse, the patient and the wife was the reality with 'the problem' located within it. That reality and that knowledge were products of the interaction.

The nurse worked on the basis of understanding typical consequences of not acting. Nurse Val had a 'recipe' for the appropriate action:

> N: That was really the idea, to, to, get them out of the house, in a neutral, (laughs) neutral place, right? (laughs) With a referee, (laughing) and see what happened, and, and it worked, so that was the main thing..

The practical knowledge was the knowledge needed to 'get out of the way' the problem which stood in the way of the patient going home. There was an unspoken assumption that getting things out of the way and getting the patient home was the aim. Arranging the confrontation of father and son can be seen as 'therapy' in that it created the conditions necessary for development of the story to one in which the patient was restored to his place in his home. The tacit assumption was that the paramount reality was one in which the father's place was in his home, not in the ward.

The validity of the practical, working knowledge was evident: 'and it worked, so that was the main thing'. This may be read two ways, both valid. That it worked was the main thing; and what 'the main thing' was, was seen through how 'it' worked.[21]

This may be read as a paradigm of socialisation and social construction of reality in Site One. Reality was modified through conversation in which the patient, his wife and the nurse negotiated a realisation of the problem. The nurse and the wife were led to grasp what the patient understood and to act as the patient did toward the symbols which objectified the patient's understanding. The objectification of the main thing, however, depended on one more process: that through which the intersubjective understandings, when acted upon, were seen to be meaningful in their consequences. The main thing was the objectification of what worked through the intersubjective process of conversation. This, in microcosm, was the process of socialisation into the main reality (Berger and Luckmann, 1967). Socialisation was the development of subjective and objective realisation through interaction.

'The main thing' emerged through a circle of interpretation and realisation The development of the interaction and of the stay was accomplished through a process of interpretation. The nurse came to interaction with background understandings. Through the process of 'reading', interpretation and 'handling', understanding was changed.

The nurse went out from a circle of understanding - the case review in which the staff said there was a problem in the marriage. She went out to 'see what she could pick up'. She picked up what was embedded in the patient's talk - not only what he said but how he said it. She picked up 'the real problem' through hearing more than was said. The reality of the problem as constructed through the interaction was a product of a process in which the subjectivity of the nurse was involved, as were the subjectivities of the patient and others. Through the process of interaction a new intersubjective reality was constructed.

The circle of understanding was a general feature of nursing accounts, and the above analysis may be taken as paradigmatic of a process which can be represented graphically (see Appendix 6).

The circle represents the form of the nurse's knowledge in practice. This process of interpretation and understanding had its counterpart in the nurse's method of explanation. She led me to understand 'the point' of her story about P3 by picking out key features of the interaction. She highlighted and related the elements of the story, and drew on shared background understandings (note her reiteration of 'right?'), so that I was led to understand 'the main thing'.

This was an account of nursing work, told from the point of view of the nurse. The account related a form of nursing practice: the practice of realising and doing something about 'the main thing'; that is, the practice of assessment and treatment, 'therapy'. The point was that 'the main thing' was realised (got into the open, objectivated), that it was got out of the way, and that the patient and his wife felt better. The point of Nurse Val's story was the recognition and remedy of problems. The nurse in interaction and in accounting for interaction drew on and constituted features of the context in order to render her action accountable as action meaningful and warranted as right ('right?') in the site.

In the above account can be see the typical form of nurses' work with these patients. In doing their routine work, the nurses 'picked up' worries and troubles. They picked up what worried the patients through noting the signs of worry. The nurses understood in a pragmatic way that patients' shows of feeling were signs (see Hochschild, 1983). A show of feeling signalled to the nurse some worrisome or troublesome aspect of the patient's reality, interpreted as the 'problem'. The concepts 'problems', 'worries' and 'troubles coping' were common to all three frames of meaning: 'ordinary talk', 'talk of illness and problems', and 'work'.

The interaction was thoroughly contextualised. It 'came from' a history of interaction with this patient and fed into further interaction. The concept 'getting things out of the way' implied action in a direction, teleological action. 'Getting things out of the way' implied resistance, tension, the work of the site. What has to be 'read in' is what was at the end of the 'way': home, the place to which the patient was restored through the work of the site. The nurse gave as her rationale: 'So I felt that to get that out of the way would be beneficial to him'. In this can be read an implicit maxim: 'when a problem is found, it is good to get it out of the way'. Nurse Val's action is not presented as a rational, planned process but as the exercise of judgement in the situation, representing knowledge of context and response appropriate to context.

Knowledge of the meaning of the interaction was knowledge got by 'looking back': 'looking back it was a good idea'. The teleological meaning could be grasped only in a new context. The maintenance and repair of reality was confirmed in time. The image that came through this account was an image of the knowing nurse in the situation, working on the basis of both 'in order to' and 'because' motives (Schutz and Luckmann, 1974), in light of pragmatic knowledge of the patient and the illness, in the context of the stay. It was sometimes necessary to look across accounts to see lines of sense: Nurse Val related that P3 said that talking lifted a weight from his shoulders; another nurse said that in their conversation P3 had 'lifted a stone'.[22]

The point of the various kinds of work the nurses did was the maintenance or restitution of unproblematic reality. The various kinds of work included: policing of reality, and encouragement of self-policing by the patients[23]; 'reinforcement'; 'reassurance'; 'putting the reality back to (patients)'; 'picking things up', a kind of putting things in order, or hoovering of reality. Reality work was done on a routine or emergency basis. Tools and skills required for reality work were stories, metaphors, shared understandings, knowledge of the normal. The main tool and resource was common sense.

Validity and reliability of the nurses' practical knowledge The validity of Nurse Val's knowledge, the usefulness of the recipe, was not divorced from the context of the situation and the other knowledge she had. She got the patient and his son together in the site on a Saturday morning so that they could sort things out with her there as a 'neutral body': '...But the idea of neutral territory was based on the type of person he was. Maybe with someone else I would have said...'. The nurses' claims for the validity of their work were always claims of validity in context. They claimed that what they did made sense in the context in which they did it, and that they could never exhaustively account for that context. The nurses' claim for the validity of their action was implicitly that its rationality[24] consisted of the method of interaction, including interpretation.[25] The validity of their knowledge rested on the process of developing understandings through interaction.

These aspects of the nurses' methods and rationality could not have been 'caught' by use of methods which decontextualised accounts of interaction.

'Picking up the vibes': intersubjectivity

Nurse Val's accounts omitted the chain of reasoning, the 'deliberate, rational' accounting, that might be expected in defence or explanation of professional conduct (see Chapter 2). However, it is like typical accounts given by experienced practitioners.[26] 'Seeing what happened' was 'guided' by the ongoing sense made of and in the interaction: knowledge in practice.

Pressed for how she knew he was the type of guy who needed support, Nurse Val referred to previous interaction with him: 'Because a lot of times he said he couldn't do things and if I had said could he do it, he would have said he couldn't cope'. Typification was the sedimentation of what happened 'a lot of times'. The nurse's knowledge was contextualised in time, place, and in relation to her own and the other's subjectivity. The type emerged from its documentation, each document marked by features of indexicality, with the type freed to feature as taken for granted in explanation. The rationality of the nurse's action was the method by which she acted. This method could not be exhaustively documented (Garfinkel, 1967). Nurse Val interacted with the type of guy whose typicality could not be questioned.

The terminus of Nurse Val's accounting lay in 'feeling', not ratiocination:

> N: Eh, and I'm sure if (?I had) said to him, 'Could you do it at home?' (?) '(? I) couldn't cope with that sort of thing.' eh.. So you sorta get that, sorta feeling. That what you want?
>
> R: Mnmn, yeah. Yeah,
>
> N: Right.
>
> R: that's what I was (?looking for)
>
> N: Right. (mock whisper) The vibes. (laughs).
>
> R: Right (laughs), the vibes, right (laughs), exactly
>
> N: (laughs)
>
> R: This is the kind of thing,
>
> N: (laughing) Yeah.
>
> R: that actually..
>
> N: But a lot of stuff is like that, you know,
>
> R: Well, that's what's unclear..
>
> N: You get feelings, right? Eh, and you just, maybe something people have said and you just sort of latch onto it, and it's probably more than they're saying.

The 'theory of data' implicit in the nurse's claim to knowledge relies on acceptance of intersubjective understanding. It specifically refutes a theory based only on the content of what is said. The end of explanation was the nurse's appeal to what was 'more than they're saying'. This is a claim about reality and a move in the social construction of reality. 'It' had to be latched onto. The nurse's active participation in the interaction was necessary: this was practical knowledge. The 'more than they are saying' had to be pulled up from what was said. This was a form of 'handling' in conversation. The nurse handled assessment by latching onto something, picking 'it' up and handling 'it'.

Insider knowledge: the problem of the order of knowledge That picking up the problem was unproblematic to the nurse highlights the problem I faced in trying to understand how the nurses practised. The ultimate appeal, whispered and thus drawing me deeper into insider status, was to 'the vibes', to something that was - you had to take the nurse's word for it - present in and informing the interaction. The appeal to 'you know' highlights that I was called upon in interaction to use insider, indexical knowledge to make sense of what was said. Intersubjectivity was an essential characteristic of my recognising as knowledge what the nurse claimed as knowledge. I had to draw on a common sense in response to Nurse Val's frequent 'you know?'s. I knew by taking on trust that her knowledge was informed by the same kind of understanding that I would have had in the situation she described. The nurses' accountability, in terms of this research, was tied to intersubjectivity. The same is true of the patients' accountability. The order of knowledge was that established by the intersubjectivity which formed the ground of interaction: the starting point was the nurse's or patient's understanding.

This 'more' that was understood through embodied interaction was crucial in distinguishing between what the nurse could tell (and her hearer could 'tell') in her account of talk - the heart of interaction - and what was recorded in the nursing Kardex. Nurses knew that in the Kardex they were to record as if they were not interpreting the patient and the interaction in which they were involved. The nurse, to explain as well as she could what she actually did, had to refer to the 'more' that could not be pinned down, an intersubjective 'more'. The unit of analysis on the basis of which nurses' knowledge in practice can be considered valid is thus the 'nurse with the patient in the context'.[27]

Articulation of rules, frames and stories

I have discussed devices - maxims, frames of meaning, accounts as stories - used by nurses and patients in making sense in and of their interaction. In this section I describe the relationship of these devices.

Maxims and resocialisation

The maxims told how to act accountably and provided guidelines for constructing accounts which would count as knowledge. They were vital ingredients in 'recipe knowledge'. Some of the maxims were useful for 'ordering' the relevance of elements of stories (for example, 'attend to the main thing at the time'). They provided the basis for giving accounts of action, for displaying competence through shows of knowledge in action. 'I was listening to the patient's story' was accountable, as long as no other patient was unsafe or unfed at the same time (Site Two) or causing anxiety (Site One). I will show in the following chapters how these maxims guided accountable action, and the consequences of violating the maxims (deviance).

The maxims contained the knowledge needed for constructing reality in the sites. They contained the knowledge needed to sustain the sites as sites of re-socialisation (Berger and Luckmann, 1967). The metaphors of resocialisation, 'healing' and 'problem solving', were subsumed under the metaphor of 'work'. The maxims told how to keep the work going, maintain the main reality. The articulation of the nurses' and patients' maxims (enforced by the nurses) enabled nurses and patients to take their parts in the work of the site. Taking part was resocialisation.

By following the maxims of the site nurses and patients took part in its reality, with the consequences for selfhood that implied. An implicit rule for all taking part in the site was thus 'change yourself in following the maxims'. I have noted how the maxims for patients in the site contradicted some patients' 'personal maxims'. This was probably the case for all patients. The patients' stories told of 'rule violations' (Smith, 1978; Scheff, 1966; Goffman, 1967), violations of common social 'maxims' like 'feed your family' (S2P6), 'do something, don't sit like a lump' (S2P4), 'don't talk nonsense' (S1P5, S2P2), 'act your age' (S2P4), 'be a good stepfather' (S1P3). The maxims patients had violated were 'residual rules' (Scheff, 1966) whose violation featured in accounts of illness or problems.

The logic of maxims, frames and stories

Nurses and patients used the frames of meaning and the maxims to guide and legitimate action, to do the work of the sites. Articulation of the maxims and frames was accomplished through stories. The 'logic' of case development was not the logic of deductive argument but the logic of story, of the documentary method (Garfinkel, 1967). The patient's story, and accounts of conversation mediated by understanding of the staff's story about the patient, were 'documents' used by the staff in the work of developing the story. Interaction was guided by the ongoing developing sense of the story as that was shared by staff and, through the course of interaction, by the patient. Thus a methodology based on story or the documentary method was needed to 'follow' the logic of case development, assessment and treatment. The method of enquiry and form of analysis of this study revealed previously unrecognised aspects of the nurses' and patients' knowledge in practice.

The logic of case development was the logic of the work of the sites. It was the logic of keeping the work going and of how to go on. The logic was implicit in the metaphors which broadly guided work in the site. 'Healing' (the metaphor in Site One) implies a story, as do 'detection' or 'problem solution' (Site Two). The logic of case development was also implied in the metaphors which guided (were used to guide) the 'development' of patients' stories: the metaphor of 'development' itself (child development, S1P2), or 'struggle' or 'challenge' (S1P3). The metaphors told how to 'go on'. They were metaphors apt for admission wards, whence the patients would have to 'go on', to 'do it themselves' after discharge. Some of the skill in assessment and treatment (an experienced nurse in Site One called it finding the 'right word', being able to 'tell it all in a wee story') lay in knowledge and use of the metaphor apt for the admission ward, and knowledge and use of metaphors apt for use in admission wards.

Stories shaped by metaphors, frames or meaning and maxims were all devices for defining the situation. They enabled construction of 'capsule versions of reality' (Bennett and Feldman, 1981) ordered in relation to the paramount reality. They were the tools needed to 'place' people in settings and guide action in doing the work of the sites.

These were the common-sense devices used in the practices of assessment and treatment; that is, in the maintenance and repair of reality. In the stories there had to be an 'illness'/'problem'/ 'personal thing': there had to be an act. There had to be some part for the patient to play: agent or agency; and there had to be some part for the nurses and other staff: again, agent or agency. There had to be a motive: 'getting better' or 'working out the problem'. And there had to be some role for the site itself: setting.

Accounts and stories were thus the devices with which nurses and patients managed the work of assessment and treatment, managed personal states in public places. With these elements of dramatic action (Burke, 1969a), the stories provided the means for answering the questions: 'why (motive) is she (agent/agency) here (scene) now?' and 'what do we (agent/agency) have to do for her?'.

They provided the commonsense vehicles for assessment of need and for treatment. They contained the knowledge needed to manage private states (what was revealed in the patient's own story) in public places.

The frames and the metaphors accommodated the distinction of 'special' and 'ordinary' knowledge; and understanding of the roles appropriate to those who possessed these kinds of knowledge was provided for in the frame ('illness' or 'detection or problem solving'). These kinds of knowledge and understanding were also implied by the metaphors in individuals' stories: the 'development' of a 'child' implied the wisdom of adults, 'sitting like a lump' contrasted with sentience.

Metaphor and role

The nurses' role with these patients was not only the role they played in a given patient's story ('mother' to 'child', for example) but also the role they played in keeping the patient's story in the 'library'. Articulating the realities of ordinary talk and illness talk through the frame 'work', they kept the patients in two 'libraries', those of the community and the site. The nurses maintained the symbolic environment (including that of ordinary life) in which the stories of patients in the sites developed. The nurses anticipated and 'fed' the development of the stories. Their doing so can be construed as a process of 'person growing' (Shotter, 1984; Harre, 1983; see also Barker, 1989; and Peplau, 1952). The implications of this analysis for nursing theory will be developed in Chapter 8.

In their talk the patients and nurses articulated frames of meaning, in the course of developing and maintaining 'working relationships'. This articulation will be explored in the next chapter, 'Power'; and Chapter 7 will focus on the hazards involved in telling and being told about in the 'Moral Order'.

Summary

Maxims, stories and frames of meaning were the social resources (Harre, 1979) nurses and patients drew on and reconstituted in their interaction. By following the maxims and by interpreting action through the frames of meaning, and by telling their story and understanding the story about them and the story of the work of the site, the patients could play their parts in processes of resocialisation intended to return them to the community. They came to recognise that their personal knowledge and maxims placed them somewhere in the frame of 'illness' or 'problems' (though also in the frame of 'ordinary life'), and they took part in work to 'restore' themselves to the community.

Knowledge was not monological. Nurses' and patients' knowledges were different and often disputed. Nurses sometimes disagreed among themselves and with what others knew about the patient. I have argued that the differences between nurses' and patients' knowledge provided the occasions for assessment and treatment intended to restore the patient to common sense. In the next chapter I will argue that the work of the nurses with the patients in this study comprised a form of rhetoric.

The implication of this analysis for understanding nursing knowledge is that psychiatric nursing knowledge is context dependent and inextricably related to ordinary understandings. It can be challenged or developed in the contexts within which it is used for 'work' and which it (in part) reflexively establishes, but not from without. It is essentially practical, not theoretical knowledge, intended to maintain and facilitate the work of the site: answering the questions 'Why is she here now?' and 'What do we have to do for her?'. In the final chapter of this monograph I will explore how this understanding of nurses' practical knowledge - construed as situated, dialogic and dynamic - relates to definitions of nursing.

Notes

1 See discussion of the 'pentad' in Chapter 3.

2 In claiming that in ordinary talk the patients talked about the ordinary things of day to day life I am claiming not only that the patients saw these as the ordinary things but that they are the ordinary things. To talk about ordinary talk is to claim membership in the society in which these things are ordinary and to call on the other to recognise this as ordinary.

3 The reader will note that no distinction is made between 'illness' and 'problems' at this point. However, the distinction will be noted and addressed as relevant at various points hereafter.

4 See also Appendix 4.

5 The patient's view corresponded to a working definition used by a consultant in the site: 'neurotic' meaning an extension or exaggeration of normal emotions, so that they 'rule' social life (Site Two).

6 Issues related to responsibility will be discussed more fully in Chapters 6 and 7.

7 See Goffman (1963, 1967) on interpretation of behaviour in 'public and semi-public places'.

8 By 'experienced nurses' I mean 'more senior members of the nursing staff', either in terms of grade or in terms of length of time in nursing practice, particularly in the site. I use the term in part to avoid identifying nurses by grade, in accord with agreements of confidentiality.

9 This may have been due to the empirical links between knowledge, power and moral order.

10 By 'charge nurse' I mean both 'charge nurse' and 'sister'.

11 It would be possible here to construct an account, using further data (a junior doctor saw P7 as 'a lonely old lady, really'; she was regarded by medical staff as depressed due to her situation), on the basis of which to argue that the student nurse's account (and her knowledge) of the patient's stay was 'valid' or warranted despite her uncertainty. However, the point I am making here is that knowledge of stay was, pragmatically, whatever 'passed' for knowledge in practice and accounts. This nurse thought that the patient's lack of social life outside the hospital was reproduced inside. She therefore went out of her way to arrange activities for S2P7. The 'stay' was shaped by interaction mediated by such understandings of 'the stay'.

12 The relevance of Foucault's (1979) analysis of knowledge produced through practices of power is relevant, and will be explored more fully in later chapters.

13 The ordering is construed in this monograph from the perspective of the social construction of reality, not on the basis of any claim about the ontological status of the 'appearances'.

14 There is some ambiguity in this account. 'Everyday' might mean 'everyday in the working life of the nurse', including patients going to day centres; or encountering unexpected situations and dealing with them without getting panicky. What is important is that the nurse used her grasp of the 'everyday', whatever that means, to comprehend what the main thing was for the patient.

15 It will be seen in Chapter 7 that different understandings of 'it' were consequential in terms of rights and obligations in interaction, and in terms of according respect or lack of respect.

16 The game involved patients and staff imagining that they were in a lifeboat. Only if one person were to leave the boat could the

rest survive. A nurse chose the difficult patient to be put out of the boat, justifying her decision by saying that the patient was acting as if she did not want to be in the site.

17 Discussions with MacLeod (personal communication) indicated the relevance of some of Heidegger's concepts.

18 See Teasdale (1989) on the concept of 'reassurance' in nursing.

19 Further discussion on this will be found in Chapter 7.

20 See Burton (1978) and Eco (1979) on 'telling'; see also Marks (1981) on meaning in psychiatry.

21 The nurse accomplished 'face' validity and reliability by getting feedback from the patient and his wife.

22 For a fuller account of the metaphors involved, see Appendix 2.

23 This will be discussed more fully in Chapter 6.

24 Mead's (1934, p. 334) concept of 'rationality' is appropriate for understanding this: 'Now if the individual can take the attitude of the others and control his action by these attitudes, and control their action through his own, then we have what we can term 'rationality'.'

25 See Burton (1978) on participant observation as a 'theory of data' (Chapter 4).

26 See Dreyfus and Dreyfus (1986); and MacLeod (1990).

27 This may be compared with Benner (1984, 1985) and Kasch (1986).

6 Power, or 'the working relationship'

Introduction

In Chapter 5 I discussed the knowledge on which these nurses and patients drew in their interaction, and with which they reflexively constituted the wards as sites of assessment and treatment. I explained how the nurses' first order concept 'the main thing' conveyed the meaning of 'Why is she here now?' and 'What do we have to do for her?', and how nurses used the frame of meaning 'work' to understand and order interaction involving 'ordinary talk' and 'illness talk'. 'Work' constituted a 'working ideology'.

In this chapter I argue that the nurses' first order concept 'the working relationship' conveyed important features of the nurses' and patients' interdependence in accomplishing the work of the sites, construed as power ascription (assessment) and power development (treatment). I interpret nurse-neurotic patient interaction in terms of the practices in the working relationship which constituted responses to 'Why is she here now (am I here)' and 'What do we have to do for her (I have to do)?'. The concept 'power' was inductively derived through analysis of patients' talk about, among other things, nurses' 'authority' or support; and analysis of nurses' talk about, among other things, patients rebelling or thwarting the nurses, and patients' abilities and liabilities.

Empirically, the production of knowledge was related to practices of power and relations of power. Knowledge of 'the main thing' was produced through and structured 'the working relationship'. The reflexive relationship between knowledge and power[1] is analysed by exploring aspects of the working ideologies of the two sites: the ideology of responsibility in Site Two, and the mixed ideology of responsibility and character in Site One. These were the ideologies drawn on by the nurses in their work of 'therapy', re-socialisation of the patients intended to enable them to return to the community.

I will elaborate conceptual links between the concepts 'powers' and 'power'. The need for a conceptual tool to handle this distinction arose from analysis of nurses' and patients' accounts of interaction in which interpretation (determination) of the patient's ability to do, her 'powers', was structured by relationships of power grounded, for example, in the 'authority' of nurses in relation to patients. Thus what was often at issue in these accounts was conflict over whose interpretation of the patient's action (and what interpretation of her powers or liabilities) would 'stick' and structure future interaction. This analysis enables re-examination of the complex concept of 'opportunity'.[2]

By the concept 'power' I mean the capacity to intervene in courses of events to influence them (cf. Giddens, 1976); and in particular the power to intervene in events by influencing the action of others (cf. Foucault's, 1982, 'action on action'). The concept 'powers' means those abilities or capacities to act which are taken as signs of agency; as distinct from 'liabilities', which are taken as signs of patienthood. 'Powers' are thus involved in determination of the kind of person or being one is. The relevant empirical distinction is explained further below.

As interpretation was a continuous process, and knowledge not something fixed, so power was an ongoing process of influence, strategy, push, resistance. It was not one-way, but multi-directional. What happened between a nurse and a patient could be part of a long chain of interactions involving, from the nurse's point of view, action by doctors, psychologists, other nurses; and from the patient's point of view, other professionals, family, the wider society. Nurses had greater power than patients to order interaction and to convey definitions of interaction that influenced the course of a patient's stay in hospital; but that power was limited, and the features of power were determined by resistance as much as by assertion.

The plan of this chapter is first to introduce concepts needed to follow the argument; then to describe nurses' and patients' powers in getting into working relationships and working in them; to explore the tensions and conflicts related to power in interaction; and then to describe features of discourse relevant to analysis of power.

The working relationship: response and responsibility

The conception of psychiatric nursing I have developed through the analysis is that of interaction as pragmatic 'response' to the questions which guided nurses and patients in their interaction: 'Why is she here (am I here) now?' and 'What do we have to do for her (do I have to do)?'. I use the concept 'the working relationship' mindful of Peplau's (1978, p. 44) claim that the definition of mental illness can be construed as the definition of 'the work the patient is expected to do to become a more fully functioning person'. The sense of 'response' implied in the analysis presented in this chapter is related to Peplau's (1952) 'drama of pushes and pulls'.[3] It is also related to Mead's (1934, p. 78) notion of 'adjustive response', construed as the interpretation of gesture as a social act:

> Meaning arises and lies within the field of relation between the gesture of a given human organism and the subsequent behavior of this organism as indicated to another human organism by that gesture...Just as in fencing the parry is an interpretation of the thrust, so, in the social act, the adjustive response of one organism to the gesture of another is the interpretation of that gesture by that organism - it is the meaning of that gesture.

This perspective implies the reflexive relationship between knowledge and practices of power involving action and interpretation. It implies that power is always contextually related to the social situation in which action is constituted as socially meaningful.

This conception of power is related to Foucault's (1982, pp. 220-221) concept of 'conduct'[4]:

> Perhaps the equivocal nature of the term *conduct* is one of the best aids for coming to terms with the specificity of power relations. For to 'conduct' is at the same time to 'lead' others...and a way of behaving within a more or less open field of possibilities.

In this chapter I will argue that nurses' and patients' interaction is interpretable as a relationship of 'action on action' (Foucault, 1982). Through their interaction the nurses and patients realised each other's power; negotiating the basis of their relationship, 'service' or 'work' (Stacey, 1976). Their interaction is construed in terms of the administrative aims of the sites: assessment and treatment.

Patients' accounts of inability to make sense or to do

In the course of their accounts of interaction with nurses, the patients typically told of inability to do what they normally did, and inability to make sense. One felt groggy, depressed, not able to cope, wanting to cry; another had come to the end of things; another sat like a 'lump' staring at the walls. The patients also told of failures of their ability to do for others or to get others to do for them. They could not talk to their children or spouses, or get others to dress and care for them, or house them. Not 'thinking toward things', not understanding, not talking, wanting not to hear, not knowing but wanting to know who was from where, not taking part or joining in; these were some of the ways in which the patients characterised themselves. For example, S2P2 said:

> P: But I didn't do anything today (?) (?thank goodness) I'm tired, **I cannae sleep, if I could just sleep**. Anyway, who was I talking to, nobody I think I was so tired (laughs).

In their accounts patients often told of their loss and recovery of capacity to share and take part in ordinary life with others, in intersubjective reality. They told of not being able to understand what had happened to them.

Much of nurses' work with these patients was based on responding to such accounts in interaction, making sense of liabilities and getting patients to 'take part' in working relationships intended to restore them to the community.[5] In this chapter I will explore differences between nurses and patients' interpretations of complaints and liabilities, and the relevance of the empirical data to a theoretical definition of nursing.[6] Before exploring aspects of power in nurse-neurotic patient interaction, I will elaborate the conceptual understandings which facilitated analysis of the empirical data.

A conceptualisation of 'powers' and 'power' relevant to the analysis

I will clarify the distinction between the concept 'powers' and 'power' as they will be used in this monograph. I have noted that patients gave accounts of inability to do what they normally did. This observation was the empirical source of the concept 'powers' as I am using it. By 'powers' I mean a person's ability or capacity to act, taken as expressing the agency of the person; or, in the case of 'liabilities', her patienthood. This empirically grounded notion of 'powers' is related to Harré and Secord's (1972, pp. 77-82) notion of 'powers'. In their analysis (see Chapter 3 or the quotation in the footnote[7] below), attribution of powers to another is attribution of agency - it is the other as agent who is the source of the action which is evidence of a power. Action need not be displayed for power to be attributed (see Chapter 3 or the quote in footnote[8] below). Claims of powers or liabilities are linked to moral status and personhood; to the status of agent or patient, respectively.

An example of what I construe through this meaning of 'powers' will be used as various points in this text. S1P2 claimed that her difficulties at the weekend were due to her medication.[9] The relevance of this notion of 'powers' to analysis of nurse-patient interaction is seen by grasping that responses to the question 'What do we have to do for P2?' hinged on interpretations of her powers and liabilities, and the nurses' powers to act in relation to her (for example, to take part in altering her medications, or slowing down plans for her discharge). It will be clear from this example that questions of nurses' and patients' powers were closely tied to issues of rights and obligations to act.[10]

While Harré and Secord (1972) (see Chapter 3 and below) note that moral status as a person - agent or patient - depends on the balance of powers and liabilities in peoples' accounts, they do not note a point of crucial importance to nursing as interpreted in this study, namely that the social reality of powers or liabilities depends on interpretation of the account in which the powers or liabilities are claimed, and on making the interpretation 'stick'. What I am referring to as 'power' in this context is the capacity of one person to make accounts about self or other - including accounts of powers or liabilities - 'stick', and by making them 'stick' direct future interaction, action on action. This 'power' is not simply a function of a person's 'powers'; it is also a function of place in social setting, of role (including rights and obligations), perhaps even of the possibility of force. An example is the 'power' of a nurse to interpret 'signs' of 'anxiety', to provide or legitimate an account of inability to act, and to act and direct action by the patient, self and others on the basis of that interpretation. While this power may depend on the nurse's 'powers' of perception, etc., it also depends on having the 'power', the 'authority' to maintain that interpretation against others (including, as I will show from the data, the patient's interpretation). I used the terms 'powers' and 'power' in interpreting accounts of interaction in which nurses spoke of trying to get patients to see or to do something. According to this analysis patients were unable to do something - they lacked 'a power' or 'powers', that is, they had a liability; and the nurses exercised 'power' in acting to try to get them to do or see differently. 'Power' in this context was not one-way. The patients' exercised 'power' in giving accounts that obliged the nurses to reply to their claims of agency, if upheld.

When P2 said her difficulties at the weekend were due to her medication and the nurse said that they were due to her, I interpreted the difference in terms of 'powers' and 'power'. The interpretation in terms of 'powers' was that the patient was claiming liability rather than agency: something other than herself was responsible for events and for what she did. The interpretation in terms of drugs made her claim particularly relevant to nurses. The nurse claimed that the patient was responsible (at least in part): she attributed to the patient powers rather than liabilities. It may be claimed that the nurse's claim was based on her own 'powers' (e.g. of 'observation'). Whose interpretation of the P2's 'powers' got accepted as social reality and structured future interaction depended on relations of 'power', and the ability of the nurse to command resources, including those of other staff, to act on the basis of her interpretation of P2's 'powers', rather than on the basis of P2's interpretation.

The link between 'powers' and 'power' relevant to the argument of this monograph is that 'powers' were 'read' from accounts. The ability to get accounts read in such a way that they structured interaction according to one's interpretation depended on having the power to give an account of powers and make it 'stick'. Because the power to get accounts of powers and liabilities accepted was also the power to define the person (as agent or patient), one aspect of 'power' was the power to define the other and self.

Accounts were the vehicles through which I grasped patients' complaints, and the devices through which, in their interaction, nurses and patients negotiated their 'working relationships'. I found in Harré and Secord (1972, pp. 247-248) conceptual tools useful in interpreting relationships between accounts, powers and liabilities, and agency and patienthood. The example Harré and Secord give to illustrate the idea of agency is that of someone who cannot speak. If the person is aphasic, he is said to lack an intrinsic enabling condition. If he does not speak in response to a question because he is deaf, his failure to speak would be due to an extrinsic enabling condition (p. 255). Failure to speak because he is gagged would be failure due to external circumstances. An example of failure of agency is given by S2P2:

P: You need your brain triggered off, (?). Because you're lying there and not thinking of what you could do to rectify the situation. You're just, (? even of ? you're in) sorta, tunnel-like, you know you're not

R: Right.

P: sorta, (? lyin' in your),

R: Right.

P: which possibly before it was a piece of cake to you know like, not even, even **thinking** about, you just **do** it. But in **this** state, you need, you need to be, you know, a...

In this chapter I have interpreted the data in terms of claims of agency and patienthood. Issues of power in nurse-neurotic patient interaction often centred on whether failures of powers (liabilities) were due to circumstances, including 'illness', or to failure of 'will'. Harré and Secord (1972, p. 243) argue that two sorts of account can be given if a person does not display a power when conditions appear satisfactory. Accounts of 'not wanting' and 'inability to bring oneself to' were common among patients' accounts to me and to nurses in interaction. Thus S2P2:

R: Um, (Note: researcher is reading text of first account) w-w-, yeah, when you were ill, here, you felt dizzy on your feet, and you couldn't do much, you didn't feel like doing much.

P: Well I didn't **want**, well,

R: Right.

P: **couldn't**.

R: Right.

P: (?)

R: Couldn't.

P: Couldn't.

Disputes between nurses and patients often centred on 'can't do' or 'won't do'. Thus a student nurse said of P2:

N: ...(When) P2 was first in and **was** actually quite ill, she wouldn't lead a conversation, and she required a lot of prompting which, now, and from that conversation in particular she certainly didn't need.

Harré and Secord's conceptual distinction helped me interpret differences in nurses' and patients' interpretation of action. The distinction focused analytic attention on the role of accounts in establishing patienthood, and in management of issues of responsibility for failure to act, or for inappropriate action. This conceptual analysis enabled me to interpret nurses' and patients' construction of themselves and each other as nurses and patients, and their interaction based on those constructions. I came to understand that, as they were 'sense makers making sense of sense makers', so they were also 'actors acting on actors', whose interaction was characterised by questions of interpretation of role, 'impression management' and 'conning'.

In the analysis to follow, I will show that nurses and patients worked on the assumption that they had to 'read' and interpret each other's accounts of powers or liabilities, in order to know how to act. Thus the power to give an account of one's powers mediated the 'appearance' of the patient as agent or patient, and interpretation of the patient's account mediated the appearance of the nurse doing the work of assessment or treatment. A main finding to be elaborated below was that assessment and remedy of liabilities was mediated by processes of accounting which were themselves shaped by the nurses' and patients' relationships of power. Interaction between patients and nurses was in part shaped by the patient's power to get an account of liability accepted. Both patients and nurses could be interpreted as trying to persuade each other to versions of the world, including themselves in the world. The views to which they persuaded each other structured further interaction. I interpreted the question of whose view 'stuck' in terms of power.

The theme of 'power' emerged through the act-action-episode analysis; and through analysing acts as interpreted in the patients' accounts in relation to those in nurses' accounts. In addition, I analysed themes of 'strategy', 'conflict', and 'challenge'. These emerged from nurses' and patients' accounts, as first order constructs; and from comparison of nurse and patient accounts, as second order constructs. Thus some of the issues related to power described in this chapter were 'implicit' in the interaction, and emerged from analysis. For example, the student nurse thought that P2 had a plan in returning to hospital:

N: (My) reaction to that (Note: to what P2 said) was P2 was maybe wanting to go home and bring a sorta suitcase in and, reinforce her ideas that she wanted to stay a while....Um, without saying 'assumption', I had it in mind that because of, em, her, sort of, her unwillingness to stay **away** from the hospital while she was, actually a patient at a different hospital, i.e. the Epton Downs, she still kept coming back here. And at every given opportunity gave reasons why she should still be in hospital, as in-patient. That's why I presumed that, you know, this was another ploy of, of needing to stay in.

Because the meaning of action depended on its place in acts and episodes, I have chosen not to catalogue actions and acts. Rather, I will give representative pictures of action in the course of exploring the empirical and theoretical issues related to powers and power. The 'microphysics' of power were analysed in the microprocesses of interaction as interpreted through accounts and in the processes of accounting, and the productive and coercive effects of power in the institution were found in accounts of face to face interaction between the nurses and patients, at the 'capillaries' (Foucault, 1980, p. 96).

I will discuss the processes of power by outlining how nurses moved, or tried to move, from social to more personal relationships, in order to help the patient do the 'work' necessary to move back to the community. I will outline some characteristics of power in meetings, and then discuss power in one-to-one interaction, including variations in relations of power. I will also discuss the discourse related to power, in particular the use of metaphors of power, and nurses' and patients' rhetoric.[11]

Forms of collective power

I have interpreted the sites as institutions, structured by relations of power to effect 'therapy' (Berger and Luckmann, 1967); that is, as centres of reality maintenance and repair. They were formally organized to produce, through processes of power, knowledge in the form of 'assessment' (accounts given by staff of patients' liabilities and powers, patienthood and agency; whether given in terms of mental illness or another ideology). They produced through 'treatment' effects of power which returned 'strays' to the community.

Conversation and interaction were the main forms of reality maintenance and repair, the media of knowledge production and action on action. The social construction of the reality of the patient's illness and treatment was a process of power, exercised mainly through observation and talk. Observation and talk were the methods used to produce accounts of the patient and to exercise social control on the basis of that definition.[12]

The processes of social control were mediated by the definition of why the patient was in the site and what was to be done with and for her. Thus, interaction between these patients and nurses, and conflict in the interaction, centred on definition of reality, and on whose definition of reality was accepted as the basis for ordering interaction. The definitions related to interpretation, definition and management of the patients' private states in the public places of the wards.

Glass walls and boundaries, knowledge and defences

Observation was one form of power. In the 'Site' section above, I described the 'goldfish bowl' effect of Site One, where the possibility of being subjected to gaze was constant. One morning a patient looked at me, quickly got up from her chair, looked toward the nurses' station window and said that she had better go to occupational therapy: 'the nurses, especially Dave, miss nothing'. I noted that in Site Two there were more rooms, spaces, barriers. In both sites nurses at times placed patients on 'levels of observation', comprising specified practices of accompaniment and gaze.[13]

Questioning and the giving of accounts based on the answers - a kind of 'observation through talk' - was the second major practice of power. The kind of knowledge of the person produced through questioning was distinct from ordinary social knowledge. Both 'sides' wanted to maintain the boundaries between the domains of knowledge. In Site Two a nurse said she would not like to come to this ward with a 'nervous breakdown' because she knew the questions that junior doctors asked patients and she would not want people she worked with to know her in that way. Patients in Site One said that they would not like people 'outside' to find out what was found out about them in the site.

Ordinary relations of power could be inverted in the sites. Younger people could require older people to tell them where they were going; and patients were asked to bring out what normally they kept to themselves - their subjectivity, feelings, history. In this way they brought into the sites their stories, their problems. The nurses and other staff were privileged in being able to 'observe' the patients. The privileged practices were correspondingly privileged in the practice of discourse, in which nurses emphasised 'our words', e.g. 'anxiety'.

Thus power and knowledge were closely interlinked. The patients imputed to the nurses powers of observation and assessment, and the power to comfort, to console; for example, S2P2: 'And that's where the nurses are so understanding, so they do help you and they know how to help you, and they really do make you well.'. They often noted limits to the nurses' powers to help (see an example below).

'Territory' and boundaries: the definition of sites of practice - the ward and the patient

Social control was exercised in part by maintaining the definition of the places as sites of 'work', thus reflexively maintaining the grounds of accountability. Nurses and patients acted on each others' actions in meetings in the two sites. In Site One, the community meeting was the place where nurses and patients defined the site as a work place, where the ideology of the site was expressed. In talking about the current issues, problems, tensions, the staff and patients defined the reality of the place and the work that all had to to do maintain the reality. On an ongoing basis this included repetition that 'You have to really try to get over your problems', 'We (the staff) can do so much but you have to help yourself too', 'Share your problems'. The meetings were used to get patients to tell how they saw each other; producing knowledge of responsibility and character. The meetings were an essential part of 'the programme'. In Site One, the nurses more explicitly emphasised that the ward was a form of community in which patients could learn to cope as they would need to on return to the community.

By contrast, community meetings in Site Two were brief, formal, and mainly administrative. Whereas in Site One meetings were routinely led by nurses, in Site Two they were often led by the consultant, with nurses saying nothing. Definition of the site as a community, to the more limited extent it occurred, was done by psychiatrists rather than nurses. The power to define reality, and to act on the patients' action, was more firmly in psychiatric hands in Site Two. This was a matter of degree. In Site One, too, the psychiatrists had greater formal power to interpret action, to direct action on action, and to exhort the staff to make the programme work. When a nurse emphasised the need for the consultant to spend time in the ward, he did so indirectly.[14]

Assessment was dependent on the ability to 'command' the appearance and interpretation of the other through accounts. Later in the chapter I will discuss this in terms of assessment and rhetorical persuasion to a view of the other. It is important to note that the power to command the appearance of the other, and more generally to command the patients' time and use of space, was literal.[15] Thus nurses in Site Two had the authority to require patients to attend meetings as part of their 'programme' (see Chapter 7); and to require patients to attend the day hospital.[16] In directing appearances, the nurses could be seen as acting on behalf of medical or other staff. The typical case of this was the nurses' responsibility to ensure that patients were available to be 'seen' by the doctors at a 'ward round'.

Territory and command of sites of production of knowledge

Through observation and accounts, and especially by moving from one site to another, I construed power in terms of territory. By 'territory' I mean the space and time in the sites constituted as places for 'work'. 'Work' related to command of time and space, command of the use to which the facilities of the sites were put. Conflict between nurses and patients centred on the use of facilities, including staff. The round of meetings structured patients' time and 'work'.[17]

The meetings as 'territory' were the meetings construed as sites of work to produce knowledge. The nurses in Site One commanded the meetings as sites of knowledge production. The nurses in Site Two had no clear claims to territory, and territory was more often disputed there.

The question of use of facilities could be construed in terms of whether a patient 'should be here now'. Control of the sites was accomplished through control of definition of the sites, and control of definition of the sites was maintained by the enforcement of obligations, for example, to attend meetings, to be available to talk. The issue of whether the patient should be here was couched in terms of whether the patient accepted the staff's definition of the 'work' she had to do.[18]

Territory included the patients, construed as sites of work.[19] In Site One the main ideology was based on seeing the patient as a 'whole person'. The nurses in Site One were the staff mainly responsible for the coordination of the programme in conditions of limited space and time. In Site Two, the patient as a site of work was, in a sense, 'divided'. She was construed in terms of 'deep' and 'shallow' work. Rights and obligations regarding 'deep work' were matters for both interpersonal and interprofessional negotiation. Compared to nurses in Site One, the nurses in Site Two were more often 'middle men' in work with individual patients. The data suggest that they were less often main agents in 'deep work'. They appeared less often in patients' accounts as the professionals mainly involved in work on 'the main thing'. They mediated the work of other professionals, through 'programmes'. Nurses in Site Two conducted a small group (see below) but its work constituted a zone between 'deep' and 'shallow' work, in that it was based on 'sharing' between patients and nurses (cf. Chapman, 1987; Robinson, 1985). I construed it as a territory screened from observation, a territory in which feelings could be revealed.

There were thus a number of divisions of territory, in use of public space, and between personnel in Site Two. The divisions of territory constituted divisions in social reality.[20]

Practices of individual nurses' power: from the social to the personal

I have described the sites as places structured by relations of power. To get into the sites I had to negotiate those structures (see Chapter 4, 'Sites'). Individually and collectively the nurses had to organise their practices in order to 'get into' work on individual patients while maintaining the site as a work place. Through analysis I construed the sites and the patients as 'fields' in which work was to be done.[21] The concept 'field' conveys the idea that power was needed to get into and claim a field as a work place. The idea of getting into the field was conveyed by nurses' use of the terms 'moving' or 'making moves' to describe their work in interaction.

Using data from accounts I will describe the practices of power nurses used to get into the field to work with patients, and the work they did once in. The practices were those of starting working relationships, moving from the social to the personal, and working on problems. This will be followed by an analysis of the form of interaction, from the perspective of a powers analysis. I will present portions of patients' accounts to highlight important issues regarding interaction.

An account of starting a working relationship: the nurse's tale

In using the concept 'the working relationship' a student nurse conveyed the power involved in getting to know patients: starting from sharing the place, to noticing, to forming a social relationship, to getting to talk to the patient about her problems or illness. The nurse, new to the ward, had noticed the patient looking at her, 'obviously' wanting to 'get to know her'. She had waited for an 'opportunity' to 'chum' the patient to the canteen; not wanting to 'come on too strong, asking her direct questions and things':

> That's my general approach when I go to most wards (? acute), you don't want to come on too strongly to the patients because you're too much of a threat to them and they don't know you, you're not a familiar face. Just by wee, wee conversations like that, gradually over the weeks you can maybe then go into a working relationship but not, obviously not right away.

Students typically gave accounts of approaching patients to find what they had in common. They started indirectly, intending to 'go into' the relationship. The work was expressive. The nurse said her talk with the patient was 'sort of superficial conversation'. It was 'ground breaking', 'helping me get to know her, and maybe she got to know me slightly as well':

> So I think she sort of realised I was reasonably friendly, and that I was quite willing to get to know her, and that, well hopefully that I showed an interest in her.

The patient's tale The patient gave her account:

> P: ...just going down to the canteen today with one nurse and asking me how I was feeling and I'm feeling really well today. We went down and we got some, em, cigarettes for Lisa because once you're well, you can start doing little errands and making yourself useful again, how you were before you became ill so you get more and more responsibility...That's the new nurse, and then also I was able to take her down to the canteen and I bought cigarettes for Lisa, so it was quite good and you feel a lot better because you're helping people and you feel really good.

The episode appeared in the nurse's account as an exercise of judgement and power enabling her to take the opportunity to get to know the patient. It appeared in the patient's account as her helping the nurse and a fellow patient in a process of 'getting better', recovery of powers, and taking responsibility. The patient, having experienced a loss of responsibility, worked on getting herself better.

The metaphor of the field In using the metaphor 'field' I am construing the patient as a work place/object (cf. Stacey, 1976). To the student nurse it was obvious that, to get into the field, she had to 'break ground'. She had somehow to negotiate through the distances appropriate for strangers to ('hopefully') a different, working relationship. The student nurse thought that she was 'conducting' the patient, and the patient thought that she was 'conducting' the nurse. (See Foucault, 1982, on 'conduct'.)

In her account the student used common terms about common powers to convey aspects of the working relationship. Students typically talked about seeing what they had in common with the patients. They began by trying to establish common social ground. The common was construed as 'superficial' in relation to the 'deep'. Deep work involved penetration to the personal. The students started from the social to get to the personal. The common had to be realised through talk, sometimes talk of a particular kind (for example, 'women's talk').

The fields of 'social' and 'personal' talk (see Chapter 5) were constituted through distinct practices. Entry to the social field was based on the power to join a group of people and talk about everyday things. Entry to the personal field involved the power to get into a 'sorta' relationship with a patient, to get her to disclose her problems and worries. The nurses in Site One constituted the field of daily work when they started their shifts. They walked from patient to patient, kneeling or sitting beside patients to look at and talk to them.

Moving into a working relationship

The practices through which the nurses moved from the social into the personal appeared in both the nurses' and patients' accounts. This movement may be considered metonymic and metaphoric.[22]

Metonymically, the interaction was part of the wider field of interaction with the patient and with other patients. The movement was also, in some cases, part of a process of relationship development.[23] Metaphorically, the movement was from the social field, the common, more deeply into the patient's world. It was a movement which brought the patient's subjectivity into the realm of public discourse. These themes will be developed later in the chapter. Here the focus is on the reflexive play between the social construction of the patient and her subjective identity.

A student nurse said:

> N: ...We talked about, we talked about the other patients, just in a sort of social kind of way, for a wee while, just to get into things, and then, she started s-, she was telling me that she was feeling a lot better for having been in hospital, and that she was going to make sure she never came in again, and that, she felt that she'd, things had just got on top of her, and she wasn't going to let it happen. And, she said that, um, her (?) a very strong person, and she could cope with everything, and, I said, did that mean that she found it hard to ask people for help, and she said 'Yes', she did, she's used to coping on her own. And I said that, maybe, she **should** ask for help, because people like to help, they like to **give**, as well as to **take**. And she said 'Yes', but she found it very difficult to do that...Um, I got the impression that she was, keeping things, very much, to herself, that she finds it hard to, to open up to people, and to tell them what she's really thinking. Um, I don't, really think that she knows herself, sometimes, that she's got problems, she's just used to bottling things up...I think, she would rather help other people with their problems than be helped herself. Think she's a **giver**, not a taker.

What happened in the interaction can be seen as the problem. The nurse interpreted P5 as saying that she has difficulty in asking for help. P5 confirmed this meaning and parried with an account of what she was used to doing. The nurse replied that perhaps P5 should ask for help: parry to the thrust[24] of P5's meaning that she could not talk about personal things. P5 countered, 'Yes, but..' and gave an account of her difficulty. Through the process the nurse construed P5 as a type of person: a giver, not a taker.[25] The definition implied the action to be taken on P5's action in the working relationship: P5 was to 'give' accounts of her problems in order to 'take' help. (See Mead, 1934, on the 'parry and thrust' of fencing as a metaphor for meaning; and Peplau, 1952, on the 'dramas of push and pull' in which the nurse as participant observer takes part.)

The nurse interpreted what P5 regarded as strength - not asking for help - as a liability, elements of her former agency as the basis of her patienthood. Specifically, the liability was 'not opening up'. The nurse drew on the ideology current in Site Two that talking about your problems was good. The ideology served administrative as well as 'therapeutic' functions in that it legitimated keeping the patient open for work, facilitating assessment and location of problems for further work. It legitimated the practice of exploration.

The interpretation of patients as people with problems in communicating, in particular about their problems, was typical. Of the patients in Site One, one could not talk to his son or about his grief; one was deaf; one seemed confused and disorientated and was barely audible. Conceptualisation of 'the main thing' as a problem of not talking about problems had counterparts in a number of accounts in Site Two: a problem in saying 'no', a problem of being too 'private'. That the patients kept their problems to themselves was seen as part of the problem. The definition of the patient that prevailed was one which legitimated the nurses' challenging the patient for keeping problems to herself. It legitimated their exercise of power in knowing the patients in ways the patients did not, ordinarily, wish to be known. In effect the nurses defined an ideology which legitimated their work: talk was construed as a form of 'therapy'. Thus legitimated, talk was a tool in the production of the 'individual' (cf. Foucault, 1982).

The effect of these practices legitimated by the ideology of 'talk as work' was to structure interactions through which the patient was exposed to the view of herself held by others. The process was that of re-socialisation (Berger and Luckmann, 1967).

In emphasising the metonymic and metaphoric meanings I am arguing that in these common, often repeated interactions the nurses played their parts in the process of 'therapy'. The process consisted of practices of admission and disclosure. Metonymically, the conversation 'stood for' the admission. Metaphorically, the process was one in which the patients were asked to dis-close their (subjective) worlds (Ricoeur, 1971) in order to reach a common understanding of what was wrong and what to do about it. In her account, P5 said:

> P: ...It's, is a **help** to talk to a **stranger**, really, somebody you don't really know, who's, you know, outwith, your own, **thing**. Um, but uh, I, I felt better after it, you know.

The process of interpretation of and use of the other was thus two-way: a mutual social act. The patient interpreted the nurses as the kind of people she needed (cf. Peplau, 1952). In the process of mutual interpretation the nurses formed a more powerful field. In cases where compatible definitions could be negotiated, as above, the working relationship with those nurses who shared the definition functioned smoothly.[26] In cases where complementary definitions of the main thing and the action appropriate to that definition could not be negotiated, the relationship of patient with nurses was characterised by conflict, or discrepant definitions were 'glossed' (see below).

Power, resocialisation and the development of significance In 'personal talk' the nurses 'gave feedback' to the patients, asked what they had done or how they felt, and interpreted what the patient said. They asked about the patient's plans, 'exercising' the patient's responsibility. The nurses could be construed as constituting a 'generalised other' (Mead, 1934), treating the patient as a kind of person until she was ready to treat herself as that kind of person (cf. Shotter, 1984). Thus after talking to the nurse P5 talked to other patients about her problems:

> P: No I hadn't spoken to anyone else, about that, until, Winnie (Note: student nurse). And then, actually I spoke to one of the **patients** after that, about my daughter, which, I hadn't done before, and which, was really, quite surprised me.

The process was one of development of powers. Thus P2 in Site Two:

> P: So, and as time went on, I felt, I could **be** there (Note: in cooking class), and not have this, if I didn't go too fast myself, which I couldn't, um, I didn't feel, I can still feel dizzy so that's, but, **that's** how you can, progress and not know you are, by **their** help.

Another student gave an account of talking to P8:

> N: I remember talking to P8 at, eh, the OT, when we had to, write these things down about ourselves, and I said that I felt she had never opened up to me, that I enjoyed her conversation, but I felt that she was hiding something. And she denied it. (? Uh eh), quite annoyed, 'Oh no, I, I've told you everything, Shula, I don't know what I need to tell you'. (Note: N's voice is a 'mock innocent' voice.) But then, she came to me later and said that she had a friend up, and she had been telling her, what I had said. And the friend that's known her frae, childhood, had said that she had the same **impression** of P8, that she always held back, and didna give **all** herself, em, was a wee bit reserved. And P8 hadnae **felt** that at all. So, I was

> a bit annoyed, cos I says 'P8, I hope I didnae embarrass you, or offend you', and she says 'No, no', but she says 'It's just interesting what other people think', and she says 'I don't **think** I'm reserved'. But she says 'Both you and my friend have said that, so,' she says 'maybe I am'.
>
> R: Aye. Aye. So she, it sounds like she took what you said, and uh, thought about it, and and kind of, reflected it back, to **her** friend, who said, 'Actually, (laughs), that's right, I think the same thing'.
>
> N: Uhuh...Cos she said that she never **thought** that she was a wee bit **private**. But she says 'When **both** of you is, under that impression', she says, 'maybe I am, maybe I am a wee bit reserved'.

The patient's interpretation of the nurse's action occasioned further work by the patient on subjective reality maintenance (or attempted repair).[27] This process may be interpreted in terms of 'pastoral power' (Foucault, 1982): through the practice of self-interpretation and other-interpretation the patient took part in the production of truth about herself as the kind of individual she was.[28]

Thus I have argued that in their face to face interaction the nurses and patients organised 'fields of work'. The nurses had to get into work on problems with the patient, sometimes having to overcome 'resistance' to do so. They got the patient to open up; accomplishing the administrative aims of assessment and treatment, by drawing on the ideology and getting the patient to realise reflexively that 'talking about problems is good'. They worked at working on 'why she is here now'.

Forming the field of action: from the social to the personal

The fields formed by the nurses and patients in interaction may be described by considering typical patterns of interaction and talk about interaction, especially the metaphors which shaped it. These aspects will be described in the two parts of this section.

In the first part I will interpret an account which exemplifies important aspects of nurses' and patients' relations of power. The nurse, an experienced nurse in Site One (called 'Nurse Jean', a pseudonym, throughout these excerpts) noted that the interaction with P7 had a beginning, a middle and an end. The nurse's account had the form of a story. The patient's stay as a whole - the episode of admission, treatment and discharge - was a story subsuming the stories of interaction. The account can be read in terms of the metaphors that conveyed the work of the site: 'development of a picture' of P7; and testing and development of P7's responsibility, against the background of an intention that she would be returned to the community. The conversation which started from the social and moved on to the personal was a metonym for the stay, in which the patient came from outside into a social environment new to her, where new relationships started, and where she was required gradually to tell more of what was personal. Metaphorically, the interaction was a form of development, of the picture of her held by the staff, and of her personhood, her powers to show herself and be seen by others as ready to do for herself. A patient said that 'personal talk' usually 'started from the social', confirming nurses' (especially students') accounts of the form of interaction. Talk started with chat and moved on to (and into) the personal. The personal implied a history of interaction, prior responsibility, which the method of this study captured (see Chapter 4).

Typical process of interaction: the actions of moving from the social to the personal This set of excerpts can be interpreted in terms of the microprocesses of power, power at the 'capillaries' (Foucault, 1980) of interaction. In their accounts nurses and patients typically recounted a process of interaction. The process was that in which an episode of interaction was accomplished. In this process the nurse noticed the patient (sometimes in response to a display of distress by the patient); negotiated an understanding of 'the main thing'; acted on the patient's action, typically through rhetoric (influence); and concluded the interaction. Each such episode marked another node in the stay, a phase in the realisation of 'the main thing'. These episodes were 'the working relationship' in action. Typically in these accounts the nurse noticed the patient, approached, asked how the patient was, heard an account, responded, noted the outcome and moved on. (See Appendix 6; but note that the diagram decontextualises interaction, and that the meaning and social effect of interaction lay in the network of connections with what is not represented in the diagram.)

Noticing and being noticed The typical features of the process of power are represented in an account by a nurse from Site One. The reader will recognise that in this interaction Nurse Jean drew on all aspects of knowledge in the frame 'work' (see Chapter 5).

In noticing a patient, the nurse noted how the patient stood out from the background of all that was happening in the site.[29] 'Noticing' occurred in the context of what else was going on at the time and in the context of previous interaction with the patient:

> N: Hmn. Well, at the very start..it was a quiet point in my day, and I had, you know I had just felt I hadnae had much time with her. But at the same time my observation was that she was, you know, she was just sitting quietly, she looked a bit fed up..

In accounting, the nurses established their action in its contexts of relevance.

The patient played her part in the act of noticing, by showing distress or coming into the nurse's field of vision, hearing or action. Things that the patients did frequently were no longer actively noticed. They became 'routine', an 'ongoing thing', background in relation to which nurses noticed other things. The patients in Site One who had been in a long time and were waiting to be rehoused were not noticed as much, in handovers, in Kardexes, ward rounds, in the daily round of life in the site. The nurses ceased noticing aspects of their own work. For example, a trained nurse in Site Two said that 'rebelling' patients were 'just there' and she did not think about it 'too much'.

Approaching and being approached Generally the nurses approached patients in a group for social talk, and a patient on her own for illness talk. The patients recognised the nurse's approach as part of the act of 'illness talk' or 'talking about problems'. They knew that the nurse approached if the patient was upset. Approach was already informed by 'noticing' and was part of an intended act. 'Approaching' sometimes followed directly from 'noticing'; at others it was mediated by the setting of an agenda. Thus, Nurse Jean:

> N: Um, when it's quiet, then you can set your own, set your own scenes, you can, eh, you can go to whoever's on your agenda..whether or not you're working to everyone else's agenda for a while, so..so if there's a lot of demands made on you you have to deal with them first.

I noted earlier in this chapter that issues of power appeared as questions of use of and command of time and space. The microprocesses of interaction reflected the histories of nurses' and patients' past negotiations of time and space.[30]

In another nurse's account, approach was deliberate even if not pre-planned as part of an agenda. A staff nurse in Site Two said:

> N: Well, I was aware that I hadn't really, spoken too much er, to her since she'd come in, so, I deliberately sat beside her, for five minutes, but not with any intentions in mind, it was just, to try to get an idea, of, how she was feeling.

Nurses contextualised approach, in terms of person, situation, and manner. For example, a nurse in Site Two said:

> N: But she's been, a **fairly** isolated person, so, **I've** found it's quite difficult, cos you have to go up, and **approach** her, and she's usually either reading or, you know, just, not really wanting to talk much..

Approach was mediated by 'signals': reading a book was interpreted as a signal the patient did not want to be approached. Patients who did not or could not signal risked being ignored. Nurse Jean said:

> N: Often it's the person who shouts loudest that nurses often tend to run to..There's a terrible temptation if people don't make time, (?) don't demand time of you that they kinda get neglected..so you've kinda got to reach out to them, and, and offer them some time, and I felt she needed it, she deserved it.

I will return to fuller discussion of 'time' and the economy of attention. Approach, 'reaching out', had to be accomplished in the context of the demands of others and the nurse's own agenda.

Nurses sometimes deliberately did not approach; deliberately ignored the 'attention seeking' patient, for example. Patients had their own ideas about why nurses did not approach them - nurses were too busy, perhaps helping other patients; or they talked to 'the young ones'.

Nurses distinguished between psychotic and non-psychotic patients on the basis of how they would approach them. The psychotic patient was less predictably in 'their' reality (cf. Bunch, 1982). The assumption was that non-psychotic patients, including those diagnosed as neurotic, were in 'their' reality.

Asking and being asked The main nursing practice with these patients was asking the patient to 'tell', getting an account from her:

N: I thought OK let's just, sus out..really, more, in more detail, how she's feeling, and also, offer, try and offer her some sort of reassurance..some sort of time.

The nurses asked patients how they were, where they had been, what they would do, what their problems were. Student nurses appeared in their accounts to ask very directly: 'Early on in the conversation, I was, I was asking her what sort of, problems she had'. Nurse Jean, an experienced nurse, asked P7 if she meant she was ready to go home. She asked her because she knew that patients typically did not ask nurses whether they (the patients) were ready to go home. Thus nurses asked not only because patients typically did not ask, but also because not asking was sometimes part of the patient's problem (see above).

The 'give and take' of asking and telling was mediated by the ideology which held that 'talking about your problems' was 'good'. However, in some cases, nurses knew that they could only ask once - if the patient did not want to tell, they could not force her. Nurse and patients emphasised that patients could not be forced to talk. The practices of power were practices exercised, in these cases, in relation to people who could, and often did, resist them. Foucault (1982, p. 220) noted that:

> ...(A) power relationship can only be articulated on the basis of two elements...: that 'the other' (the one over whom power is exercised) be thoroughly recognized and maintained...as a person who acts; and that, faced with a relationship of power, a whole field of responses...may open up.

Thus S2P2 said that she did not have to talk, but the nurses 'preferred' her to. Or thus S2P5:

P: Em, if you **want** to talk about anything, you **can**, if you don't want to talk about anything, they don't **push** you. Em, you know, which is very very **nice**.

Listening and being listened to The nurses listened for 'the main thing'. Nurses' listening was active and intentional. Nurse Jean said:

N: and I was intent on listening to this cos I thought Well, OK, she's saying she's miserable here, what's her options, what's on her agenda? And then she painted a very, em, you know the picture of somebody busy, at home..

A trained nurse in Site One said that she listened, asked, asked again when P3 came back from his weekend home: '...and then again he said...'. She heard something that 'called for' more asking or that indicated more that needed to be told.

'Reading' was the metaphor nurses used for the process of listening intently and interpreting while listening. Some nurses in Site One likened themselves to detectives. I came to hear them that way: as rhetorically leading me, the hearer, to 'follow' what the patient said as the nurse had followed it; as laying trails for reasoning about what the patient said. The nurses persuaded each other in handovers, and me in account sessions, to a view of the interaction and of the patient seen through the interaction. There was a foreground/background depth to some nurses' listening. For them, listening was construed in terms of 'sense':

> N: And (?) she was very animated, you know, 'I brought up all these grandchildren, I do the cooking, and, baking'..uh, at the back of my own mind I'm busy thinking Well maybe some of this is, I've got to, I'm not going to be conned, in a (laughs) sense. I'm sure she's painting the brightest picture: 'Let me out of this place', you know 'I can do all this myself'. Sons were, a bit, perhaps when I had seen them on admission they were a wee bit more moderate in their assessment. She would, you know, she would do quite a lot for herself, but there was some support, but the way she was describing it it was really 'I can do everything'..you know. I I was weighing all that up with her eagerness to get out of hospital, of course, so she was trying to, see, she was painting her picture to me of
>
> R: Saying 'Everything was perfect at home, Let me out of here and I'll be back and everything'll be OK'.
>
> N: That's what I sensed, and I was taking what she was said with a pinch of salt, but what it was telling me was, (coughs) This woman's keen to go.

The nurse portrayed herself as responsive to P7. Nurses sometimes controlled the conditions for hearing by cutting off patients who were too loud (cf. Bunch, 1982). They put a patient in a side room when her shouting disturbed other patients.

Responding The nurse responded to the patient in the context of what she already knew, what was happening at the time, and in light of intentions. She responded in the context of 'the main thing at the time'. Response was part of the process of negotiating the main thing in this interaction. 'Noticing', 'approaching' and 'hearing' were all parts of the response guided by monitoring the interaction while developing it.[31]

The term nurses used for response was 'handling'. The nurse 'handled' the situation according to how she 'read' it. 'Handling' could mean moving the patient along or moving with her. Kinds of 'handling' included 'reinforcing', 'comforting', 'challenging'. 'Handling' as recounted in the nurses' accounts was mainly rhetorical talk. Examples of what I construed as rhetoric, meaning persuasion to a view of the world, include a nurse from Site One:

> N: Just information, really, and eh well she also felt that she told me how her weekend had gone and she felt that the drugs had a lot to do with it and I let her know that the drugs really didn't have much to do with how she had been at home, eh, it was mainly up to her, a lot of it was up to her. And she says well 'You know, do you think that's, you know, do you not think it is the drugs', I said 'No, I think I think a lot's something to do with you and you've got to try maybe to get on with Phil', cos I think they were having some difficulties with their relationship. Em..(now ?) she agreed with that,

She spoke of the 'suggestion (she) had planted' in the patient. In Site Two a patient described a nurse's attempt at persuasion:

> P: Oh, I was in a mood yesterday, I went home...Nan spoke to me, in the morning, cos I was in a mood.
>
> R: C-, can you **tell** me a bit about that?
>
> P: About the **mood**? (Laughs).
>
> R: Well, the conversation.
>
> P: Couldna tell you the conversation, I could only say that Nan was trying to calm me down. That's all. (? About l-), trying to make me, see, things in a different light, and I wasna having it, so I just marched out and that was that (bitter laugh). Went home.

Hearing and responding were part of the process of dialogue. The nurses 'read' the patients, interpreted them, 'picked up the vibes' and responded. Responding often involved remedying. Varieties of 'remedy' included 'giving information', 'reassuring', 'reinforcing'. Thus Nurse Jean:

> N: Ah! I'd already said I'll get the doctor to write these things up, so, immediately there was a doctor (?beside) ...(To) the patient, they think, Great, something's getting done now..they mean business . Th- this was another form of reassurance to her that, eh, God they're they're actually stopping whatever they're doing...to attend to me, and that always makes people feel very special, I think...when they do that, if they actually stop what they're doing, it may be something totally trivial, but, it makes them feel good because you're having to do something for them. And I just say (Note: nurse reads her own words in the transcript) 'I took the opportunity..'...

The nurse's response involved taking 'the opportunity' as perceived in the situation. This was the essence of 'savvy' in Site One (see Chapter 5): to mean business, to keep the work going through seeing and taking opportunities to work.[32]

Finishing the episode Nurses typically noted some outcome of their response or remedy. This was typically brief and related to the patient's satisfaction, for example, 'she seemed happy with that':

> N: So I thought, I'll take the chance now, plus, it'll be a boost to her that she sees something's getting done..and it'll also do something about her pain...ken, at a practical level, she was needing paracetamol, she had trouble with her ulcer..so, it meant, it it it was something tangible the client could hang on to, ken..the patient could grip on to. Um, so then I came back and says 'Well that's it, it's done', you know? Uh, (laughs) and I think she felt Oh that's great, you know? Sorta kinda Thank you very much, and I'm..I think, as well, it perhaps kinda concluded, it had, you know there was a task, a target, something on my agenda, and I felt that I rounded it off quite nicely because, there were a start, and there were a middle, and there were...a conclusion to the whole business.

In finishing the episode the nurse defined its practical meaning: 'that's it, that's it done'.

Moving on and being left Nurses moved on at the end of interaction, perhaps to the next item on the agenda, or because someone else shouted, or because the patient moved on:

> N: So I felt I could walk away from her saying, even if it was on pretext of, 'Well I'll just go and, better put this away' you know? Or 'I'll I'll go and get the drugs out the cupboard', or

> whatever...I could disengage myself, then, from her..and move on to something else on my agenda.
>
> R: Right. Right! Because, you see, that's that's a that's a point..these things start when there's, where there's a gap in your..your um, time..
>
> N: That's right..there's there's, aye, there are certain things, standard things that will happen at certain times..so, you know, whatever you're going to achieve has to be done within a, a certain period of time.

Work had to be accomplished in the setting of the moment, with whatever 'pushes and pulls' operated. Command of time and space was limited due to the circumstances in which much interaction took place, 'in passing'.[33]

The work was practical and expressive (Harré, 1979). In moving into and out of the field of interaction with the patient the nurse did the 'hidden labour' of acting politely, treating the patient with respect (Hochschild, 1983). The practical and expressive work was situated within the context of the demands and constraints of the site. The work of nurses and patients emerged in accounts of talk 'in passing', of 'sitting down with', of 'looking', 'seeing', 'handling' and 'moving on'.

From the point of view of the nurse, the interaction appeared as something to be started, gone through, completed and left behind. She moved through the work of the day. From the point of view established through the account, the interaction appeared as part of the process through which the patient was moved on, part of her passage through the site.

It was in face to face interaction that the processes of institutional power were realised. Whatever was done was what could be done in the time and in the context of all else that was going on. In work done 'in passing' the nurses dealt with 'the main thing at the time' and 'moved on'. The patient had to do her work in the time of her stay. This meant that she had to participate in the order of work in the site ('get geared up'). The nurses had to order the work and the patients, to get the work done. The nurses and patients had to get through the work in interaction in order for the patient to get through the site.

The nurses' and patients' 'dramas of push and pull' (Peplau, 1952) were varied, but in all of them the patient appeared as someone participating in working relationships in order to accomplish passage through the site. The nurses intended that the sites should not be so comfortable that patients would want to stay. Patients and nurses alike held in low regard patients who 'like it here'. The site was interaction. Passage through the site was passage through interaction in the site. That passage was a process of accounting for 'why she is/I am here?', 'what are her/my problems?' and 'what is to be done?'. Accounts could roughen or smooth the passage[34] depending on whether they were accepted as allowing the patient to 'pass' the interaction.[35]

Power and the representation of powers 'Noticing', 'approaching', 'asking', 'listening' and 'responding', 'finishing the episode' and 'moving on' were key actions in the acts of assessment ('reading') and treatment or care ('handling'). 'Picking up' and 'interpreting' were threads that ran through the actions. The actions were not mainly applications of technique, but joint accomplishments within contexts. The accomplishment was always underpinned by reference to context, and the phenomena were actions in a context (cf. Benner, 1985) which reflexively constituted the context. There were no 'technics apart from persons' (Hughes, 1951, p. 315). The acts were essentially nurse/patient acts. Intrinsic to the social acts in interaction as accounted for by nurses and patients were: the response of the other, interpreted as an interpretation; and the history of interaction.[36]

Second level accounts and the juxtaposition, in analysis, of accounts given from the points of view of the patient and the nurse provided contexts for further understanding of the complexity of power in interaction. In this part of the section I will use segments of P7's account and Nurse Jean's first and second level accounts to emphasise the centrality of claims about the patient's powers as interpreted in interaction, and the power involved in making these claims. Thus I am exploring issues related to nursing assessment.[37] It will be clear that the issues addressed here relate to those of meaning and knowledge, addressed in Chapter 5; and to the concerns about moral order addressed in Chapter 7. Empirically, the social construction of reality was mediated by relations of power and positions in moral orders. The issue I highlight in these accounts is that of 'readiness to go home'. I have interpreted the relations of power in terms of efforts to get the patient 'ready'. Determination of 'readiness' was accomplished in face-to-face interaction. What I am arguing in this section is that the process of determination of 'readiness', the interpretation of the patient's powers to cope at home, was mediated by relations of power.

The first section is from the patient's account. She began by saying that she had spoken to a nurse that morning:

> P: Oh, she was talking about, eh, my own condition...About, eh, I, you see, I have an ulcer. (I'm) (?) in here with a sort of complication thing. (Note: the patient discussed changes in medication and their effect on her.)...And then I talked, we spoke about, em, I've had depression before of course, you see, on and off, but I've always fell back on (Note: an antidepressant)....Oh, I was just talking about myself, how I was trying hard to fight it, you know...Trying not to give in to it...but it's so difficult... Just, they can, they help you, but you've sorta got to help yourself to a certain extent. I'm plenty old in the day, seventy-seven,[38] to help myself, amn't I? ..You see?
>
> R: We- were they saying that you had to help yourself, or was that what you.. ..?
>
> P: No, (?) That's what they meant, really, you know what I mean, that I'm not, not (?) to give in to it...See?..Oh yes. (sighs) Oh yes. But I think I, I, this young nurse too said that that I'd get on better (?) my own home.
>
> R: This nurse said that?
>
> P: Yes.
>
> R: Yes, uhuh, right. And you understood them to be saying you had to do, to get over it yourself (?) part of it..
>
> P: Well, (?) they didn't say it straight out, but deep down that's what they really mean (?)...But, as I say, at my time (?)
>
> R: Yes, aye.

The patient construed the nurse as discussing with her 'why she was here now' and implying that, despite her age, she had to 'get over' and 'fight' her depression herself. She understood that the nurse had suggested that she would be better off at home, after stabilisation of her medication ('what they were to do for her'). P7 can be construed as drawing on common-sense understandings (age) and understandings from 'within' illness, in interpreting to me (persuading me to her view of) the nurses' attempts to persuade her to a view that she should deal with her depression. Hers was an account of the limits of her personal power to 'fight' depression. My interpretation of the interaction from her point of view was structured by her capacity to articulate these frames of meaning in the interview setting.

Portions of nurse first level account were as follows:

> N: ...she was telling me about her hiatus hernia. This led us on to saying, 'What else do we need to do while you're here?' ...Eh, and I think at the same time she was saying how fed up she was you know. I said 'Well maybe you'd be better at home', said 'Once we've got your medicines at a status quo'...
>
> R: Uhuh..she was fed up being in here..?
>
> N: Oh aye...Yeah: (Note: imitating patient's voice) 'I'm..sitting in this chair from morning to night, seven o'clock in the morning' she says, um 'If I'd a been home I could be dusting my window sills..'...she was really giving a picture of a busy wee woman in her ain hoose...who's really quite happy in that situation..and I was quite pleased to hear her say 'That's what I want to go back to'...Cos I was just testing the water (?)
>
> R: Did you have it in mind that that might be good, already, or just when she said that, you thought..
>
> N: Oh I think that, I think that was, perhaps on the cards..because she had, she did respond pretty well, I think, I personally think and collectively we felt that it was, a virus that she'd had, eh, that brought all this on..that she had..changes, and she took changes very badly...But I felt she was really quite stable..and the next step would be to, to get her back home. So I was just testing a wee bit, to see (?)

Nurse Jean recounted features that corresponded to the patient's account: the review of reasons for her being here ('why she is here now').[39] She related that she checked if there was anything more 'we have to do for you'. She heard the patient's complaint of boredom at being in the site and of what she would be doing at home, and responded by 'testing the water' to see if the patient agreed that she would be better at home. The nurse anticipated that, now that a view had been formed of what had occasioned the patient's admission and how to treat it, 'the next step' would be to get her home. Interaction in the institution was always interaction towards an end, towards moving the patient on, back to the primary reality. Nurse Jean worked to 'keep the work going', drawing on metaphors of business ('agenda', see below).

In her second level account, Nurse Jean said:

N: We didnae really know what would happen, but, we surmised things would settle down, but we werena really, we couldna be a hundred percent certain. Uh, so I was testing the, I said here (Note: nurse reading first level account) ...'testing the water'. I was testing her motivation tae, kinda draw herself (ourselves?) together and find out what's on her agenda...She's put on her agenda 'I'm I want to go now'...you know, 'As soon as possible let me get things back to normal...and, send me home'. Um..

R: But you actually say that first, right? Am I have I got that right, I mean, that, was that because you had sensed that, or..?

N: I think I had sensed th-, aye, I say I was testing the water...Just the previous conversation...was setting the scene. She was saying to me, I was sussing this out, 'I'm orientated, uh, I can (?do away?) for myself...I'm bored in here, I need to be out, this is the life I present outside, I can..', uh..so, I mean she was saying all these things to me, and I was picking them up and thinking Great, this is, you know, this is, this gave me heart I think, then, eh, to say, em (Note: looks at transcript), you know she was telling me all about the gran-, busy wee woman..

The 'test of motivation' was one of the exercises of power practised by the nurses. The processes of developing a picture of the patient as ready to go home, and development of readiness, went hand in hand. What was developed was an understanding of the patient as agent, able to give an account of herself as the source of her action (Harré and Secord, 1972). In developing this picture the nurse developed an understanding of her role in relation to the patient. The nurse went on to characterise the conversation as 'mutual reassurance', highlighting the emphasis throughout on response to the patient.

This set of accounts illustrates the complexity of interpreting the interaction of these patients and nurses on the basis of their accounts; of analysing the social construction of the reality of (powers related to) readiness to go home. The interaction, action on action, appears different as interpreted by nurse and patient. 'Readiness to go' can be interpreted, in light of P7's account, in relation to what she perceives as the claim that she is 'fighting hard' and that, while 'they can help', she's got to do it herself, in part. In the patient's account and the nurse's first level account, the nurse suggested that the patient was ready to go home. In her second level account, the nurse explained that the way that the patient 'presented' meant to her that the patient was in effect 'saying' that she was ready. Therefore the nurse 'tested the water'. The patient's response confirmed her readiness. The patient appeared in her own account as still disheartened, while the nurse in hers appeared heartened by 'mutual reassurance'. The 'ratio' of the pentad (Burke, 1969a) is different in the two accounts: the nurse as agent in P7's account, P7 herself a struggling agency; the nurse as agent in her own account, enabling P7 to act to get home.

The question related to power in these accounts was: given that the interaction was constructed by 'sense makers making sense of sense makers' and 'actors acting on actors', which interpretations structured further interaction? These accounts highlight the complexity of an analysis of the social reality of power in the interaction. Two analytic issues - accounts between nurse and patient as interpretations of the (social) reality of P7's powers, and accounts as exercises of (rhetorical) power to construct that social reality - are closely related and important to the interpretation of this as nursing action. The nurse was able to 'authorise' a version of the conversation, and of 'what happened' in the conversation, by speaking in the patient's voice and by calling on the hearer to respect the nurse's judgement that the patient's 'presentation' had been correctly interpreted. The authorised view was that the patient was ready to go home, as indicated by her readiness to resume her ordinary activities. Elsewhere in the second level account the nurse portrayed the patient as trying to 'sell herself' in order to get home. The nurse rhetorically constructed a picture of herself as a detective able to determine the true picture in the context of a possible 'con' by the patient. The nurse was engaged in interpretive work intended to reveal the validity of claims of readiness or ability to do.

In her account, Nurse Jean can be construed as interpreting P7 on two 'levels'. P7's ordinary powers - to clean, to bake - were interpreted in light of her power to give an account of herself as an agent. Nurse Jean also construed P7 as a rhetorician trying to persuade the nurse to her view of herself and her powers, displaying her knowledge of and command of the social resources needed to cope at home.

The power in interaction can be considered by thinking of Nurse Jean's interpretation of powers as determination of powers. This construction highlights that, regardless of how interpretation structured the interaction, the interpretation that structured further interaction was the claim that P7 was ready. The nurse's determination of P7's readiness was made on the basis of interpretation of the powers that could be exercised at home, as construed in light of the power to manage appearances or to 'con'. The patient likewise interpreted the nurses as 'really meaning' something else about her powers to help herself. The passage of patients through interaction and the sites was passage through the screen constituted by the nurses interpreting the 'reality' of the patients' powers on these two levels.[40] The nurse's 'testing of motivation' (realising determination) constituted a discipline which required patients to produce accounts which 'passed' at both levels of interpretation:

> I've got to kind of see her..(laughs) through her words uh uh what she's doing...

The nurse's accounts can be interpreted as a rhetorical claim of power to see what the patient was really doing in interaction through interpretation of the patient's rhetorical claims.[41] The rhetoric of patient and nurse alike drew on understandings of ordinary powers of a 'wee woman in her ain hoose', or of ordinary liabilities of the elderly. These claims were underpinned by claims of power to interpret what the other was really saying. The point to be emphasised here is that the patients and nurses construed each other as trying to persuade to views of the world, and structured their parts in interaction on that basis. The interaction was shaped by the 'test' of motivation, the test of readiness to adopt the nurse's 'picture' of the patient's readiness.

Power and the right to say Interaction was a dynamic process structured by relations of power. Nurse Jean elaborated why she suggested that the patient was ready to go home:

> N: ..It's a powerful reassurance. You know, if you're kinda sitting around miserable and dour, wondering when things are going to happen, and next thing, you know, somebody in authority comes along and is kinda talking to you about you going home..without it being totally explicit like you're going tomorrow..I suppose, similarly here people often tend to just, (laughs) they wait for that wee bit reassurance that everything's well, they're all well...You're often better doing that, rather than waiting, because, people, patients being ordinary people often have difficulties with authority..people they see in authority, 'Oh I couldna ask them, I couldna ask the doctor'. You know, they'd rather go along in ignorance

thinking 'They know what's best for me, they'll tell me'. Um, so in a way you've got to kinda make moves towards them..

Through the rhetorical device of contrasting the patient, one of the 'ordinary people' who 'wait' in 'ignorance', and the nurses, who have authority by virtue of their understanding of why the patient is 'here' and judgement of when the patient is ready to leave, Nurse Jean legitimated her 'move', on the grounds that she must, as the authority, 'author' or authorise the patient's readiness to return to the community.

The general point to be made on the basis of this analysis is that display of a power by a nurse or patient had to be interpreted in the context of the local system of rights and obligations to display powers. The nurse, interpreting the interaction in light of her background understandings of the power relations of nurses and patients, used her power to prompt a 'response', interpreted as how P7 'presented', and to move toward moving the patient on. Nurse Jean in effect reified the practices of power by attributing responsibility ('presented') to the patient. She reified the relationship of P7 as one of the 'ordinary people' to herself as 'someone in authority' 'without it being totally explicit'. The site, the nurses and patients, were maintained in part by the interaction mediated by these relations of power, sustained by inexplicitness and silence. The nurse directed attention to the power of the unsaid.

The administrative decision that P7 'would be better at home' can be seen as 'fitting' with both 'it's up to me' and 'she was ready'. The nurse had the power to give an account which drew on claims made on the basis of ordinary powers and the power of 'observation' to reach a 'determination', a view which 'stuck'. The view of 'readiness' was fed into the processes of decision making that led to P7 returning home. This analysis has highlighted that the 'determination' of P7's powers, her readiness, was the outcome of a process of complex interaction in which power was realised at the 'capillaries' of interaction.

Thus while the interaction can be interpreted through the accounts as structured by complex 'readings' and 'responses' of patient to nurse and nurse to patient, the nurse's command of the definition of the patient's readiness[42] structured the action of others in moving the patient toward discharge, the 'next step'. Nurse Jean's interpretation of herself and P7 as 'working' well together, mutually reassuring, can thus be interpreted as command of the discourse used to construct the patient for administrative purposes. In the process of interaction, Nurse Jean set the agenda.[43]

Interpreting what happened in the frame of meaning 'work', the nurse construed the patient's dissatisfaction in terms of the patient's 'options' and 'agenda'. She interpreted the patient as, in effect, 'working' to get out. She commanded the development of the 'next step' toward discharge, and authorised the definition of the patient as 'patient ready to go', drawing on the commonsense typification of a 'nice wee woman in her ain hoose'.

It is impossible to provide a monological account of power as microanalysed in this episode of interaction. This impossibility can be interpreted in terms of command of the definition of powers. Nurse Jean 'commanded' the definition of 'readiness' by claiming that P7 'commanded' her: 'send me home'; while P7 claimed that the nurses implicitly 'commanded': 'you've got to get over it yourself'. My argument is that the interaction was mediated by both actors' interpretations of relations of power. The parts played by the patient and nurse were mediated by their places in larger systems of (reified) power in interaction in the institution.[44]

Power, powers and opportunity

Having highlighted the difficulty of trying to provide a 'monological' account of the power involved in assessment construed as ascription of powers, I will now discuss other interprofessional and institutional factors which contribute to the complexity of analysis of the 'working relationships' between nurse and patient. These factors can be considered in relation to the concept of 'opportunity'.

Any discussion of 'opportunity' has to be read in the context of the current 'enterprise' culture's preoccupation with 'opportunity'. Nursing researchers have stressed that psychiatric nurses 'miss opportunities' in their work, especially with neurotic patients.[45] 'Missed opportunities' have been considered wasteful of time and money (MacIlwaine, 1980). The theoretical perspective of this study led me to consider how the concept 'opportunity' functioned in nurses' and patients' interaction and in their accounts. In this study nurses in their accounts interpreted their interaction in relation to a context of deprivation of time, space, opportunity.

Nurses and patients were engaged in the practical work of powers ascription: determining for practical purposes what a patient could or could not do, and what was to be done to enable her to do what she could not do but needed to do in order to return to the community. To determine powers the nurses attended not only to what they saw but also to the patient's accounts of her powers. The concept 'opportunity' figured in nurses' power ascriptions. The nurses spoke of 'taking opportunities' to work with patients[46] and of how various features of context - lack of time and lack of information from other professionals - limited their opportunities to work. Nurses understood that different nurses perceived different opportunities for work with the same patients.[47]

I have highlighted 'opportunity' because the construction of opportunity was empirically and conceptually related to the practices of power in nurse-patient interaction. Understanding of nurses' and patients' accounts of interaction was facilitated by analysis of their management of the concept 'opportunity'. The concept 'opportunity' as used by these nurses articulated with the concept 'opportunity' as used in the context of powers ascriptions (Harré and Secord, 1972). The logic of power ascription is that a person's powers are located in his accounts of action and are based on balances of conditions, circumstances and claims of agency. Failure of powers may be accounted for in terms of failure of will, wrong conditions, circumstances or lack of opportunity.

The perceived existence of an 'opportunity' may determine whether an account is called for if something is not done. 'Not doing' is only apparent if someone else is present to claim that something 'could have been done'. 'Opportunity' linked the concepts of 'responsibility' and 'definition of action'. The clearest example was the claim that a patient was 'hiding' from 'work', a claim that could be sustained only if the patient had had the opportunity to 'work'. Conversely, the nurses' accountability for provision of opportunities for patients to work on their problems, and their power as evidenced through their action, depended on how they handled claims of 'opportunity'. Thus 'giving and taking' opportunities to work was central to nurses' and patients' interdependence in doing the 'work' of the site.

The importance of the concept 'opportunity' was implicitly recognised by patients and nurses. Patients in effect excused nurses for not talking to them on the grounds that nurses were dealing with other more important matters: they did not have the opportunity. In their accounts nurses told of not talking to these patients, but provided the context that indicated that they had not had the opportunity to do so. They also emphasised that opportunities to talk had been provided but not taken through no fault of the nurse. Thus an experienced nurse in Site Two said of S2P4:

> ....Uh if, if you, put a question, over, and in the question you'd, in-built, you know, an **opener**, let u-, say (? you), 'Do you not feel that it, could be, situation at **home** that might be..adding to, your anxiety?' If you get a straight 'No' from that, then obviously you can, **not** move any further. Whereas, if, 'Well, there are some things that are **problems**' and (chuckles) then you say 'Well, what **kind** of problems?', then you can move in, from there, but, as long as 'Everything, at home is **fine**, there is nothing wrong', then obviously, she's not willing to look **at** that. (?We) may get rid of her symptoms, the things at home **may**, continue on, but, she **might** not develop any psychiatric type symptoms, she might just (laughs) end up with a broken marriage, which, a lot of people, encounter without actually engaging in, contact with the psychiatric services.

The definition of the patient's 'willingness' and the definition of the patient as a kind of agent or patient, depended on the nurse's definition of an opportunity.[48]

This excerpt highlights nurses' perceptions of patients' power to 'block' work. The nurse, in accounting for the working relationship, used a frame of meaning based on 'willingness', casting the patient as an agent who 'does not want to' talk about problems (cf. Stelling and Bucher, 1973). The nurses were willing to work (to 'move in'), and provided opportunities; the patient was not. The appearance of the nurse as a worker correlates with the appearance of the patient as a non-worker. The talk of these patients and nurses often centred on whether patients' failures to work on problems were due to (*pace* Harré and Secord, 1972, p. 257) 'not wanting' or 'not being able to bring oneself to'.[49] In Site Two, especially, where patients were construed by the consultant and nurses as having problems due to failure to talk about or resolve personal problems, the proposed remedy was talk. There, not taking opportunities to talk amounted to not complying with efforts to remedy illness or problems.

The offering of 'opportunities' thus implicitly created the potential for non-legitimation of and by both nurse and patient: of the nurse, if the patient declined to talk; and of the patient, if that refusal were interpreted as due to the patient 'not wanting to' (cf. May and Kelly, 1982).

These accounts may be read as interpretations of the microprocesses of interaction, as accounts of the 'microphysics' of power (Foucault, 1979), power at the capillaries. In face to face interaction the nurses and patients negotiated whether to talk or not talk, give or not give: the dramas of 'push and pull' (Peplau,

1952), 'parry and thrust' (Mead, 1934). In their interaction the nurses and patients negotiated not only the definition of opportunity but also definitions of each other as kinds of people. The nurse's account regarding S2P4 (see previous page) was also an account of the patient's personal power. In bringing 'will' into the account, the nurse shifted the account from one of inter-personal power to one of intra-personal power. The patient was interpreted as resisting the nurses, her 'not looking' attributed not to disability but to unwillingness. The nurse's power to give an account of the patient's powers, the patient's willingness or unwillingness, depended on the offer of opportunities. The provision of opportunity was a 'litmus test' of willingness. The offering of opportunities was therefore centrally important to nurses' management of their own and the patients' accountability. In the microprocesses of interaction (including the microprocesses of interpretation), the nurses realised, in the double-edged sense of the word, the patients' 'knowledge, will and power' (Henderson, 1966) and their own responses to these.

I have noted elsewhere patients' comments that nurses were 'available' to talk if the patients needed to and wanted to, but that they knew that nurses' time was limited. In general, in talk in which patients were defined, the nurses' definitions of the provision of opportunity and of the patient were the definitions that 'stuck'. However, other professionals' definitions sometimes competed with those nurses, and nurses sometimes disagreed among themselves. In the latter case, a nurse who could command resources could create other opportunities to 'test' a patient's willingness to talk, and rescue the patient from the moral judgement attendant on being judged unwilling to talk. Thus a staff nurse in Site Two said of another patient (S2P5):

> N: I deliberately asked...one of the other students, if they could spend some time with her, cos Nurse Julia, had been under the impression that she'd been trying to avoid us...and I didn't really think so, but, she had had a lot of visitors, so I asked if one or two of them, could, have chats with P5, (? just) to see how she was.

The construction of the patient as a patient was thus based on interpretation of her powers, and that interpretation was based on practices of power, including strategic operations like the above. The interpretation of the patient that 'stuck' depended on who commanded resources for 'reading' and 'handling'; that is, on who commanded the frame of meaning ('avoiding') that was applied, and who commanded his or her own and other nurses' time.[50] It depended on 'who says?' (Berger and Luckmann, 1967).

The dialectic of personal and social: metaphor and the main social acts of these nurses and patients

I have suggested in this chapter that nurses' accounts related reflexively to their practices of power in relation to the patients. That is, in the working relationship they practised getting into the patient's 'field' in order to keep the patient 'open' for 'assessment'. They commanded resources to generate accounts which then structured further work; the nurses 'withdrawing' from the patient who 'signalled' unwillingness.[51]

In this section I will outline an important way in which the nurses' language and their practices of power were related. Nurses and patients ordered their interaction through use of metaphor to create shared understandings of what they were doing. The interpretation occasioned by use of metaphor mediated the 'work' they did. The metaphors they used were metaphors of relations of power which provided 'scripts' for interaction. 'Work' was itself the main metaphor used to coordinate interaction with the aim of getting patients back to the community. 'Work on problems', in the form of talk, was the 'therapy' through which the patients returned to the community of language which mediated their return to the community structured through language. Metaphors were used to structure accounts which 'smoothed the passage' (Harré, 1979) of the patients back to the community. What I present here is a summary of some of the key understandings about metaphor in nurse-neurotic patient interaction.

Nurses used the metaphors 'reading' and 'handling' (conveying the acts related to power ascription and development) to account for their work. Here I will outline the metaphors they used to account for their working relationships with patients. The metaphors the nurses used to account for their handling of patients included: 'managing dependence', 'controlling', 'guiding', 'supporting', 'challenging'. The metaphoric terms the patients used included: 'getting to know others'; 'taking a break'; 'getting responsibility back'.

The metaphoric quality of acts The terms the nurses used all had literal as well as metaphoric meanings. The concepts 'dependence', 'control', 'guidance', 'support', and 'challenge' referred to acts in episodes. They also indicated features of the nurses' talk about action, or accounts. For example, some patients literally depended, falling to the floor if not supported. Whether or not they were literally supported depended on whether their accounts of inability to support themselves were supported by the nurses' accounts. If nurses did not 'support' a patient's account of need for support, instead construing the patient as 'playing the sick role', then they might literally not support her. This is no play on words. The concepts conveyed the meaning of the patient's and nurse's behaviour construed as action in an act legitimated as appropriate treatment. How the nurses and patients managed their use of the concepts to name actions and acts related directly to how they defined and organised their working relationships. The legitimation (or non-legitimation) of patients' accounts was accomplished in nurses' accounts.

The concepts conveyed aspects of the nurses' and patients' relationship as agents and patients, that is, as persons.[52] The metaphors in use were vehicles for common understandings. They enabled nurses and patients to coordinate their 'work'. The metaphors conveyed relations of power: 'weaning', 'working on an agenda', 'supporting', 'guiding', 'pushing', 'challenging', 'thwarting'. The common terms conveyed complex and multi-layered understandings about power in the working relationship: the world of the parent who had power to require that the child control her feelings or transfer to another source of support, the power of the nurse in her role as parent, the power of the nurse to use the metaphor of nurturing and maternalism to command definition of what she and the patient were and did; the world of the business man with power to set agendas, the nurse to act as business man, and the world in which a nurse could use the metaphor of business man to define what he and the patient were and did. I understood the work the nurses and patients did through interpreting the metaphors they used in their accounts of interaction. Appendix 2 contains two examples of the way I understood the power of nurses and patients in interaction through analysis of their accounts.

Common sense and metaphors The metaphors were common-sense terms referring to common experience, not terms of a specialist discourse. They were the vehicles through which the nurses and patients co-participated in the construction of a cognitive-emotional intersubjective reality (Denzin, 1989). They occasioned interpretation of interaction in the realm of the site in terms of something the patient or nurse knew from another realm, common relationships and typical acts. Use of metaphor was a practice, not describing or talking about but realising aspects of intersubjective reality. Metaphors enabled nurses and patients to draw on common sense, with its tensions and ambiguities, to order, direct and conduct their interaction.

The metaphors told of the work the nurses and patient had to do
The metaphors of power 'told' the nurses and patients what to do, what the problem or drama (Harré, 1979) was, and the roles they had to play for each other. S1P2 was like a child, and like ground for the seeds of ideas: she needed to grow and develop. The nurses had to tell her what to do and to plant the seeds of ideas; they weaned her from the hospital. S1P5 was a coiled spring: she needed to be released. The nurse had to let her release her tension in tears and cries to God. S2P5 was bottled up, not knowing what she felt: she needed to open up, give and take, let others help her. The nurse told her what she needed to do. S2P2 could not think for herself: she needed nurses to trigger her. A nurse suggested which dress she might buy. S1P3 had a heavy weight, a stone, blocking him: he had to shift it. The nurse listened and shared his own grief. S1P4 was tormented by 'voices' and shouted at them: she needed to tone down to live with others. Nurses told her the voices were not real. S2P4 'put anxiety off' into panic attacks, was frightened to go out and could not adjust to her family leaving home: she needed to challenge her fears and to learn to cope on her own. Nurses went out with her and tried to get her to look at what was frightening her. S2P6, overcome with panic and depression, sat like a lump: she needed to talk with others and start doing things again. Nurses tried to get her to assert herself to her family and went with her when she went to the Day Centre. S2P7 could not look after herself: she needed to learn to live on her own and not depend on her daughter. Nurses helped her in the shower and urged her to do more for herself, and made plans with her and her daughter about where she would stay. S2P8 had a hole in her life after her husband died: she needed to fill it. Nurses suggested that she be less private, and that she go out with a friend. S2P10 was anxious and dependent on alcohol and drugs but gave conflicting accounts to different professionals: she needed to reduce her dependence on alcohol and drugs and learn other ways to manage her time. Nurses suggested she take a break, get a job.

Metaphors bridged the personal and the social To say that metaphors played vital roles in the interaction of the nurses and patients is itself a meta-metaphor. The metaphor is social action construed as drama (cf. Harré, 1979; Burke, 1969a and 1969b). Nurses and patients needed to know how to act with each other, how to conduct themselves. Metaphors defined the dramatic action and the roles nurses and patients were to play. They defined problems and implied solutions. They implied the 'objectives' of nursing action.[53] Thus the metaphor of 'dependence' of S1P2, with the notion that she was 'like a child', implied the kinds of action that were appropriate. Thinking of S1P2 in this way, it made sense that an experienced nurse would 'sow a seed' of an idea of how P2 should act.[54] The metaphors did not define in detail the action the nurse would follow, but rather the 'main channel'.[55] One of the 'main channels' defined by the metaphors used in the sites was the 'objective' of 'going home': the 'child' developed until weaned; the 'agenda' taken care of and the meeting finished; the 'block' removed so one could go on one's way.

Examples of the metaphor of dependence - stories of dependence In Chapter 5 I discussed how common sense provided the 'seeds of arguments' relevant to understanding the knowledge in the nurses' and patients' interaction. Here I suggest that common metaphors provided 'germs of action' (Stanislavski, 1980) through which nurses and patients realised their power. The metaphors were key terms in the shared language used to accomplish the work of the sites, particularly in Site One.

As common sense comprised a set of terms which could both occasion and resolve dilemmas, so the metaphors of action were used in different ways to accomplish different practical ends. The concept 'dependence' was used by nurses in accounts about most of the neurotic patients in Site One. However, the meaning of dependence was different for each patient, in the sense that nurses' action with patients considered dependent was not uniform. Dependence was always negotiated, in a context in which the implications of dependence had always to be taken into account.

Sick role and acting: In Kardex notes on S1P1 a nurse wrote: 'P1 appeared to be trying to slide further into the sick role, e.g. ...trying to slide off the seat on the ambulance because her legs wouldn't hold her'. This may be read as a discourse on powers, in which the nurse attributed responsibility. P1 was seen as actively trying to accomplish (agent) what others might have thought was just happening to her (patient). The claim that P1 was trying to play a role implied both an intention on the part of the patient and resistance on the part of the nurses. In the discourse of medical and nursing staff the playing of a sick role was interpreted as a sign that P1 was insecure and looked for support from the nurses. The nurses helped her, but 'pushed' her to do more for herself because they understood that they had to make her less dependent in order to move her on.

A nurse said that from the nurses' point of view 'she was dependent, (therefore) our aim was to make her less dependent on us' by encouraging her (with 'firm physical management' at times) to do for herself: dress, walk, and care for herself. The immediate translation of 'her dependence' to the nurses' 'making her less dependent' made sense in the context of the challenge by nurses and doctors to the patient's claim to be unable to help herself; and in the context of their intention to move her on.

A second account of dependence The relationship of powers and power can be seen in an account of a nurse taking 'a tough line' with S1P2:

> N: We decided that, we'd, stop being as supportive, eh, changed our attitude in a way that, although we were still being supportive, we're really, weaning her off us, if you see what I mean, so, like she was saying, 'I cannae cope with any more passes', and I was saying, 'Well you're going on pass, (? like more) sort of thing' (laughs). Sort of more, strict (?) the tough, yeah, more the sort of tough line you sometimes have to take if, they're too dependent. It, it's (? a line or ? one) we, occasionally take, with over-dependent patients, eh, so that they'll go back into the community.

The metaphor of 'weaning' conveyed the harshness and necessity of 'deciding to stop being supportive' (cf. Pollock, 1989). The metaphor conveyed a sense of 'natural' action which elided consideration of ways in which supporting a dependent patient by taking a tough line was unlike weaning a child. Use of the metaphor elided questions of how the community or home might not nourish or sustain the patient. The ward's place in the community was reified in part through a discourse in which the nurses 'had' to take the tough line as mothers have to wean their children. In some instances, the nurses' use of metaphors appeared as rationalisations of practices of power which might have appeared less accountable had they been expressed more explicitly.[56]

Tensions in the metaphors - a third case of dependence: A third example of the nurses' management of dependence was found in a trained nurse's account (Site Two):

> N: I suggested that she get up for her shower, and she said she needed help, and I said 'Where do you need help?', and she said 'It's getting in and out of the shower, it's the steps', and I said 'Well, if you get yourself to the bathroom I'll help you in and out'. But she did it, all by herself, really. And (?). So um, all I said to her was, 'We'll have to start practising a bit more' for when she goes home, or else, we'll have to start looking around for, alternative ideas for her when she **does** wash herself. If she's going to be on her own without any support.

The nurse considered what she needed to do and acted within a frame of awareness that the patient was going home, that she would have no support, and that she would thus be 'dependent' on herself. From other data it was clear that the nurse acted in awareness of a larger context: P7's daughter's inability to cope with her mother; P7's reluctance to limit her demands on her daughter; limits on choice of accommodation. The nurse worked with the patient and family to try to get the best accommodation for P7, but directed her action on the basis of what the patient would need 'if she is going out without support'.

The nurse worked to advance P7's passage through the site. Peplau (1952, p. 240) asked[57]:

> What are the obligations to society that a nurse needs to consider: to get the patient out of the hospital as quickly as possible in whatever way seems most direct or to help patients to use experiences such as illness as stepping stones to further development of personality?

Neither term in this dichotomy fits this nurse's exercise of power. She acted within a working relationship to help P7 adapt to the scarcity of resources on which she could depend, the nurse being one of these resources (cf. Pollock, 1989). The nurse managed in face to face interaction the definition of what the patient needed to manage in the conditions likely to face her in the community. In such microprocesses of power at the 'capillaries' (Foucault, 1979) the nurses managed the resources of the larger society. The metaphors which guided practice functioned also as terms in ideologies of caring (cf. Pollock, 1989).

Negotiation of responsibility: agency and the requirement to talk

In previous sections I discussed ways in which the nurses used metaphors, and concepts including 'need' and 'dependence', to organise their working relationships. They negotiated in face to face interaction responses to the question 'What do we have to do for her (do I have to do)?'. The metaphors and concepts were terms in ideologies of care or treatment which functioned to direct action toward the administrative end of returning the patient to the community. In discussing the concept 'opportunity' I suggested that the nurses participated in a 'politics' of opportunity provision, negotiating with patients the terms of responsibility to provide and to take opportunities to use the facilities of the site, to 'work'.

The thrust of my argument has been that power ascription and power in interaction were reflexively related. Responses to the question 'Why is she here now?' were produced through practices of power in assessment. Responses to the question 'What do we have to do for her?' were structured by the frames of meaning developed in interaction. The practices of interpretation were structured by relationships of power ('diagnosis' was the province of doctors; student nurses were restricted in their interaction with patients). In turn, 'what we have to do for her' was structured by power ascription.

The institutions were these practices, dynamically structured and realised. The 'working ideologies' were clusters of terms, including 'dependence', 'community', 'work', 'responsibility', 'kind of person', drawn on to order work and accounts of work. In this section I will argue that it was through the patients' 'responses' to the practices of power in the sites that they were known as kinds of people, patients or agents, and characters. Thus the 'politics' of the institution were reflected in the 'politics' of person and self, as patients took on or resisted taking on their roles in the processes of 'work' on themselves.

Patients in Site One knew that they did not have to talk. P5 said:

> P: They, they don't put you in a sort of position that you **are** embarrassed. Em, if you **want** to talk about anything, you **can**, if you don't want to talk about anything, they don't **push** you...you know, which is very very **nice**. You, you do it in your

> own **time**, when you want to, you know, which um uh, I think's really nice.

Nonetheless, patients risked being considered 'unwilling' to be helped if they did not discuss their problems. The claim that patients did not have to talk was part of an ideology of 'work' according to which the patients were regarded as (agents) responsible for their decisions to talk or not to talk. That definition of them was maintained by nursing practices. Management of opportunities to talk was the point where the politics of site and the politics of the person and self intersected.

The ideology of 'responsibility' was more strongly expressed in Site Two and was related to institutional factors.[58] Some nurses there had worked in a ward specialising in treatment of neurotic patients, and vestiges of that different style of work and ideology may have survived in their working practices. These nurses emphasised the need for staff and patients to take responsibility for their actions.

The ideology was not monolithic, nor was it a monopoly. The staff drew on the ideology flexibly to control and order work. 'Responsibility' was sustained if nurses, having asked if a patient wanted to talk, and having picked up 'signals' of unwillingness to talk, did not ask further. The politics of opportunity provision reflected the distribution of power among staff. Student nurses in Site Two were told that they should not tell patients what to do, but 'just listen'. The rationale, based on the ideology, was that patients had to work out for themselves what to do. Structuring the work on the basis of the ideology may have functioned both to control the number of competing negotiations going on with one patient, and to protect students, and the staff supervising them, from the consequences of working on issues for which they could not be held responsible. It maintained the divisions of work: 'deep work' for psychologists, social workers and psychiatrists; and 'being available', support, and 'talking if you need to or want to' with nurses.

While the ideology may have been functional in ordering work, some nurses found it inadequate. Students had to deal with some of the most difficult situations identified in accounts. When a student had, from her point of view, to tell patients what to do, she drew on an alternative frame of meaning ('if you empathise, you have to suggest something'). Perhaps because she was not authorised to deal with these issues, she did not discuss them afterwards with trained nurses.

The ideology of responsibility was an ideology of personhood. It was used to construe the patient/person as agent or patient, in terms of powers and liabilities (cf. Towell, 1975). Specifically, it was used to define the patient in terms of agency: willingness to work on problems, including problems related to self ('giver or taker'; role; 'private person'). The ideology was expressed in terms of the rights and obligations of nurses towards the patient as a person. It was a 'working ideology'. The reflexive play between ideology and moral order, and the ways in which the ideology was used to legitimate practice will be more fully addressed in Chapter 7.

Conflict between patients and nurses

Nurses and patient sometimes gave accounts of interaction in which they disputed interpretations of events or powers. This aspect of accounts will be analysed in Chapter 7. Their interpretations of each other's powers also differed in the accounts they gave to me (e.g. Nurse Jean's and P7's accounts, above). Discrepancies between accounts were typical (cf. MacIlwaine, 1980; and Llewelyn, 1985). I interpreted power and resistance to power in the practices of accounting through which responsibility was attributed to patients, other nurses, and the nurse himself.

The resistance could be construed in terms of the patients not producing, in their work with nurses, a discourse interpretable as 'work' (a discourse on their own responsibility). An experienced nurse in Site Two said that various of the patients in the study did not want to work on their problems, or 'hid' from the nurses (avoided talking about their problems). In their accounts the patients said that they were working with other professionals or did not know what work was required. Nurses and patients disagreed over whether responsibility for patients' liabilities was due to failure of conditions (including the exercise of the nurses' own powers), to circumstances, or to the patients themselves.[59] The result was that they disagreed about the patients' powers. For example, S2P4 appeared, in an experienced nurse's accounts, to be holding something back, 'not working'; while in her own accounts she appeared to be 'working', but with a psychologist. Their disagreements reflected the distribution of power and their relative powers to give accounts. The last public word lay with the nurses and other professionals.[60]

Management of accountability

In describing the nurses' and patients' 'working relationships' I have discussed their 'working practices' ('getting into work') and the ideology of responsibility which reflexively shaped the relationships. The work in which nurses and patients were (asymmetrically) interdependent was management of accountability. Accountability here means both the ability to give an account, and responsibility to tell others what is done in work (Thompson et al, 1983). I use the latter sense of the concept to include not only nurses' obligation to provide accounts to managers and doctors, but also patients' obligations to provide accounts to nurses. Management of accountability was linked to character: the 'giver, not taker' was someone who did not give accounts of troubles or take offers of help; the 'private' person was one who withheld accounts; as was the 'hider'. Empirically, character was appraised on the basis of how patients managed their accountability in working with the nurses.

The concept 'accountability' ties together themes related to knowledge, power and moral order. In Chapter 5 I considered accounts as forms of knowledge, devices for defining, maintaining and repairing reality. In this chapter I have considered the processes of accounting that structured and were structured by 'working relationships'. Accounting refers to the practices of interpreting self and the world to explain what is happening and to attribute responsibility for action. In this chapter I have described those practices. By accountability I mean the obligation to participate in those processes. The work for nurses and patients in both sites had certain features in common, despite the finding that Site Two operated on the basis of an ideology of responsibility and Site One, to some extent, on an dual ideology of responsibility and character. Nurses' power to play their parts in the systems of accounting in which they were bound with each other and doctors, depended on their ability to get accounts from patients; that is, to manage the patients' accountability.[61]

Discretion and the relationship of patients' and nurses' powers A thread that runs through this chapter is the ordering of appearances in nurses' and patients' discourses. The interdependence of nurses and patients can be understood in terms of the nurses' ability to command the appearance of the patient as an accountable subject. The patients' appearances were literally ordered through, for example, requirement of attendance at meetings and refusal to let the patient lie in bed during the day. Equally important was the ordering of the appearance as agent or patient. This was part of the larger project of reality maintenance and repair in the sites: ordering (in terms of the paramount reality) illusions, delusions, and ordinary misperceptions. I have already suggested that nurses commanded a discourse in which their powers to order the appearance of the patient were privileged. Terms like 'presented' and 'observed' amounted to second order constructs used by nurses to warrant claims that what they had seen was what was there to be seen (cf. Raffel, 1979). This discourse 'ordered' a warranted view of the patient.

The power involved in use of this discourse is indicated by noting that when a nurse said that a patient 'presented', the patient was construed as participating in the observation through which she was defined as a patient. The nurse's interpretation was elided, recalling Foucault's (1979, p. 187) analysis:

> Disciplinary power...is exercised through its invisibility; at the same time it imposes on those whom it subjects a principle of compulsory visibility. In discipline, it is the subjects who have to be seen.

This visibility was accomplished through a discourse in which patients were construed as 'presenting' the features which, in nurses' accounts, characterised them as patients (cf. Atkinson, 1977).

A second way in which the discourse enabled the nurses to claim and disclaim accountability lay in the nurses' use of 'we' rather than 'I':

> N: ...Well in a way, the kind of conversation almost got to the point of...discharge, ..I was kinda sorta saying to her 'I think this explains your illness..I think this explains why you're the way you are.' And I think I probably, I may have used the term 'we'...'We think this is what's happened to you, this is why we want to put you on the stat-, back to status quo.' You know, so it's almost talking to someone as if they're just leaving that they're having everything explained to them...what's happened.
>
> R: Right, right, right, right.
>
> N: '(?) this is our opinion.' It's like when you know the surgeon says 'Goodbye' to you after taking your appendix out..

Through use of 'we' the nurse legitimated acting in a role usually played by doctors. Nurses could also challenge a patient's claim that (the patient's) 'I' could not do something. Through command of the discourse the nurses managed the appearance of and socially constructed self and patient as accountable subjects.[62]

The nurses practised limiting accountability through management of their own appearances (appearances of themselves as accountable subjects) in written records. These practices had to be learned. Thus, a student was told that when writing the nursing Kardex (the daily written record) she was to put in 'facts not impressions'. The nurses excised from written records the interpretations which mediated their practices of power in interaction. Accountability was also limited through subscription to the understanding that each nurse was an 'individual', that each individual had her own style, and that moreover, one nurse would 'pick up' more in a given situation than another and hence 'handle' things differently (cf. Pollock, 1989). This provided a general account that different nurses would do things differently; and its corollary, that one nurse could not be expected to account for another's action (Hughes, 1988b). The nurses limited accountability by working on the understanding that it was in talk, not writing, that necessary interpretation was conveyed; and where rhetorical skill, style and character were displayed. The nurses' practical accountability was founded on an oral discourse. Their practices maintained the privileges of talk (cf. Grypdonk, 1987)

The reader will recall that in Chapter 5 I explored these issues in terms of knowledge. Here, in reviewing them, I want to emphasise the power involved in interpretation and in enforcing the frame of meaning 'work' to define the paramount reality ('my (Note: the nurse's) reality'). The ideology of 'responsibility for work' was drawn on reflexively to sustain the relations of power in the sites.

Responsibility, administrative accountability, and the 'middle man'

I have noted that the working ideologies of the sites were not monolithic, and that working practices were not uniform. In Site Two especially, different views of the same patient in different nurses' accounts were common. The differences can be seen in portions of accounts about P4's stay as seen from the nurses' points of view. An experienced nurse said:

> N: She originally came to us...after having, a, panic attack, uh which was in fact so, disturbing to everyone **around**

her...(Note: there follows an account of her first period of admission, during which the patient was treated with drugs, with 'problems in coping' apparently resolved; followed by discharge; followed by further panic attacks and readmission.) When she came in, the panic attacks had then dropped, so obviously there was something out there that was a little bit **too** challenging for her. So we tried to talk with her, to try and find out what this **was**. And, between ourselves and the medical staff came up with this idea, that uh, **probably** it was something fairly long-standing..and, there was a lot of anxiety that she had which was put off, on these panic attacks so, so (? it was) thought, to bring in the psychologist to try and handle it from there, and, basically we then saw it as being simply a management of building up her confidence, and having nurses available to work with her, on her programme.

Nurses' and patients' accountability in Site Two entailed reference to a body of knowledge (a 'working ideology') about responsibility for problems. This entailed an account of what was responsible for the appearance of the patient at the time ('Why is she here now?'); and the articulation of that account with an account of the staff's responsibilities toward the patient: an analysis of the patient's powers[63] and liabilities and the staff's powers. On the patient's readmission, the nurse's interpretation was that anxiety was 'obviously' displaced from something 'too challenging' 'out there' ('Why she is here now'). The staff 'tried to find out' what 'this' was. They shared a theory that 'it' was 'something long-standing' that was 'put off' to 'panic attacks'. The response was to 'call in a psychologist' to 'handle it' ('What do we need to do for her?'). Nursing management followed: 'then' 'simply' 'building up' and 'being available to work with her'.

The working ideology was drawn on to legitimate allocation of professional and interpersonal responsibility: allocation of responsibility for the patient's work and for work with the patient (cf. Peplau, 1978). The work and the working relationship were reflexively related to definition of 'it'[64] and work on 'it'. The nurses' role was construed in terms of availability for work. The patient was correspondingly constructed as someone who was to be available for work on her problems. Provision of the resources of the site, couched in terms of 'time', was dependent on the patient's availability for work.[65] Availability as the basis of accountability provided the basis for strategies of work management and accounting practices.

The working ideology of responsibility entailed theories of the patient as a person (agent or patient) and the appropriate working relationship. The ordering of work depended on how the terms of the ideology were used to structure face to face interaction. The nurses' role related to the structure of power and territory. Knowledge of knowledge was knowledge of power and territory. 'Deep work' was someone else's territory:

> And, from there on, really as I say, it's just been, a kind of supportive role we've had since she does **not** seem to be willing to look at the issues, which we suspect, of, a marital nature which is the **real** problem. (? Um), she's not willing to do anything exploring **that**, to any depth, therefore we're just looking to ease her off her symptoms.

When the patient was perceived as being unwilling to do 'deep work,'[66] the metaphors of work changed: from depth to support, from 'exploring' to 'easing off':

> N: Um..broadly speaking I have to admit, uh, no, um, she tends not to relate to us, except in a conversational thing, so I'd suspect that she sees the doctor and now the psychologist as the **curer** and ourselves very much as **hotel services** and somebody to talk to...just that we're **nice people** (Note: the latter spoken ironically).

I have noted that the nurses in Site One were more often the main agents in work with the patients in this study than was the case in Site Two. In Site Two nurses more often appeared, in their own and patients' accounts, as 'middle men'. Their role in 'support' was that of supporting the definition of the work of others and others' definitions of 'it'. They faced problems associated with this role: working in the dark when ignorant of what others thought 'it' was; managing conflict when they did work which they could not openly acknowledge, and when they disagreed with others' definitions of 'it'. There were risks that, because they did not command the definition of the patient as 'work object' (Stacey, 1976), the nurses would be relegated to a service role.[67] The extent to which this happened depended, to an extent, on how well the patient 'supported' their work role (cf. May and Kelly, 1982).

In a system in which accountability was based on availability, one could be always potentially and never actually responsible; while the other could always be held responsible. An experienced nurse in Site Two continued:

> N: (Our role has been) **initially** assessing. And then, as I say, reassurance and generally trying to engage with her, to give her the opportunity to talk over these issues, which **have** been raised, but which she is **not** wanting to do any **work** on. Um, involvement also with the support group, again, to give her opportunity to vent her feelings and think through the issues, which again have not really been taken up. Um, latterly, as I say, we've withdrawn a bit to a more broadly supportive role...She's **signalled** to us she's not really wanting to engage in anything terribly **deep** in the way of conversation, so, time for exploratory work you could say's now no longer available, so (?that) it's just building her up emotionally.

In the nurse's account the patient was construed as an agent signalling unwillingness to work[68]; the nurses as accountable for provision of opportunity, as having the 'potential' to help. They and the patient were portrayed as agents tacitly agreeing not to work. This can be construed as an account of mutual non-legitimation (cf. May and Kelly, 1982): of the nurses (and perhaps the other staff) as 'deep workers' by the patient, and vice versa.[69]

I have emphasised throughout this analysis that nurses in their accounts sometimes offered alternative definitions of the patient and interaction, including alternative conceptions of the powers of the patient and the nurse. An alternative view of what P4's stay had been about was given by one of the nurses active in the support group:

> N: In the support group...there were things, I don't think she said, in the **family** situation, that she didn't always express her feelings outside in the, family, and that was one thing we talked about in the group. And...she was always a mother that was sort of, was inclined to, continue the child's **childhood** maybe a bit too **much**..She's probably a woman that's going to have to try and **find** her, her **role** when her child leaves home, or, or goes to university. In the support group...she also found that she could talk, **through** the support group she learned that she could, **talk** to other patients as well, you know, other people...saying that, uh, that it was sorta **good** to be able to talk to other, people and share experiences **here**...

In the first nurse's reality P4 'did not want to look too closely' at the marital conflict. In the second nurse's reality P4 learned through the support group, talked about feelings and shared experiences.

The accounts can be interpreted in terms of the power of different nurses in face to face interaction to bring different frames of meaning ('responsibility' versus 'sharing') into play to structure interaction differently. The frames of meaning could be based on common experiences (literally, here, 'sharing'; or in the case of a student nurse, the experiences of difficulty in asserting herself to relatives); as well as on the ideologies of the sites. Specialist frames of meaning related to illness (anxiety, depression) were drawn on in structuring other forms of action (relaxation therapy, an agoraphobic 'programme'). The patient, as person, appeared different(ly) through the different accounts of 'working relationships'.[70]

Control through signs

I have emphasised that practices of power were not monological, and that power was an aspect of interaction and relationship. In the first nurse's account above, the nurses were construed as responding to P4's 'signals' of unreadiness to work. The processes of power in interaction were mediated by typification ('giver not taker') and common-sense understandings of willingness and readiness, as noted above, interpreted in the context of 'opportunities' offered by the nurses. The sites could be construed as processes of power mediated by signification and interpretation, where what mattered was which interpretations 'stuck' and ordered further action (recall Nurse Jean and P7). Thus in P4's account:

> P: Yeah, well I would tell the nurses more than I would tell the doctor. Because I feel the doctor is, that bit higher up and, and awfully busy, they've got a lot of work. I feel I would, as I thought convide, confide in a nurse, or especially a young nurse, uh, tell them how I **really** felt...They are a bit easier to talk to. Some of the older ones, and the ones which are higher up and been here longer, I sometimes feel I can't approach them, (?very easy)...I think I've actually said to some of the young nurse I wish I could talk to, the ones higher up, maybe hoping that she will relate it to the, the senior staff. I think maybe that's my way of, giving them information, right enough. But I think I haven't realised it before...I hope that when I'm talking to the student nurse that, that she tells the, the higher up ones, (?and) I don't want them to come running to, me, probably I've been crying, I've been so upset and, I think to myself Well I hope she (Note: said forcefully) tells

someone higher up, but I don't actually say it, I don't do it for that reason. I don't expect the senior staff to come running and, hand me paper hankies you know for my tears, (?), but I just would like the doctor to know of how I really felt sometimes. I don't like to go to him and say, 'Did you know I was crying at eleven o'clock last night?' or 'I couldn't sleep during the night'. But I hope that the staff that are on, and I feel they do, would put it in, on a report, and the doctor eventually sees it.

I have used the concepts 'power' and 'powers' to highlight aspects of the social construction of the reality of interaction between the nurses and patients. P4 can be seen as trying to get her view of the world recognised and acted on; in a site structured by relations of power mediated by the availability of time[71], to convey through the nurses an account of her liabilities so that the doctor can know how she really feels.

Interaction between the nurses and patients was mediated by action based on the patients' and nurses' understandings about each other's knowledge. Articulation of frames of meaning and structuring of interaction were thus related. I noted that P7 thought that Nurse Jean and the other nurses thought that she should 'get over it' herself, when she knew that she could not. She thought that they ignored her because they thought she was not 'to give in'. The interaction ended with an interpretation of her consistent with what she saw as the nurses' view of her.[72] I will explore further in Chapter 7 issues related to who could know best and who could enforce claims based on that knowledge.

Actions

I have discussed the 'middle man' role of nurses in Site Two, and P4's mediated communication. What I have not done is to list the actions and acts derived through analysis. I have not done so because the meaning, the social effect of the actions, depended on their place in the context of interaction mediated by the actors' interpretations. For example, the meaning of 'building up emotionally' related to its distinction from 'exploration'; 'just supporting' to its relation to 'deep work'.

For purposes of explanation, however, it is important to note that the forms of work the nurses said they engaged in with patients in the sites included, in terms used by the nurses: 'exploration', 'reassurance', 'reinforcement', 'support', 'ventilation'. These actions comprised recipes: 'wee bit reassurance'; 'usual five minutes'. The work with patients was varied. In Site Two much of it centred on liaison with family and discussion of problems within the family; discussion of social problems and roles; and planning or actual practice of action to develop or recover the ability to shop, travel, socialise, talk about problems with others and sort out a multitude of practical problems. In Site One the work included discussion of illness; work with families or liaison with agencies regarding ways of coping after discharge; and exploration of feelings and experiences related to illness or problems. In many of the accounts in both sites, nurses referred to the patients' problems or illnesses; and they recounted sequences of interaction and interpretations of their own and the patient's actions. While comparison with accounts reported in other studies (e.g. Altschul, 1972) is difficult, it may be concluded that the nurses indicated through their accounts command of 'social resources' including knowledge of recipes, strategies, tactics; and practices of assessment and treatment, including group work.

Summary of the chapter

In this chapter I have interpreted power in interaction between nurses and neurotic patients, interaction construed as responses to the questions 'Why is she here now (am I here now)?' and 'What do we have to do for her (I have to do)?'. I have interpreted the power in 'working relationships' based on knowing and acting on 'the main thing'.

'Work' had to be accomplished by ordering interaction in light of competing demands and interpretations of 'the main thing'. It involved structuring interaction in order to accomplish production of accounts of powers and liabilities ('assessment'), and to accomplish action to remedy liabilities and effect the patient's return to the paramount reality of the community. Some practices of power were standard and collective: observation through ward design, community and small group meetings, and the daily talk 'in passing'. Others were based on the repertoires of individual nurses. Practices included the routine 'demand'[73] that patients 'open up' their view of the world and self for 'work', interpretation by nurses and others. Patients knew that in the end they had to do the 'work' themselves; that is, assume responsibility for interpreting what was wrong and working to get better.

Command of resources of the sites, interpreted generally in terms of 'time', was negotiated in face to face interaction. Deployment of resources was dependent on the nurse's interpretation of the patient in the situation and on her command of resources. I explored differences in practices of power between the sites and within sites, and emphasised that the relationship between working ideologies and practices was not fixed. Interaction between patients and nurses depended to some extent on the resources of each. However, there was a reflexive play between the institution and individual working practices. Nurses working as 'middle men' in Site Two reflexively realised divisions in 'territory'. Patients were construed in terms of division of 'work' more clearly there than in Site One. The analysis does not allow firm conclusions to be drawn regarding relationships between the broader organisation of working practices in the sites and face to face interaction between individual nurses and patients. However, there were suggestions that nurses negotiated working relationships that structured patients' views of self (e.g. the small group in Site Two, P8's understanding of her 'private self'). The patient as known by others and self in the site was the person known through the practices of assessment and treatment. Working relationships, especially in Site Two, were directed toward return of the patient (responsible for herself) to the community. The analysis indicates the relevance of considering the 'politics' of the nurses' and patients' work in relation to the 'politics' of the patient's work on self ('willingness') and the wider processes of power in the community.

I described the process of interaction; aspects of nursing discourse, including metaphors; and some of the forms of nursing practice ('support', 'challenge', 'persuasion', control of 'time'). Interaction structured and ordered by these processes was construed by nurses in terms of 'opportunities for work'. Different nurses offered different accounts of whether patients were offered and took 'opportunities'. Thus there were different perceptions of the 'working relationship' and of the patient as a 'worker'. This analysis does not extend to interpretation of relationships between the ideology of responsibility and the valuation of patients on the basis of their 'willingness to work', the patients' view of self, and ideologies which structure interaction in the wider community.

I highlighted through the analysis some problems associated with interpretation of power on the basis of accounts of interaction given by 'actors acting on actors' and shaped by rhetoric. In this chapter I have offered understandings of nurses' and patients' understandings of interaction. 'Order' in both nurses' and patients' first order understandings and my second order understandings was an order imposed on and in the flux of interpretation of and in interaction. The analysis has perhaps reproduced some of the complexities faced by nurses and patients: the problem both nurses and patients faced, of accounting for what was done, and saying what was responsible for what was done in interaction; and the nurses' problem of accounting for the patients' and their own action, or failure to act, when their accounts were 'dependent' on patients' accounts. Questions of 'can or cannot do' and 'will or will not do' were practically important because interaction was based on patients taking 'opportunities' dependent on the 'availability' of nurses.

Construing the interaction from the perspective of the social construction of reality, nurses 'diagnosed' deviations from normal powers (or the absence of powers) and worked to restore the patient's powers through 'work', including 'work on self', intended to restore the patient to the community. They worked to restore and maintain (through exercise) the patient's powers to act and to account for herself as an agent.

I have analysed some of the empirical relationships between knowledge and power in the nurses' and patients' interaction. In the next chapter I will consider issues related to legitimation of the practices of power in interaction.

Notes

1 The relationship between knowledge and power was reflexive: practices of power mediated articulation and imposition of frames of meaning whereby power and liability ascriptions were made to 'stick' (cf. Giddens, 1976).
2 It enables re-interpretation of the concept of 'missed opportunities' (Altschul, 1972; MacIlwaine, 1980)
3 I will address the relevance of Peplau's (1952, 1978) work more fully in later chapters.
4 An interesting discussion of 'conduct', in the context of a critique of psychotherapy, can be found in Smail (1987). The control of others' conduct through control of the 'definition of the situation' was the central concern in Goffman (1969).
5 For example, see Appendices 7 and 8.
6 See Henderson's (1966) definition of nursing as doing for the other in matters of health and illness what the other would do

for self if she had the 'necessary strength, will, or knowledge'. Also, see Peplau's (1978) claim that the work of the psychiatric nurse depends on the definition of the work of the patient.

7 Harré and Secord (1972, pp. 246-8) argue: 'One who has a generic power is an agent; he is one who initiates his own performances, that is explanations of their genesis terminates with such items as the wants, needs or intentions of that individual...(Being) an agent...has to do with the balance between and changes in external and internal, intrinsic and extrinsic conditions in the accounts that are given of the genesis of action...One who is an agent must figure as the source of his action in his or our account of it, while he who succumbs to a liability may either have 'only himself to blame', as we say, or it may be that in accounting for the manifestation of the liability, we look for the source in circumstances external to himself.' One who 'succombs to a liability', is regarded as a patient, (Harré and Secord, 1972, pp. 247).

8 Harré and Secord (1972, p. 243) argue: '1. "Not wanting" is the back-stop which preserves our status as an agent when we fail to act when the enabling conditions have been fulfilled. 2. "Not being able to bring oneself to" claims the complementary status of a patient, but preserves the conceptual system intact. 3. All those items, the non-obtaining of which prevents the exercise of powers in action, but which lie outside the person, we lump together as circumstances.'

9 See also Appendix 4 for another of P2's accounts of inability and recovery of ability to do things.

10 See Chapter 7.

11 I used Szasz's (1979, p. 12) definition of rhetoric as 'a certain kind of conversation', which he says, citing Aristotle (cited in Szasz, 1979, p. 13), is 'concerned with such things as come within the ken of all men and belong to no definite science'; a kind of conversation the good or harmful effect of which depends on the intention of the speaker (1979, p. 13). The concept of rhetoric is used to convey speech intended to persuade others to a view of the world. Szasz cites Weaver on the base rhetorician, who mis-portrays the world by depicting 'cause without consequence or consequence without cause, acts without agents and agents without agency (thus blocking) definition and cause-and-effect reasoning' (Weaver, cited in Szasz, 1979, p. 20).

12 The nurses did control some of these patients' bodies - removing one from a room, supporting others in walking or showering. Patients in both sites saw other patients being controlled physically. They distinguished themselves from patients who were in the site involuntarily (on Mental Health Act 'sections'). However, the main form of social control for these patients was talk, rhetoric.

13 For example, nurses were to be aware at all times of the whereabouts of patients on 'close observation'. Those on 'special observation' were to be accompanied, even to the toilet. While patients in the study were not 'on observation', a nurse could still construe them as 'not on any special observation'. That is, they were construed from the perspective of the power of 'observation'. That power formed part of the 'background' of power in nurse-neurotic patient interaction. 'Observation' was more often emphasised in Site Two nurses' and patients' accounts.

14 'Command' of time and space was a key factor in definition of the sites. It could be argued that the nurses had greater power to command use of time and space because collectively they were in the sites 24 hours a day.

15 However, the nurses' power to command time and space was limited, most obviously by their inability to control admission and discharge. Much of the conflict evident in the accounts could be read as evidence of the limits of the nurses' powers in relation to the patients.

16 Thus S2P2 said: 'And of course, Joan was, I didn't want to go to the Sacred Heart today, because I wasn't feeling well. However, eh, I went down there in the afternoon.' R: 'Huh'. P: 'Got my dinner down there, and, eh, here I am (laughs).' R: 'That was after speaking with Joan, or was it..' P: 'Well, Joan sorta, probably, took her orders from Dr Philps, maybe. You know, "Dr. Philps **said** so. You've, got to go." So by this time my headache was, I was feeling a bit jaded...'

17 Thus S2P4: '...I said that, I wanted away, a lot earlier last Friday, to, so's I wouldn't have to rush, as I felt, eh, Phyl said I had to stay to a, support group meeting, which quite honestly I felt, in this case, was a waste of, my time... so I stayed very much against my will... But, I feel it probably did help me, and I'm quite glad I did stay, now.'

18 I found useful Foucault's (1979, 1980) analyses of the ways in which power produces knowledge and the subjects constituted

by knowledge; and in which knowledge is drawn on in the practices of power.

19 See Stacey (1976) on patients as work objects and service objects.

20 The 'reality' of 'sharing', the power of sharing, was constituted in the small group in Site Two. Thus N: 'But, eh, I think that, she also found that she could talk, **through** the support group she learned that she could, **talk** to other patients as well, you know, other people, uh, in a similar way, cos she once sort of, opened the support group by saying that, uh, that it was sorta **good** to be able to talk to other, people and share experiences **here**.'

21 The conjunction of this analysis with Barker's (1989) adoption of the metaphor of gardening in understanding psychiatric nursing as creating conditions for growth and development will be discussed in Chapter 7.

22 By 'metonym' I mean a figure of speech in which a term for part of something is used to convey the whole; for example, 'sail' for a ship. Selden (1985) uses the example of a close-up in cinema. By 'metaphor' I mean a term used to speak of something as something it literally is not; for example, nursing as 'work in the field' or Barker's (1989) 'gardening'. Metaphors enable one to draw on meanings in one domain to inform understanding of another domain.

23 The pair of accounts can be construed in terms of developing responsibility. The nurse and the patient were engaged in what each construed as a socially meaningful act. If 'breaking ground' is regarded as a metaphor for work to develop the possibility of growth (of relationship, intimacy), their interaction may be construed as development of social accountability through action and accounts of action (cf. Shotter, 1984; Vygotsky, 1978).

24 Mead (1934, p. 78): 'Just as in fencing the parry is the interpretation of the thrust, so in the social act, the adjustive response of one organism to the gesture of another is the interpretation of that gesture by that organism - it is the meaning of that gesture.'

25 The nurse's discourse may be read in terms of what 'people' do. It is a form of social construction of 'people'. See Foucault (1979, 1982) on individualisation and population construction.

26 I argue below that nurses sometimes had competing definitions.

27 In personal work the patient's authority on definition of self was at stake. Personal work involved violation of ordinary

social relations, occasioning the sort of expressive 'face work' illustrated by the student's apology (cf. Goffman, 1967).

28 See Foucault (1982) on 'pastoral power'. The 'recovery of strays', may be interpreted as a form of 'pastoral power'.

29 See Altschul (1972) on 'the ward at the time'.

30 Thus Nurse Jean recalled having admitted P7. N: 'I'm just even thinking on the night she was admitted she didn't come in till about ten to nine. So again, obviously your agenda's a, different things, you want to reassure them, get all the information, get all your paperwork...convey things to the night shift. So I, really had to kind of say to her, "Here is the agenda.."' R: 'Mnhmn.' N: '"I I don't have much time for you.."' R: 'Mnhmn.' N: '(laughs) "with you.."' R: 'Yeah'. N: 'not "for you"'. R: 'Yeah'. N: 'You know, but being as apologetic as possible, I I put the reality to them that "I finish at such and such a time, if I don't get out, well, I won't get home, um, I'd like to spend a lot more time with you and I've got lots of questions to ask you". It immediately sets the scene that the person and the relatives have to gear themselves up...so that's what I did with her then..' (Note: Getting the patients to 'gear themselves up' can be interpreted as a metaphor for the work nurses did with patients generally: the work of enhancement of the powers of the patient as agent.)

31 A nurse noted in a second level account that the difficulty of making sense while thinking of what he had done was like the difficulty, in interaction with the patient, of paying attention to what was being said and his own feelings while trying to direct the conversation. This may be seen as a counterpart to the problematic of participant observation.

32 See below for analysis of 'opportunities'.

33 A student nurse highlighted the problems: 'A problem which, em, I think maybe nurses aren't so aware of, like, things which are incidental to the conversation like, if another patient passes, and even if they're just saying "Hello" or, if you've maybe turned to say "Hello" to them, em, I know that whilst I was talking with P2 I, I did that in fact with one patient, a "Hello", which maybe, throws the patient that you're speaking to off, off their train of thought or whatever, or, makes them (laughs) maybe even feel secondary, like you're not giving them their full attention.'

34 Harré (1979) emphasised that accounts 'smooth rough passages in social life'. My conclusion based on the empirical data is that

accounts given by patients to nurses could be two-edged. Giving an account that was judged inappropriate could roughen the interaction and occasion further work by the patient to repair the social reality. See Foucault (1979) on 'moral accounting'.

35 See Foucault (1979) on 'examination' in the 'disciplines'.

36 I have focused on the history of interaction between these patients and nurses. This monograph does not address the question of the place of this interaction in the history of interaction in psychiatric hospitals. The 'archaeology' of practices, and interpretations of power and respect in psychiatric institutions are topics in Goffman (1962), Foucault (1971) and Scull (1982).

37 I am interpreting assessment in terms of doing for the other what the other would do for self, in matters of health and illness, if she had the 'necessary strength, will or knowledge' (Henderson, 1966). However, the issue of what is meant by 'health' or 'illness' is not addressed here.

38 The patient's age has been changed to preserve confidentiality. She was elderly.

39 The nurse had noted earlier in the account that the staff had debated how much of the patient's problems was due to her 'histrionic' character, and how much to the physical consequences of medication changes.

40 Compare this analysis to that in Inoue (1980).

41 See Atkinson (1977) on the 'clinical gaze'.

42 This was based on the nurse's command of the facilities (including rhetoric) of assessment and the institutionalised practices of accounting.

43 The nurse acknowledged elsewhere that patients could set the agenda by 'demanding'.

44 A student highlighted the limits on her power to act with a patient: 'But um, often you feel like, you're passing the buck, but, because you're a student, you're gonna really get, well not slammed for it, but, it's not going to be appreciated if you just go ahead and, and make, authority decisions.'

45 Other nurse researchers' accounts can be construed as having pointed to nurses' failure to provide to patients opportunities for display (assessment) or development (treatment) of powers.

46 See Nurse Jean, above.

47 I have noted that nurses accepted that different nurses 'read' patients differently, an implication being that some would see 'opportunities' others missed.

48 Note Site Two accounts of nurses' 'availability'.
49 See above the discussion of Harré and Secord's (1972) conceptualisation of agency and patienthood in terms of accounts.
50 It was also related to whether the consultant told the patient to 'talk to the nurses'. In Site One, a member of staff asked the consultant to tell patients what the staff member did and what the patient's responsibilities to the staff member were, because the consultant 'was seen as the authority'. In Site Two, a consultant told a patient that his (the consultant's) job was to tell the patient what to do to get better, and hers was to do it.
51 See Appendix 7.
52 The concepts 'guide' and 'support', for example, could meaningfully be used to describe aspects of parent-child relationship.
53 'Every objective must contain in itself the germ of action' (Stanislavski, 1980, p. 123).
54 'A grain of truth must be planted under the falsehood, eventually to supplant it, as a child's second set of teeth pushes out the first' (Stanislavski, 1980, p. 131)
55 Stanislavski (1980, p. 114)
56 The dilemmatic and ambiguous aspects of the metaphors which informed the 'working relationships' may have reflected nurses' ambivalence with regard to the exercise of power (cf. May and Kelly, 1982). The central ambiguity and ambivalence inhered in nurses' work with patients whom they construed as having the will, not to work, but rather to remain dependent.
The nurses legitimated limiting dependence by arguing that the patients had to be returned to the community. Submerged in this claim was another: that the patient had to be returned to the community because the nurses, and the sites as admission wards, would not accept her dependence. The nurses sometimes reified through use of metaphors their role in management decisions in face to face interaction involving exercise of power. Whether the ward was the right place for the patient, and whether the patient had a right to be in a place, were questions negotiated in face to face interaction, from positions of unequal power.
57 The lines that follow this - 'Who should decide what a nurse should do in relation to the patient's ability to participate or his lacks in skills required for building a democratic society'? (Peplau, 1952, p. 240) - should be kept in mind in this and later

discussions of the 'politics' of self and society in nursing practice. While Peplau's discourse is rooted in broader American discourses of her time, the theme of micropolitical action is relevant today.

58 Towell (1975) analysed differences in psychiatric nursing as practised in wards with different psychiatric ideologies. He found that in a therapeutic community ward nurses' judgements of patients' responsibility were mediated by ascription of 'illness'. In the therapeutic community patients were held to be responsible for their problems. My analysis of the data of this study likewise indicated that judgement of 'illness' was reflexively related to ascription of responsibility and treatment; 'really ill' constituting the basis for ascription of non-responsibility when the making of an illness/problems distinction was problematic. However, my data also suggest that in both sites the nurses' practice was not based, at least explicitly, on diagnosis; beyond the practical distinction of 'psychotic' and 'non-psychotic'. This conclusion might have been altered with fuller analysis of the nurses' use of concepts like 'histrionic'. In addition, my data indicate more overt and covert differences in interpretation and practice, more competing definitions of the patient and practices based on them, among nurses and between nurses and other staff than were indicated in Towell's study. The concept 'responsibility' enabled the nurses to manage varied and sometimes competing strategies.

59 This will be discussed more fully in Chapter 8.

60 One consequence of the method of this study was there could be a competing last word to me, as in the case of a patient who told me what she could have said to the nurses, but did not say to them because she did not want to create problems prior to discharge. The effect of what she said was to recast the reality constructed through previous accounts by nurses. The final version of the conflict lay with me.

61 Nurses and patients were interdependent in that the authority of each depended on legitimation by the other (cf. May and Kelly, 1982).

62 Peplau (1952) understood that claims of agency related to patients' use of pronouns ('I', 'we') to claim or deny agency. My analysis suggests a further development of Peplau's insight: namely, that by claiming the patient-as-subject ('I' in the patient's discourse) as subject (topic in the nurse's discourse), the nurse managed the appearance of himself as an accountable

subject. He did so by managing the appearance of the patient through command of the discourse.

63 Regarding the patient's 'panic attack' disturbing other, see Bott (1976); Towell (1975); and Goffman (1967) on the relationship between mental illness and violations of social order.

64 Note: by 'it' may be meant, the problem, illness or otherwise defined focus of defined work.

65 Accounts of non-responsibility ('she doesn't know herself') were given for other patients.

66 The nurse's view of the deeper reality was of a kind of dynamic process: 'That (Note: the marital problem) seems to be the, the energy, comes from that, and just, putting the anxiety off to, things in the environment on a general not-coping basis.'.

67 The nurses resisted patients' attempts to impose a service role on them. Injunctions not to treat the sites like hotels or holiday camps served this function, as did disparagement of 'bed and breakfast' patients (who were admitted by duty doctors on Friday nights and discharged on Monday mornings). They resisted it most strongly by expressing the ideology of work and responsibility.

68 Harré's commonsense typification of 'not wanting' is 'bloody mindedness'.

69 See Pollock (1989) on psychiatric nurses' management of appearances.

70 The discourse of the first nurse can be read as an account of the patient's resistance to the nurses' 'pastoral power' (Foucault, 1982) through which she would have been subjected, or would have subjected herself, to the truth of herself as an individual.

71 I will discuss in Chapter 7 the concept of 'time' as the currency of respect. The availability of time was linked to the patient's willingness to take the offered opportunity to work. S2P5 noted that the nurses did not 'push', but let her do things in her 'own time'. Claims of work and command of rights in the territories of site and self were expressed in terms of time.

72 In general, the nurses had the last public word. However, in Site Two, the consultant occasionally elicited from the patient an account of conflict with nurses, and provided a mediating account.

73 The 'demand' was based on obligation to respond, rather than on force (see Hochschild, 1983, on different family control systems, which correspond to styles of getting people to manage their feelings).

7 Moral order, or 'the kind of person' and 'taking the right attitude'

Introduction: accounts, accounting and accountable subjects

In Chapter 5 I used the empirical data - in particular accounts construed as devices for accomplishing intelligibility - to describe and explore the interaction of the nurses and neurotic patients in terms of knowledge, 'the main thing'. In Chapter 6 I construed their accounting practices in terms of the 'working relationships' through which they acted on each others' action.

In those chapters I described the complexity of negotiating common frames of meaning and coordinating action. In this chapter I will use the data to explore and describe the nurses' and patients' interaction as participation in moral orders. In doing so I will emphasise the role played by accounts in ordering action, and in warranting and legitimising views of the world and ways of being and acting in it. In particular I will address how some people are accorded lower cognitive status and rights to act. I follow Harré's (1983, p. 245) criteria for identifying a moral order when among a group of people: there are rituals for 'public marking of respect and contempt'; actions, including practical ones, are 'treated as displays of character'; actions are accompanied by talk in which 'interpretations and warrants of what is going on can be negotiated'; 'rituals, confirmations of respect and contempt and displays of proper character and moral commentary - are permitted only to those who in this or that collective, have the right to perform them'. I will therefore be examining how certain ways of thinking and acting in the two sites were accorded respect or contempt, and discuss the moral commentary that accompanied or followed those shows.

Two of the nurses' first order constructs conveyed the most important aspects of the interaction as it related to moral order: 'the kind of person you are' and 'taking the right attitude'. Through this discussion I will show how people got to be known as the 'kinds of people they are' and how the 'attitude' taken toward them was legitimated as 'right' and, thus legitimated, ordered action. I will highlight the reflexive play between 'the kind of person' and 'the attitude taken toward them'.

In interpreting the interaction as moral order, I interpreted nurses' responses to the question 'Why is she here now?' which were couched in terms of 'the kind of person (including patient/agent) the patient is'; and responses to 'What do we have to do for her?' which were couched in terms of taking 'the right attitude' toward the patient. Producing accounts 'as if' in response to these questions was work done in the sites on behalf of the wider community. The accounts were occasioned by something that had happened in the community that had 'brought the patient to the door'. In doing this work the nurses and other workers interpreted the patient's character or being in the context of a moral order. The act of interpretation reflexively reconstituted the legitimacy of the moral order. In acting to recover 'strays', to return patients to the paramount reality of the community, the nurses reflexively realised a moral order in which both were accountable subjects: they put 'everything in its place' (Berger and Luckmann, 1967).[1]

The moral order in Site One

I will compare and contrast the moral order in Site One with that in Site Two by discussing the distribution of rights to moral judgement and commentary (Harré, 1983) in relation to a situation referred to in Chapter 5. Nurses and patients in Site One knew that it was wrong to talk about a patient in a meeting if the patient was not there. This 'rule' was, however, suspended on occasions when the patient's behaviour had occasioned her absence. Then nurses in a community meeting sought some common understanding of what the patient and nurses were doing, and how to understand and judge it.

On one occasion, S1P6 - nominated as suitable for the study, though she declined to participate - was present but resolutely unresponsive when the nurses took the extraordinary tack of discussing her in front of the other patients. P6 had been verbally and physically abusive toward staff. The question the nurses posed to the group of nurses and patients was whether P6 was 'putting it on' or whether she was 'really ill'. In asking the patients what they thought, the nurses revealed the distribution of rights to moral judgement and commentary. In asking, they presented themselves as accountable in advance, to the patients, for action which might otherwise have appeared unwarranted; namely, treating P6 as responsible for her actions. Secondly, they enlisted ordinary judgement in assessing her and determining whether to hold her accountable.

This episode illustrated two aspects related to the centrality of moral evaluation in nursing these patients. The nurses could not act accountably without a judgement of responsibility (cf. Parsons, 1951). Responses to the questions 'Why is she here now?' and 'What do we have to do for her?' were responses dependent on judgements of responsibility. Moreover, nurses acknowledged that they did not have a monopoly on judgement of responsibility. The context for moral action was not supplied, in this case, by 'professional' knowledge alone. The professionals reached across to ordinary judgement to find the authority for what they were doing (cf. Hughes, 1980).

The judgement concerned the intentionality of P6's action. The nurses could not act appropriately without knowing what kind of person P6 was - agent or patient. The ritual concluded when a nurse asked P6, who had remained mute and impassive throughout the enquiry into her actions, 'I wonder what you think, P6?'. P6's reply - 'Who's P6?' - transformed the tension to laughter, due, according to my interpretation, to her having succeeded in using the occasion to reproduce the problem, by defining herself, in two words, as responsible and non-responsible.

Talk was the occasion for appearance of the actor in the symbolic order. In talk one subjected ('I') oneself and was subjected to the moral order as a moral subject. Language was the medium for locating others, and relating to others, in the moral order. It provided, in pronouns and other indexical particulars, the devices for attaching to persons the consequences of judgement; hence the struggles over whether 'I' or 'it' was responsible. The nurses' and patients' work in this meeting was to hold accountable the person located by the name 'P6' and by 'I' as spoken by P6. P6's talk countered that move.

The nurses asked the patients whether, in their view, P6 was 'ill' or, instead, knew what she was doing. This was a complex action on the part of the nurses. It was, explicitly, a move to get the patients and nurses to show P6 how they saw her. By asking, the nurses also implied that 'nursing' judgement overlapped ordinary moral judgement, specifically concerning questions of whether the patient was a person who knew what she was doing and could therefore be held accountable for her actions. On other occasions, too, the nurses in Site One elicited the patients' views on aspects of what could have been considered 'professional' judgement. The implication was that judgement of intention was not, at least in some cases, a matter of expert decision only. There was thus in Site One an implication that, though the right and obligation to make judgements on intention - to make them stick and to act accordingly - was generally accorded to the nurses; in difficult situations the nurses and other professionals were obliged to take into account, if not accept, the patients' judgements. The limits of professional judgement were negotiated with the patients in practice (cf. Webb, 1981, on 'framing').

By asking the patients, the nurses acknowledged that professional judgement had its home in the wider community of ordinary judgement. Reflexively they established that community in the professional mental health setting. The contexts of judgement were bridged (or breached, from the point of view of the resisting patients) through the shared (professional and ordinary) understanding that a judgement of 'illness' rested on judgements of responsibility and agency. I have indicated at several points in this monograph that the problem of determination of 'illness' was complex. In resolving particularly problematic cases, nurses as well as medical staff used all the knowledge to hand to make a judgement (Hughes, 1988a).

The patients appeared irritated at being involved in such a judgement, one saying that the nurses should know whether P6 was ill.[2] The nurses used the meeting to provide a context for judgement on P6. Their doing so may have been strategic, in that they had to act toward P6 in ways that might have appeared unkind, had she been judged 'ill' and therefore not responsible (cf. Hughes, 1962, on 'dirty work'[3]) . Had they not accounted in advance they could have been judged by the patients to have acted unfairly or unwisely.

The work of the sites generated problems of determining responsibility through the incessant giving and getting of accounts. From this perspective, the work of the site could be regarded as the definition of moral order on behalf of the community 'outside' as well as in the wards. The question posed by the nurses was whether

P6 could be regarded as part of the community, treated as competent to give an account of herself; and whether the community could be regarded as competent to give an account of her.

Places in the moral order were thus realised and negotiated in practice, and the order defined in practice. Though P6's case was exceptional in Site One, the sharing of views that a patient was 'ill', 'not herself', and so on, was not unusual. That is, while the constitution of a 'court' of judgement on P6 was unusual, nurses and patients in Site One often referred to issues of agency and responsibility. They did so because these issues appeared as practical problems of sharing the site: with someone who stripped off, or broke windows, or refused to eat. In Site Two, such matters were rarely discussed with patients in the community meeting.[4]

The appeal to the patients reflected features of Site One which distinguished it from Site Two. When nurses in Site One told me that the patients knew what was really going on at any given time, and that they therefore watched or asked the patients when they could not get a feel of the place, they made a point about both the distribution of knowledge and the moral orders in the site. If the patients could really know as well as or better than the nurses, then in problematic situations the nurses incurred an obligation to ask the patients. The reality of the sites was, practically, a moral reality reflexively structured by judgement.

Justification and excuse

The case of P6 can be interpreted as a case of exceptional accounting occasioned by P6's behaviour. The nurses asked the patients if there was a valid basis for excuse - was she ill? They could also be seen as preparing a justification of their own action in response. They used the meeting to define the moral context of action, to 'tell the code' (Wieder, 1974) of the site. Telling the code defined the moral order and at the same time constituted an enforceable claim. In another meeting, a patient who was 'really ill' spat on the floor and was told by a nurse 'you wouldn't do that at home'. Telling the code called on others to enforce it. This was the case with P6. Implicit in telling the code was a claim that the right to be in the site ordered by the code was contingent (to an undetermined extent) on abiding by the code.[5]

The case exemplifies an important feature of moral order. In explaining, excusing and justifying their action to each other and with each other the patients and nurses defined, maintained and repaired the moral order by locating responsibility for action which violated it, including failures to honour rights and obligations. In locating violations of the moral orders inside and outside the sites the nurses played their parts in defining the moral orders, legitimating the realities sustained by compliance to the moral order. They did so in order to establish their claims to respect in the moral orders they inhabited and constituted. But in doing so they also played their parts in the work of the sites. That is, they played their parts in defining 'Why is she (am I) here now?' and 'What do we have to do for her (am I to do)?'.

There were two aspects to taking the right attitude. The nurses showed that they were taking the right attitude toward P6 by interpreting her explicitly as a responsible moral being, regardless of what specific judgement and attitude they took. They also needed to take the right attitude toward her in order to treat her appropriately ('treat' implying moral treatment as well as 'therapy'). The excuses and justifications the nurses negotiated were meaningful, had their effect in the moral order they reflexively constituted. That moral order was constituted by themselves and the patients in the process of requiring and giving excuses and justifications.

That the patients were irritated suggested that the nurses' action was differently interpretable. By implication, the moral order was not monolithic or monological. In the moral order, rights to require accounts and to excuse and justify were asymmetrically distributed: the patients could not have initiated such a meeting; and in the end the formal judgement on illness, with consequences for psychiatric management, had to rest with the staff. As I will argue below, this distribution was not static but subject to tensions.

The meeting did not take place in a vacuum. The process of moral judgement also occurred in meetings with the medical staff and occupational therapist, and among nurses afterwards. The meeting was a moment in a process of definition of P6 as a moral subject. The process of social judgement was not accomplished by a single nurse as a single moral being. Rather it was a social act in a social setting which, as part of a dynamic process, it reflexively defined.[6]

I will summarise some general points on the basis of this example. Firstly, 'work' on P6 was considered 'called for' because she was held to have violated the moral order in the site. The violations were cited as wrongs, reflexively defining the code of the moral order - 'don't abuse the nurses, not only because they are nurses but because they are ordinary people who do not like being sworn at or punched'. (If 'really ill' a patient could be excused breach of the rule.) The nurses ordered the work of the site to deal with the violations. The work based on the code involved negotiating a definition of the actions and the actor in terms of the moral order, defining occasions for excuse or legitimation. In the moral order, the terms for the actor ('ill', 'not ill') were used by those with the rights and obligations to use them. Use of the terms occasioned moral reasoning ('she wouldn't do it if there weren't something wrong'). In the work the nurses and patients defined the patient as a moral being by coordinating a point of view toward her, an attitude. This provided a working definition of her as a moral being toward whom certain actions could legitimately be taken. It therefore legitimated further work: by the group, to get P6 to see that what she was doing was wrong; and by the nurses, to deal with her aggression, possibly through prompting discharge. The categorisation of P6 thus implied roles for workers in the moral order. The allocation of warranted work was based on warranted work: P6 had to be judged in the appropriate way and treated as if capable of responding as a moral agent before a decision could be made to treat her otherwise. Thus, warranted nursing action in Site One involved knowledge of types of people as interpreted in the common moral order, and the power to order moral work. The work produced knowledge of types of people and ordered further work.

Individual moral work in Site One

These features of moral order were also found through analysis of interaction between individual nurses and patients in Site One. Thus when S1P2 had a difficult weekend before discharge, blaming her drugs, an experienced nurse interpreted her action using the concepts 'dependence' and 'institutionalisation':

> N: What I'm thinking is, sh-, she had been at home, right, she'd had, a bad pass, and that she'd come back and, she was talking about suicide and couldn't cope, things like that, and it had been discussed, and, we decided (?) it was a lot to do with P4 being institutionalised and, dependent on the ward, and that(?), what she needed was, a wee bit shook up, (? you know), for us to take, for her not to be so dependent on us.

Seeing P2 as a 'kind of person' in categories meaningful in the moral order of the site, the nurse could legitimate taking a 'tough line' (see chapter 6). Taking the 'tough line' was further legitimated by reference to the need to get her back to the community. The nurse 'ordered' P2's action in compliance not only with the moral order of the site but also with the moral order negotiated with the family, and more broadly with an implicit order recognised in the wider community:

> N: I (? really) said to her that, you know, the drugs (? just) (? didn't) have anything to do with it. It was just up to her, how her passes went, and, eh, in **her** (?) she did at home, it transpired that, (?), other things were, like her husband who had been used to, coping in the house with the two young kids, had set up a routine...and with P4 coming home, he couldn't cope with her, you know, (?), she couldn't cope with him, (?) criticising...Sh-, she didn't, go into that much depth, but what, how it came over was, eh, you know, she said Uh, "Mike looks at things different from how I do at home." Em...He gave her a row about breakfast and, (?), things like that, right?
>
> R: Aye.
>
> N: And th-, and that's the way I took it and I , you know I says (?) Well I (? broke it down) to how **I** saw it, and she agreed with it, (? in or ? it was) that way...And eh, (?), to **her**, she hadn't really been a mother, or a wife for, over a year. And, the guy had had to take over these roles...So, in a **way** I was giving them (? maybe), construc-, constructive criticism..

The order of the patient's home had been threatened through her admission and return home, and the nurse acted to facilitate restoration, through 'constructive criticism'. She used forms of rhetoric, persuasion, casting P2 in the role of agent, asking her to 'try hard'. The nurse warranted her action ('right') through appeal to a common recognition of common problems and their remedies:

> N: (? But), (? the way I had) worked out how the weekend had gone was, yeah, collectively it was (?) (? decided) at the Kardex that P2 was coming up for discharge...(?). Em, (? actually) the (?) of it was the fact that, although that probably was a big issue, a smaller issue had been that Mike had nagged her (?)...Yeah, that, there's not, there wasn't very much I could do about, her coming up for discharge...Em, but I could do some-, I could offer her some suggestions towards, coping with, eh,(?)...her attitude to (?) her husband and (?),..which, which (? she took), you know, (?), she, she had a (?), (?), the only way we could really (? do anything about it) was to put her back on pass and

> (? see how) she coped...I just kept reinforcing (?) about the relationship with her hubby, em, but, I put that in too because, her husband tried (? really hard), eh, to (? get back) with P2, but she, being so immature, eh, he had to, he had to sort of guide her...(?), she was the type of person you had to, had to guide. If you im-implanted a suggestion, it would grow (? for a wee while) sort of thing, so, so I was, (?) implanting the fact that she had (?), (? responsibility?) (?), it couldn't just be all one sided, um, she couldn't take everything from her husband, she had to give also, eh, so I was sowing a wee seed..So eh, (? you know) she took that, says 'Oh yeah yeah', sort of thing. So she was the right type of person, but that was (? the) individual, you know, that, that (?) individual thing.

The nurse worked within an order of work structured by rights and obligations - unable to affect discharge, she worked on marital problems. She established P2's obligation to cope. She worked on the basis of her view of the 'type of person' P2 was, with implicit rights and responsibilities in the marriage, and legitimated her own action on the basis of that. The action was ordered through definition of P2's place in the moral orders of home and hospital, and reflexively reproduced the order: moving P2 back to home, to the paramount reality. Throughout, the action was warranted by 'the way things are'. Through the work P2 was called on to treat herself as the kind of person she was seen to be, to take the common attitude toward herself. P2 did take this attitude toward herself, sharing the metaphor of 'weaning' from the ward, expressing her 'responsibility'.[7]

Work, the moral order and emotion

I have thus argued that nurses and patients structured and legitimated their work, ensuring its intelligibility and warrantability in the moral orders they reflexively defined. The 'moral work' of these patients and nurses was not 'extra', or 'about' the 'real work': in many cases it was the real work. P2 was called upon to manage her feelings at home. She was also given help with caring for her children and with re-learning how to cook. All of that was interpretable as action in the moral order, structured to 'guide' her back to her place.

Admission and subsequent moral work for P2, as for most of the patients in this study, had been occasioned by some experience of and display of emotion coupled with inability to act socially accountably, some 'personal state' interpreted as problematic in the moral orders of home and community. The interpretation of emotion as a moral phenomenon was described by Harré (1983, p. 257):

> By the presentation of self in public one creates one's social being. One's personal being is the product of appropriations and transformations of social resources...For example, emotions are not feelings, but interpretations of personal states, *within a moral order*. (Note: italics in original.)

On a day to day basis the nurses and patients in Site One interpreted personal states as emotions and provided or failed to provide relief on the basis of the interpretations.[8] Legitimations which had been available to P2 in the past were now withheld. P2's 'personal state' was now interpreted as due to excessive 'dependence' and a 'line' that might have appeared harsh in the past was now warranted.

Different nurses interpreted different patients' states in different ways and responded in what they took to be the appropriate way. A student nurse's account of S1P5's distress can be found in Appendix 9. The student responded to P5 in the moral order they constituted in a side room. P5 had been placed in the side room because, in the view of trained nurses, her displays of emotion were 'attention seeking' and she was disturbing the other patients. Her having been put there could be interpreted in terms of her violation of norms embodied in the maxim (see Chapter 5) 'keep the place anxiety free'. Reference to her excessive 'demands' legitimated her being 'managed' through placement in a room away from others.

The relationship between work and interpretation of emotion in the moral order was reflexive. The more senior members of the nursing staff recorded, as evidence of 'attention seeking', their observation that P5's cries grew louder as they approached; while the student nurse interpreted the distressing crescendo as evidence of P5's need for emotional release. Each legitimated action toward P5 in a different moral order.

I have noted that in Site One patients' and nurses' interpretations of the warrantability of action, their interpretations of the action in a moral order, sometimes coincided and sometimes differed (see Chapter 6).

The moral order in Site Two

I will follow the theme of the previous section, interpretation of personal states as emotions, in using the example of S2P4 to describe and explain aspects of the moral order(s) in Site Two. I presented at the end of Chapter 6 an experienced nurse's account of S2P4's stay (see Appendix 7). In that account can be read features of the structure of rights and obligations related to interaction with the patients in this study. (Another account which may be read for further explication of the same argument is presented in Appendix 8.) The moral order of work in Site Two centred on establishing the basis of the appropriate working relationship with the right professional. The institution offered services which the patient was expected to use in doing 'work' (cf. Stacey, 1976, on patients as 'work objects' and 'service objects'). The patient's obligations to cooperate in treatment were explicit, and unwillingness to 'work' constituted grounds for withdrawing help (cf. Parsons, 1951). Patients who had been offered services and had rejected them were construed as 'hiding'. The moral order was structured around the rights and obligations of patients and staff in provision and use of appropriate professional services. The obligation on the part of the staff to offer active help existed only as long as there was a prospect that they could 'go' somewhere with the patient. If she 'stopped' them, it was legitimate to 'just support'. The medical staff had the power to dispose of cases through discharge, re-referral or demotion to voluntary services (see Appendix 8).

Some background information frames the excerpts to follow, which will be interpreted in terms of control, power and legitimation. The excerpts highlight that through becoming a patient, one became subject to social control of everyday activities. One's time and activity could be ordered by others, and the ordering legitimated as 'work', 'therapy', the 'programme'.

S2P4 had asked the nurses if she could leave the ward early, complaining that she was anxious at not having enough time to get to a wedding. The nurses refused on the grounds that she was obliged to attend a meeting. She complained that staying back another hour would make her more anxious. The nurses refused to accept that this delay could account for her anxiety. A trained nurse knew, because she came from the same area, how long it would take to get to the wedding. She said:

> N: I told my colleagues, and...they were of the impression too, that, there was **more** to it than just the fact, that she wasn't

getting, away early,...she was, **overly** upset over, such a, seemingly (sniggers) trivial fact.

....

N: what we were trying to do? Trying to get her to, to **recognise**, the fact her, her worries (?), that, there's, there is nothing **wrong** to be, in being **worried**, or apprehensive, about what she was, (? about face), although it was a happy occasion, being a wedding, uh, but e-, even I think for **most** people, large gatherings, weddings, parties, it can sometimes be, quite nerve wracking, for a lot of people, it can, and there's nothing, wrong with a-, admitting it. Trying to focus in, on, what it was.

Through use of the terms 'wrong' and 'trivial' the nurse established a context of justification, namely that of the paramount reality. P4 was called on to recognise the paramount reality including the interpretation of her in the paramount reality, with its implications for action in the moral order.

In their interaction with patients the nurses judged whether the patients' emotions were appropriate in degree or kind,[9] or whether they constituted violations of public order. They interpreted the personal states in a moral context founded on the paramount reality. The event as understood by the nurse did not account for the patient's feeling. In face to face interaction P4 had failed to constitute with the nurse a moral order in which her personal state was interpretable as appropriate; had failed to interpret reality competently. In the absence of a valid account of the reason for her personal state, P4's feeling did not justify her missing a meeting. Judgement of inappropriateness was based on the nurse's construction of reality, grounded in an appeal to common sense[10] rather than the patient's sense.

I highlighted in Chapter 5 that there were different frames of meaning in the sites - 'ordinary talk' and 'illness or problem talk' - with the frame 'work' 'commanding' the two. In Chapter 6, I emphasised that the 'command' of the frame of meaning 'work' was never absolute, that patients could 'rebel' or defend themselves against the demands of 'work'; that is, against interpretation and the consequences of interpretation in a frame of meaning. Among the consequences were those due to the fact that interpretation took place in and had consequences in a moral order. I noted that the nurses and patients knew that every action could be observed and interpreted in one or more moral orders: as 'illness', 'problem', or 'ordinary life'. The work done on 'illness' and 'problems' was work occasioned by interpretation of 'simple facts' in a moral order: the act of recognising tearfulness as depression and legitimating relief from responsibilities. In the nursing of these patients the activities that were interpreted in moral contexts included: showering, washing, buying clothes, cooking, managing marital conflict, relationships with children and parents, paying bills, fighting, decorating Christmas trees, eating meals. In short, everything related to daily life was potentially available for moral consideration (cf. Bloor and Fonkert, 1982; Bloor and McIntosh, 1987; Chapman, 1987).

The fact that the same action could be interpreted in different frames with different consequences meant that the 'right' frame had to be applied, to ensure order. Hence, the right to interpret and to impose interpretations was of central importance. In difficult cases the nurses (and in some instances doctors) relied on understandings rooted in the common moral order of everyday life. The case of P4 illustrates how that right was allocated and negotiated in Site Two.

The interpretive process was never-ending, and further interpretation was predicated on perception of the already interpreted moral action and actor. The nurse did not warrant P4's reason, and required instead a different interpretation, some reason for the patient's irritation and anger, something 'more'. Interpretation of this case is complex because, according to this analysis of the accounts, the actors were interpreting each other on the basis of past interpretations. The further interpretation the nurse sought was an ordinary explanation, on the basis of which P4 could have been regarded as an ordinary actor upholding the primary reality: 'most people would feel anxious' because of the size of the gathering.

However, P4 thought she was being interpreted and being required to interpret herself in terms of the frame of 'problems'. The 'simple fact' was rendered complex through interpretation in the moral orders of the sites. In her account P4 claimed that she had been anxious:

> P: Uh, so Nurse Donna knew how long it took to get to this town, and she tried to persuade me to, not to be upset and, she felt I was, because I was so upset she, I think she felt I was, there's something I haven't told them, that I was hiding, I was using this as an excuse for my tears, and I, I quite honestly I did, the doctor knows this, I, I had diarrhoea and I **was** sick, it, affected me so badly. Um, Donna did say, that she felt, all this

was because, there was another reason why I was fright-, why I didn't want to go out there, you know, and, I just tried to convince her there wasn't, because there honestly wasn't, I, you can't hide very much in here...But I found Donna, I felt she was being a wee bit cruel to be kind the way she spoke to me, but I, I very much appreciate it now.

and repeated the point:

P: I really did have diarrhoea (?)

P4 interpreted the nurse's questions, construing them as a charge that P4 was 'hiding', that she hid 'another reason'. P4 attempted justification by appeal to the higher authority of the doctor and the reality of her diarrhoea. In later accounts she emphasised that she had thought over and over again, to see if there was another reason; and she implied that she may have thought that the nurses thought that 'the reason' might have related to marital conflict, which she denied (to them and in the account). The point I am making on the basis of these accounts is that interaction in a moral context was part of a continuous process of interpretation, carried on between nurses and patients; and by the patient herself, treating herself as the kind of person she thought she was construed as by the nurses.[11]

Another experienced member of the nursing staff gave her account of this episode:

N: We had persuaded P4 to attend the support group and then go through to, to uh, Glasgow, after the support group, which still gave her plenty of time...And, when we got to the support group, in fact, P4 still had some anxiety, 'churning in her stomach' as she called it, but, was saying how, she would in fact at that point in, on the Friday afternoon, might have been quite happy if somebody had told her not to go at all. So I think this sort of indicating her, ambivalence or her, her desire to be told what to do...

R: Right. Um, and, she was saying she, had to go early, in order to ge- to get there, earlier than..

N: In, in in order to get herself settled down, she was afraid she would have nausea and diarrhoea, as she's had the weekend before. And it was actual, literal diarrhoea and nausea, vomiting that she had had the weekend before. I think she said she, that she vomited, on the Friday morning, prior to the support group, but there was no, more symptoms than that.

But there were times that she looked quite tense, and almost a bit hostile I thought.

R: Mnhmn. And um, you were saying, that it would be better to stay, till the support group..

N: Well the reason for staying for the support group would (?be) that it's, is a group where we would expect people to have a sort of ongoing commitment, to the group, and to the oth-, other group members in the group, being quite a small group.

Interpretations and warrants were required at every point. The reality of diarrhoea had to be affirmed. This nurse interpreted P4 as a 'kind of person' (one with a 'desire to be told what to do') and a patient (who had obligations based on the 'programme'). Participation in the moral order entailed numerous rights and obligations, some of which conflicted: those related to 'getting herself calmed down' and those of 'commitment to the group'. In face to face interaction the conflicts occasioned by the patient's participation in the moral order were realised: they were the subject of ensuing interaction and accounts. In these ways the nurses and P4 sustained the social reality of each other's responsibility.

The rights and obligations of nurses and of patients were different. The nurses could oblige P4 to stay; their apology was discretionary. In their accounts, patients judged, excused and justified the nurses, reasoning about their own and sometimes the nurses' emotions in a moral context. P4 concluded that the nurses were being 'cruel to be kind':

P: (Note: name of one of the nurses) actually thanked me for staying on, which said a lot for her, and, I was quite honest as well, I said that, Well I had stayed on but I did admit that I was, very upset and I was quite angry **at** Phyl, so I told her that...So I, I feel the air was cleared a bit and, I'm glad I did get on OK and, everything's back to normal again. With the staff, not that they were, they possibly were angry with me as well, and thought I was being, acting a bit **young** for my age, but, it's just it was pure emotion and excitement.

This set of accounts highlights the complexity of the processes of interpretation in a moral order in which claims about 'trivial facts' and 'pure emotions' were moral claims subject to dispute. In Site Two the interaction of the nurses and patients was characterised by the nurses requiring the patients to give reasons. The nurses interpellated them into a moral order based on a discourse of individual responsibility, in which they (the nurses) claimed greater power to interpret and warrant reasons.

The conduct of the nurse in the moral order based on responsibility

Through rhetoric - appeal for the recognition of a 'trivial fact', and by implication, the triviality of the judgement that considered the fact significant - the trained nurse worked to persuade others and me to share her judgement, to participate in a common sense not (at least initially) shared by P4. Thus these excerpts can be interpreted in terms of the relationships between knowledge, power and moral order. In the paramount reality there was an implicit claim that the nurses could know P4's emotions better than P4 herself did because they had the knowledge, power and right to interpret her feeling in a moral order they maintained. P4's reasons, and by implication her reason, were treated as less worthy of respect. The questions about her reason arose in interaction but were re-presented for judgement through the nurse's rhetorical account.

Implicit in the conflict over interpretations were issues related to power. The nurses required that P4 manage her emotions in order to act like the others acted; to be the same 'kind of person' as the rest, for the practical purposes of the site, and to take the same attitude toward herself as others did (cf. Hochschild, 1983). P4 faced the problem of maintaining and repairing her subjective reality - feelings, emotions and the fact that 'it was diarrhoea' - in a context in which she was required to manage feelings in order to act appropriately. What was at stake in the interaction was reality - what really was making her nervous - and the question of whose reality P4 would have to act in, in order to gain respect and avoid contempt. In the accounts, claims about self and reality were inextricably linked.[12] The struggle was essentially moral, about what sort of people oneself and the others were. In that struggle the facilities of power, and the rights to have one's view of reality accepted, were related.

The rights and obligations related to management of emotion were related to place in moral orders. Hochschild (1983, p. 172) cites Dale on the 'doctrine of feeling': 'The lower one's status, the more one's feelings are not noticed or (sic) treated as inconsequential'. Hochschild (1983, p. 173) notes a:

> corollary of the 'doctrine of feelings': the lower our status, the more our manner of seeing and feeling is subject to being discredited, and the less believable it becomes. A person of

> lower status has a weaker claim to the right to define what is going on; less trust is placed in her judgment; and less respect is accorded to what she feels. Relatively speaking, it more often becomes the burden of women, as with other lower-status persons, to uphold a minority viewpoint, a discredited opinion.

The patients' places in moral orders had been threatened, in many cases due to their problems in managing emotions. In their accounts they related 'being here' to their failure to control their 'states' or 'moods'. These states and moods were linked to their obligation to participate in the moral orders of the sites; entailing, in Site Two, deliberation on reasons for the emotional states.

The nurses relied on moral reasoning to structure the reality in which they defined their working relationships. Central to this description of reality was the allocation of responsibility: 'can't do or won't do?' and 'need help or want help?'. S2P2's claim that she 'needed' the nurses to 'trigger' her because she could not think for herself yet because she was still not well enough was countered in a nurse's account:

> N: ...when P2 was first in and **was** actually quite ill, she wouldn't lead a conversation, and she required a lot of prompting which, now, and from that conversation in particular she certainly didn't need.

P2's claim that her untidiness had to be excused was not accepted by the nurse:

> N: ...she seemed quite willing to lead conversation and very quickly (? for) around to 'I'm fed up being in these clothes' and I said 'I sympathise with that, because (?they of ?we) don't like to be in the same clothes all the time but at least, you don't need to have dirty clothes' and reminded her of the washing facilities.

In their work the nurses enforced the ordinary morality regarding the mundane matters of everyday life, the paramount reality (Chapman, 1987; Bloor and Fonkert, 1982). They could also be construed as maintaining the system of rights and obligations related to the 'residual categories' of work not done by other professionals.

A common theme in the moral orders: legitimation and motive

As can be seen from the above account and that of S1P6, the relationship between excuse and judgement of illness was in practice reflexive (cf. Turner, 1987; Freidson, 1970; Kelly and May, 1982; Towell, 1975; also cf. Smith, 1980, on reflexivity in the way the concept 'need' is used in social work practice). This was also the case for medical staff.[13] Patients likewise reasoned about the connection between their conduct and their illness. Indeed, moral judgement of self was part of being ill and of getting better. Thus P4 in Site Two said that she had been 'bad' lately, having outbursts, not wanting to take part in things, making excuses, saying that she was not well enough in order to get out of doing things.

The moral reasoning related to responsibility thus centred on judgements about 'because' motives and 'in order to' motives (Schutz and Luckmann, 1974).[14] The reasoning about 'in order to' motives and 'because' motives centred on questions of whether the patient's action was willed. 'Bad' was a moral judgement made by P4, based on her discovery that she could really do things, having been made to do so against her will. Previous nursing researchers concerned with 'the bad patient' (Stockwell, 1972; Kelly and May, 1982; May and Kelly, 1982) have not considered the patient's view of her own 'badness'. I am arguing that the patients were interpellated into participation in the moral order in which work was structured on the basis of decisions geared toward doing for the other who could not do for herself, and not doing for those who wanted not to do in order to rest or otherwise wrongly to claim the rights of patienthood. To 'pass through' the system of accounting which practically constituted this moral order the patient was called on to take the role of the nurses and acknowledge the good of doing for herself as she was able, and by implication the bad of not doing so.

P4 came to know what she had been doing and that she could have done otherwise. These are (McHugh, 1968) the commonsense grounds for a judgement of deviance. P4 could be seen as responding to a commonsense recognition of herself as a deviant patient by acting differently, adopting an appropriate role in the moral order of Site Two. The patient's part in the construction of her own or other patients' deviance in illustrated by P4's comments:

> P: I just feel a great load's been lifted off me and I can see now, probably a lot of my outbursts in here, because I have been quite bad, of late, just crying and I didn't want to take part in

> anything, and I've told the staff now I made excuses that, for not going to OT, I could have been there I just didn't want to go, and I said I wasn't well enough and I've been, and it's so annoying then when I hear other people, not to mention any, patients' names but, you must know the one I mean, going on and on about his past, I, I feel sorry for him, John, I mean, you have met him, I've heard this story dozens of t-, you hear it half past eleven at night, seven o'clock in the morning, goes back to when he was nineteen, if I went back to when I was nineteen, it wouldna paint a very pre-, pretty picture either probably, but it's nothing to do why, with why I'm in here. That, I admit he's, he's got nothing left, but he's still got time to, make a life for himself I think, think he quite likes it here (laughs).

The patient demonstrated her knowledge of the main moral order of the site by telling (the laugh) what was 'wrong' with another's story, as she had done with her own. What was wrong was that the patient 'wanted to be here'. His being here was motivated: it was not the case that he could not leave, but rather that he would not. The knowledge the patient and I shared was that one was not meant to like the site. If one liked it one might want to stay. The site was not the primary reality. What one had to do was get back to the paramount reality. The nurses, in enforcing a common-sense view of the patient's problems, provided a destination for the patient en route back to the paramount reality.

P4's remarks provide the grounds for considering the meaning, for different patients, of taking part in the system of commitments and accountability of patients to nurses, entailed by being a patient in the site. The meaning of interaction was its meaning as interpreted in the local community, which was a moral order. The meaning of interaction was therefore its meaning as moral action. It was also meaningful for the patient or the individual nurse in terms of the other moral orders she inhabited.[15]

By working in the paramount reality maintained by the frame of meaning 'work', the nurses ordered the moral orders of various patients and themselves, principally through determination of responsibility and motive. The work regarded as legitimate in Site Two required searches for motive, on the basis of compliance with which the patient was accorded respect or contempt. The ideology of the site thus facilitated the work of the site by ordering patients' and nurses' work. The work in Site One was based on display of character, with patients generally regarded as 'ordinary people'.[16]

Participation in this work entailed hazards whereby the patient could achieve respect only by giving up participation in reality ordered by her own devalued frame of meaning.

Through compliance with the requirements of the moral order structured through the systems of excuses and justifications, the patient mapped the paramount reality: 'I can see now'; 'I made excuses...I could have been there but I just didn't want to go'. Thus the patient's subjective and objective reality(ies) were reflexively structured through interaction mediated by interpretations in the moral order. Through a change of account a patient could change the moral reality in which she acted. The map of social reality enabled her to function because it was the map followed by others, legitimated as the map through enforcement of the moral order.

The reality mapped in the two sites could differ, according to the above analysis: being structured by reasons in Site Two, by shows of character in Site One. As I had to map the interaction of the patients and nurses as moral orders, in order to understand and take part in it, so did the nurses and patients. Just as through participation I explored the reality as mapped, so did the nurses and patients. I am suggesting, then, that the sense articulated by the nurses, regardless of its truth value, may have provided the basis for the moral deliberation and other work needed to reach with the patient a common understanding on the basis of which she could go on and be counted competent (Garfinkel, 1967).

Here, Altschul's (1972) argument can be recalled: that interaction based on nurses' 'lay understandings' may have been no less effective than what the patient had experienced before coming to the site, but was unlikely to have been better. However, that analysis omits two features I have highlighted: that what may matter is the fit, or lack of fit and possibility of negotiation of fit (Llewelyn, 1985), between nurses' and patients' understandings. Thus, what matters may be the requirement that another map be drawn, regardless of its scale or theme. Secondly, it was centrally important to understand that the sites were stages of passage between the common-sense world before and the common-sense world after the patient's stay. It may therefore be argued that insofar as the nurses founded their practice on common sense with all its contradictions, and sustained a moral order based on the legitimations of common sense, they might thereby have provided a bridging sense and legitimation to be used by patients on their returns to the community. Thus a patient worked out with his family, while on weekends home from the ward, the reasons and responsibility for his having 'been here':

> P: Well, my wife sort of feels that she was sorta responsible for my being up here. And I've, I'm gonna have to have a talk with (Note: relatives) to reassure them, and myself, and my wife that, they never really had anything to do with my coming up here, it was just a culmination of, eh, two or three things that I've bottled up for so many years...

Maintenance of the site as a reality which articulated with the world of common sense and the community was a moral activity shared by nurses, patients and doctors. Altschul (1972) noted that nurses and patients talked mainly about matters in the daily life of the ward. This could be read in light of the argument advanced above, that what mattered was the significance of 'being here' and 'here'. Thus in Site One P1, who rarely talked to the nurses because they 'had their work to do' and who had difficulty distinguishing between nurses and patients, asked all of them whether they came from her town, and whether they had mutual acquaintances. She spoke to patients who were lonely or distressed, trying to find out through the talk what they had in common. She thus constituted the moral order of the community from which she had come in the context of the moral order of the site. She played a part in the moral order based on character, by trying to identify the characters of those she spoke to in the site.

The articulation of the reality in the site with that outside was accomplished when a doctor in Site Two said that a patient had gotten a new kitchen from her husband partly because she had been ill. She joked that perhaps she, the doctor, ought to have a breakdown because she needed a new kitchen. The joke maintained the boundaries between those who could and those who could not get what they wanted in life otherwise than through the obligations imposed on others by their illnesses. It maintained a claim that what the patient did was somehow wrong, and that it would have been wrong for the doctor to have done so. It would have been wrong for the nurses and others not to have understood what was wrong, and not to have seen the patient as wrong.

Legitimating the primacy of work

The reader will have noted that throughout this chapter, various sections could have been interpreted as being 'about' knowledge or 'about' power. Equally, Chapters 5 and 6 referred often to the warrantability of action. My argument is that the nurses structured their work so as to be able to enforce its warranted character in the sites as work places. They reflexively drew on the frame of meaning 'work' to order interaction to produce knowledge for the purposes of doing the work of the sites; where the work of the sites included enabling and requiring the patients to give warrantable accounts of their action. Schutz (1968) and Schutz and Luckmann (1974) described the 'paramount reality' as the world of work. These nurses and patients worked to legitimate the work of the site and the site as a place of work, when that work was defining, maintaining and repairing the paramount reality of everyday life. In keeping the work going, or in working to get better, the nurses and patients maintained the paramount reality. Maintaining the unproblematic character of the paramount reality was moral work.

A principle of that reality was that doubt about the reality of the paramount reality was 'suspended' (cf. Schutz and Luckmann, 1974). Normally the nurses did not reveal doubts about what they were doing.[17] The first trained nurse thought that P4 might have been 'rebelling', but said that she did not think about such things 'too much' when working. This freedom from doubt was the product of work by the nurses, work founded on common sense. Altschul (1972) concluded that the nurses thought that their account was the only one to be given, despite there being variations in accounts. The argument here is that reference to 'common sense' may have constituted a form of legitimation of the work, it being taken for granted that that work would be varied and depend only on the warrant of the speaker.

I have noted that the validity of nurses' claims could be established by appeal to 'impression' or to collective judgement, with no requirement for legitimation through deliberation. Appeals to common-sense norms were adequate to invalidate a patient's account (cf. Altschul, 1972). The reality of the site, recognition of which was necessary for accounting, was the ground and condition for accounting, as it was for practical action (cf. Wieder, 1974). That reality was warranted by other nurses, while the patient's reality could be regarded as her own. Nursing practice was organised to maintain a reality warrantable by other nurses. Because knowledge of the site was needed to work in the site, maintenance of knowledge of the site ('savvy') available for use by others, was a moral requirement. The site had to be 'handed over' to the next shift. The moral order legitimating action in it had to be readily inhabitable. The moral order of the sites as maintained by the nurses was a social order.

On occasions when nurses did doubt, they drew reasons from alternative systems of discourse. I have noted that a student nurse in Site Two was told 'you're not supposed to tell (the patients) what to do' but felt that 'if you empathise with them, you have to (tell them something)'. The contradiction is one familiar in common sense. The nurses in their moral reasoning drew on and reproduced the contradictions in wider social discourse.

When common sense was lost in illness (see Chapter 5, on S1P3), patients' doubts became the subject of their own and nurses' 'work'. Patients were often in the position, as S2P4 was, of having their accounts countered by another account of what the reality was, what 'was there'. On such occasions the patient's, not the nurse's moral reasoning was scrutinised. What the patients were not meant to doubt was the 'programme' itself or the obligation to work.

The patients sustained the legitimacy of the work with every interaction. In accounting in their day to day interaction, they revealed their agency or patienthood. The process of accounting reflexively reproduced the moral order. Those who could plan and act - agents - exercised power to require of, or to provide for those who did not or could not plan and act, an excuse or a justification. In asking for excuse or in submitting their justification for warrant, the patients acknowledged their subordinate place in the moral order (within limits: patients could and did rebel). The system of accounting thus generated a discourse which provided the topics of 'work'. In participating in the discourse the nurses and patients reflexively constituted themselves as moral subjects, subjects in and to the discourse through which they constructed the social reality of the sites as moral orders.[18]

Moral orders of honour and deliberation

As the empirical data indicate, nurses in both sites examined the accounts of patients to see whether they counted as explanations, excuses, justifications. Such examination was, however, subsidiary to answering questions about why the person was 'here now' and what had to be done for her. As I argued in Chapter 6, these two questions can be interpreted in terms of 'powers' and power: the question 'why is she here now?' being answered by an account to which the second-level concepts 'agent' and 'patient' could be applied; and the second, 'what do we have to do for her?' being answered by an account of the action on action the nurse effected to 'work' on or with the patient. I will now argue that the two questions were answered in different ways in the two sites, and relate the differences to the different moral orders in the sites.

The empirically grounded distinctions between the two sites can be elaborated using Harré's (1983, pp. 236-7) concepts 'moralities of honour' and 'moralities of deliberation':

> Moralities of deliberation can be distinguished from moralities of honour. In the former, the stress is on the reasons for the action; in the latter, on the moral quality of the actor...Honour moralities exemplify moral orders in which the assessment of persons is the primary focus of moral activity...One's standing as a person depends in part on the degree to which one is capable of actually doing what the moral order requires, fulfilling one's commitments etc. So the problem of agency enters into the moral psychology of personal being and, via the world of personal display of character, so do deserts.

It is useful to simplify complex distinctions between the sites in order to clarify important differences. Site One could be construed as a moral order based on honour, and Site Two a moral order based on deliberation. By highlighting these distinctions it is possible to explore differences in the sites that affected interaction in them.

The morality of honour in Site One was related to institutional features. In a ward in a small hospital in the country the nurses often knew the patients or someone who knew them. They knew them or their types as characters in everyday life. They felt that they (the nurses) 'could not put on an act' because sooner or later they would be found out. They emphasised being 'ordinary people just like the patients', and trying not to focus on the 'illness' or 'problem' but on the person. The rhetoric of individualism extended to their emphasis on personal style in talk, 'reading' and 'handling' patients. I have emphasised their oral culture and use of metaphor and story to construct and convey their work. So in their appraisal of patients they focused on personal or social characteristics: 'wee woman in her ain hoose', 'a man who liked sport too', 'a woman who likes a joke'. They stressed appraisal by the 'community' in the site as a powerful force (see above). I have described the packing of action in a small space so that all action seemed publicly available to all. Public displays of respect for shows of character were accorded in meetings and in one to one interaction. In particular, trying to get better, working on things, and exerting will were valued.

In Site Two, the dominant moral order was based on deliberation. The deliberation of experts, often one or more places in the moral order removed, was valued highly. Respect was accorded to patients who fulfilled their obligations in working out why they were 'here'. The deliberation was primarily with the expert or delegated others, and with oneself. The moral order in Site Two was likewise related to institutional features, in particular the role of the hospital as a psychiatric teaching hospital, in which rights to patients as objects of investigation were guarded, and a patient with a rare or 'classic' version of a problem was especially highly valued. I have given examples of several accounts in which patients were asked to look at or talk about why they were 'here', not only for the purpose of assessment, but because doing so was construed as an obligation entailed by their patient role. There was a subsidiary moral order in Site Two based on sharing.

Classification and ordering of work

I have also argued that there were different and sometimes competing moral orders, in the sense that nurses considered action in the main order problematic when it conflicted with their own moral code(s) (see Appendix 13). However, some conclusions can be drawn regarding general bases of moral appraisal. The nurses' card sorts (Appendix 10) can be used to answer questions about how they organised their time and attention. A main categorisation was one related to 'illness' - broadly, psychotic versus 'others', including non-psychotic, neurotic, and dependent patients. A similar, though less clear picture emerged in Site Two sorts. The second main set of categorisations were those that related to features of the work of the site, including where the patient was in her stay, plans for discharge and likely further contact. A third were features related to how much time was spent with the patients. What emerged overall, then, was a picture of the nurses considering their rights and obligations to the patients in light of the requirements of the work setting, especially those related to degree of 'illness' (principally meaning psychosis or 'other' rather than a more specific diagnosis). It may be concluded, then, that the nurses shared an understanding that legitimation of their interaction with patients could rest on a principle of helping the most 'ill' (cf. John, 1961; Towell, 1975;

MacIlwaine, 1980). This accords with the account given on their behalf by the consultant in Site Two, and by them in interviews.

How did the nurses accomplish their interaction with these patients as moral action? From previous chapters it will be clear that one of the ways they did so was through use of a discourse on responsibility (see Chapter 6). I have also suggested how responsibility was defined and sustained through the giving and examination of accounts. One of the main practices was getting accounts which indicated the ability of the patient to plan and to give feedback on action based on planning. This was a key feature of work with S1P2, S1P3, S1P4, S1P7; S2P2, S2P4, S2P5, S2P6, S2P7, S2P8, and S2P10. Two explanations can be given of why the ability to plan would have been valued and cultivated through the practices of accounting. The first is that planning implies agency and agency is generally and commonly valued in the wider culture (Harré, 1983). The second is that development of the patients' ability to plan[19] was valued because in order to do the work of the sites, the nurses had to keep the work going, which meant getting patients back to the community: 'they can't stay here'. Data presented in this and previous chapters clearly suggest that the nurses withheld legitimation from patients who 'want to be here' or who would not do the 'work' necessary to leave.

In both sites, time was the currency in an economy of respect and contempt (cf. Simm, 1978; Hochschild, 1983). The practices of power in the frame of meaning 'work' were structured in terms of time[20]:

> N: ...(S2P5) wasn't, a psychotic patient as such, if people are, psychotically ill, you know that, sometimes you don't get an awful lot out of them, but with people like P5, who have a lot of **problems,** and are, probably in a hospital **because** of these problems, then I feel that they should have, as much time given to them as possible.

Patients who threatened to stay on longer than the staff thought appropriate (S1P2, S2P2) found that time was no longer available to them. Others' entitlement to time had superceded theirs. Patients took their places in the moral order by not demanding time, by recognising the priority of those with greater needs or more severe illness. The nurses were also judged in the moral order in which time was the currency. The patients respected nurses who always had time for them (cf. Altschul, 1972).

Patients achieved respect by working to become 'capable of actually doing what the moral order requires' (Harré, 1983, p. 237) [21];

and by developing their 'rationality' through 'displaying (their) actions as being in accord with (the) socially valued discourse principle' (Harré, 1983, p. 271) of showing the kind of person one was or talking about problems.

Patients were shown less respect if they violated the discourse principle of 'keeping the work going', either passively or actively, by 'hiding' or 'acting'. Patients who 'hid' or who 'acted' made the nurses' work difficult (cf. May and Kelly, 1982), insofar as they were unavailable for observation or other assessment and treatment. Patients in Site Two who claimed inability to plan and act when they were thought not to be 'ill' were held in low esteem. Constructing such patients in this way, nurses could legitimate treating them at their discretion: 'just support'. Displays of rationality considered 'sustainable claim(s) to worth' (Harré, 1983, p. 271) were those in which the patient appeared to be practising or planning to practise some action that marked development of agency. Thus P4 (above) displayed her worth by saying that her past claims of patienthood, including insincere ones, were errors. She assumed the role of agent. In Site Two respect was accorded to patients who assumed an agent role by accepting responsibility for problems (see Chapter 6).

These moral evaluations based on concepts of 'ill' and 'responsible' legitimated ordering of work. Female nurses in Site Two gave time and opportunities to talk to those patients who made no claim of illness and who were responsible. Patients who claimed illness but who were thought not to be ill, but rather unwilling to 'work on problems', were given less time by an experienced male nurse. The same patients were specifically given time by a female student nurse, because she thought that too little was done for them, or because she 'empathised' with them. Patients who did not claim illness and were not responsible were given time if another reason could be given for or accepted from them (S2P6 as a 'lonely old woman'). Patients who were considered 'ill' were given time according to their (negotiated) needs.

I have indicated, then, that the bases for legitimating interaction with these patients were complex and varied, between sites and within sites. Different nurses could consider the same patient worthy of respect and of contempt. However, there were commonalities in grounds for valuation, and what mattered was how the terms 'ill', 'problems' and 'work' were used by a nurse in relation to a given patient. As I have indicated, this varied systematically, in Site Two, where some patients' 'work' in the support group was legitimated by the (female) nurses who ran the group while denied legitimation by nurses not in the group.

Socialisation and the giving of accounts on behalf of the other

The task of ordinary life, of acting so as to be accountable for oneself, had been supplanted, for the patients, by the task of accounting for themselves in a new moral order, in which they also became the objects/subjects of others' accounts about them. The data illuminate the problems this posed for patients and nurses, problems of re-socialisation or 'therapy' (Berger and Luckmann, 1967). From the moment of admission, the patient's moral status was the focus of attention and work. There were broad differences in how the nurses accounted on behalf of patients in the different moral orders based on honour and deliberation.

The concept 'symbiotic accounting' illuminates features of the data. By symbiotic accounting I mean the practice of providing accounts of and for another (Harré, 1983; Shotter, 1984; and Vygotsky, 1978).[22]

Patients noted that nurses provided them with accounts of how they looked, of what was wrong with them, of what they were doing, of 'other reasons' they must have had. I am arguing that in doing so the nurses provided the patients with feedback not only on their action, but also on the patients themselves, and thus with implicit theories of persons. In nurses' and patients' accounts based on 'illness', the implicit theory was that persons could become patients through a process for which they could not be held responsible. Alternatively, patients and nurses sometimes accounted for the patients in terms of characteristics of the person held to be due not to illness but to what might be seen as traits.[23] A third kind of account was in terms of characteristics shared with those patients with whom the nurse could 'empathise' - for example, women with demanding families. In addition to these theories of person were various others illustrated in nurses' categorisations and, importantly, in the metaphors they used.[24] Implicit in the metaphors were theories of the person. Using these metaphors and acting on the basis of them, the nurses provided the patients with opportunities to appropriate the implicit theories and to use them to direct themselves.

Provision to patients of views of themselves as persons was in some cases less explicit in Site Two, as conveyed by the sometimes gnomic utterances of an experienced nurse in Site Two: 'speak if the spirit moves you'. A view of the patient as a person was also available implicitly in the Site Two ideology of not doing for the patient. In accounts given to a patient in which she was held to have 'another reason' or 'a problem' which she did not acknowledge, the implicit theory was of the person as a being capable of concealing from self the real reasons for action, and of 'putting off energy' onto other things. While this was most explicitly one nurse's view, the theory that a person could hide from herself the reasons for action was the common view in Site Two. The patient who appropriated this view took on the work of self-scrutiny and examination.

I am arguing, therefore, that the nurses treated the patients as the kinds of person they were seen to be, with the intention that the patients should come to regard themselves as that kind of person. The nurses were engaged, though not explicitly, in 'growing' persons according to the models of person they held implicitly or explicitly (cf. Harré, 1983). This recasts in different terms the argument of the monograph as a whole that the nurses' work was a form of 'therapy'. The 'therapy' as construed here comprised methods for seeing how, and showing the person how, she deviated from the ordinary, through hearing accounts from the patient's point of view, and 'remedying' the patient's understanding of self and world through provision of other accounts based on common notions of what a person should do and be. The accounts were given in the context of the moral order in which kinds of persons were privileged in terms of work: 'ill' privileged in relation to 'not ill'; 'workers' in relation to 'non-workers'. Therefore the accounts offered to others implicitly cast them in the moral orders of the sites. As with most of the conclusions of this chapter, it is important to emphasise that conflicting views of the same person were offered.

Honour: 'hiding', 'acting' and character

Closer analysis of the use of the terms 'acting' and 'hiding' reveals important issues related to character, honour, deliberation and will in the moral orders of the sites. Their centrality is related to the key role the terms played in management of work through processes of legitimation and non-legitimation, and to their articulation with both professional and common-sense understandings of the person.

The charge of 'hiding' was brought in Site Two when patients avoided talking about anything 'personal'. Implicit in the charge was an understanding of the nature of the person, and of how that person was and ought to be placed in the moral order. The person the nurses spoke to could be other than the person the patient claimed to be (authored). The 'real' person might be the one hidden as 'personal'. The charge legitimated considering her non-responsible.

The implication of this argument is that the 'push and pull' (contraditions and inconsistencies) of talk done in the course of assessment and treatment were reified as characteristics of the patient as a kind of person. This had the effect of legitimating acting toward the patient who 'hid' on the basis of the label: withdrawing from the person who was 'hiding' (cf. Scheff, 1966). It also legitimated not looking 'too closely' at the way the terms available in the local moral order reflected the requirements of work in the sites; and the limits of construing the patients through the frame of meaning 'work'.

A similar argument can be made regarding the concept 'acting', a central concern in Site One. The similarity of the different concepts in the two sites, thus analysed, justifies an argument that in both sites the conceptions of the person implied in the terms of the nurses' working ethics functioned to order and legitimate the work of the site. The kinds of person the patients came to be known as, and in some cases came to see themselves as, were reflexively related to the demands of work in the institutions. In Site Two this phenomenon was institutionalised in an argot used by experienced nurses to describe patients: 'dead wood', 'one offs', 'repeat business', 'bed and breakfast', 'cute but unrewarding', 'corridor people'.

The data may be interpreted in light of Kelly and May's (1982) argument that the terms 'good' and 'bad' as applied to patients are outcomes of social processes of legitimation and non-legitimation. The argument here is that, in constructing the patients as 'hiding' and 'acting', the nurses interpreted the patient by taking her role in interaction construed through the frame of meaning 'work', and reified that interpretation by locating in the patient the motive for her (interpreted) part.

Reputation and kind of person

The above analysis may be read in the context of the literature on reputation and deviance construction related to psychiatric nursing (for example, Kelly and May, 1982; Goffman, 1962, 1967; and Towell, 1975), as well as the literature on labelling (for example, Scheff, 1966;

Pollock, 1989). The general argument from these works is that interaction is structured through interpretation of the person's reputation or label, thus shaping further interaction. The significance of reputation is that it conveys, in advance of action, understandings of the person in terms of the local moral order.

Empirically, interaction between these nurses and patients was sometimes structured through reputation or labelling. In Site One, a student nurse told new nurses that they would not believe, seeing P2 now, what she had been like a few months before: fighting the staff, arguing with them. She was, he said, like a different person now. S1P1 appeared to me a fairly deaf, confusing if not confused old lady: where was the woman who had bitten nurses, who was still talked about as a somewhat threatening force? S2P4 gave her own reputation. All the nurses probably knew, she said, how she used to complain of pain and say that she couldn't do anything. S2P1 and S2P2's reputations as disrupters of their family doctors' working lives were retailed by hospital staff. Reputation framed how the person was to be regarded, how she had been known elsewhere or in the sites, as that was considered relevant to interaction with her now. The nurses interacted with the patient before them on the basis of the history of interaction with her. That history provided the 'personal typifications' relevant to work (Simm, 1978).

I described in Chapter 5 how character emerged from stories. Character as the bearer of reputation emerged more forcefully in Site One than in Site Two. This may have been due to the different culture in Site One, wherein nurses talked more about the patients in the course of more intimate 'working relationships' over longer periods, and were main interpreters of 'the main thing'. Alternatively, it may have been because in Site Two there was always the prospect that another story was being told about the patients by someone else whose knowledge and authority to author the patient were held in higher regard.

The view of the person in Site Two was relevant to construction of character and reputation. There was a tension between holding the patient responsible and maintaining that an 'it' could account for what the patient did. 'It' could never appear as an actor, and the patient who did not work on 'it' could only appear as a 'hider'. The person, explanation of whose action necessitated reference to 'it', was a thinner character. What metaphor brought in its wake was missed in characters explained by 'it'. In Site Two the terms of a strong institutional culture established reputation in more circumscribed, institutionally salient terms.

Multiple moral orders and the patient's view

In this analysis of the moral orders of the sites I have to an extent reproduced a feature of the sites, by privileging an account of the moral order which legitimated and structured 'work' in the sites. I have done so because that was the moral order which legitimated maintenance and repair of the paramount reality. However, I have stressed that nurses and patients in some cases inhabited multiple moral orders. I have mentioned S1P7's implication that she was too old at seventy-seven to get over her problems herself. Implicit in her account was a conception of a moral order in which age could be taken into account in relieving one of responsibility. The moral order implied in S1P2's account of having to crawl before walking was one in which adults and parents could be accorded the support needed for development. Implications of alternative moral orders could be interpreted in other patients' accounts.

An experienced nurse in Site One joked about P7's comments that she was too old for a geriatric centre. I interpreted the joke as a reflection on her command of the discourse in which subjectively meaningful terms ('too old') were subject to reframing in what an experienced nurse in Site Two called 'our words', the language of work and the nurses' practical ethical discourse discourse.

The dominant moral order of the site was thus maintained by ordering the moral orders within it through a discourse which sustained and legitimated interpretations of the main thing and the structure of working relationships. That the legitimation was potentially tenuous was made evident in analysis of the data. For every construction of the main thing maintained by the nurses an alternative construction could be located in the patients' accounts. Those alternative constructions were spoken in the terms of the patients' 'submerged' discourses: the old woman unable to cope, the patient not ready to go, the man still frightened and with more to work on, the woman unable to speak, the woman without a house.

The case of S1P4 illustrates the difficulties in interpretation of interaction in terms of different moral orders. S1P4 claimed that voices told her she would be put out of the ward. She had a diagnosis of psychosis, but at the time of the research the doctors thought that her complaints of voices may have reflected anxiety. The anxiety was thought to have been related to an impending move from the ward to new housing. In one sense, the 'reality' was that she was being 'put out'.[25] Nonetheless the view that was legitimated was that her claims were symptoms; and the validity of her interpretation was subject to regular refutation ('reinforcement'). I have selected a particularly vulnerable case for interpretation. It may be inferred that P4's diagnosis implied greater potential for non-legitimation of her interpretation. In using this case I am highlighting the general conclusion that divergent and conflicting interpretations spoken from within competing moral orders reflected the reality of work in sites which functioned to assess and treat people whose views of and conduct in the world had brought them into these systems of interpretation, power and legitimation. S1P4 was recalled to the paramount reality ('putting the reality to her') whenever she complained of voices, and the nurses interpreted her behaviour to the agency taking over responsibility for her housing. Their work to return her to the paramount reality was structured on non-legitimation of the claims spoken from 'her' reality.

Responsibility

Understanding the organisation of rights and obligations in a moral order based on responsibility is the key to understanding the work of these nurses and patients. Throughout this monograph I have used the concept 'response' in interpreting that work. I have argued that the work can be understood through interpretation of their accounts and interaction as responses to the questions 'Why is she here now (am I here)?' and 'What do I have to do for her (do I have to do)?'. In doing so I have structured the monograph as an account of the nurses' and patients' responsibility as this was negotiated in face to face contact and in accounts of interaction.

In both sites the nurses' practical concern with responsibility was expressed in their working practices, in reporting to doctors, in organising and prioritising their work so that it was accountable to senior nurses, in fulfilling their obligations to the patients. The main forms of work were those that accomplished the appearance of the patient as a kind of person, namely an agent, responsible for actions. One of the nurses' devices for managing their responsibility was use of the system of accounting to determine, develop ('exercise') and display the patient's responsibility for her actions. I have argued above that the concepts 'work', 'responsibility', and 'willingness' were used to reflexively accomplish administrative tasks and at the same time accomplish the appearance of the patient as a person. The argument is completed by asserting that the administrative work of the site was precisely that accomplishment. In the remainder of this chapter I will address some of the implications of this argument in terms of moral order.

The concept 'responsibility' as interpreted in the sites affected how patients were regarded in the moral order and how they were treated. The nurses' practical ethics were articulated through the day to day use of concepts like 'responsibility'. Used as 'working words' (cf. Smith, 1980) these concepts reflexively structured work, the working relationship and the understanding of the 'kind of person' the patient was. Local theories of the person were drawn on in work that reproduced authorised views of the local people.

In the moral order structured by the concept 'responsibility', the nurses required responsibility of the patients and withheld legitimation if patients failed in their obligations for no good reason. 'Good reason' became the subject of moral reasoning and negotiation. In challenges to reasons, what was at stake was reason itself.[26] Through this process the patient's legitimations, grounded in her conception of person, self and moral order were called into question. The moral order of 'responsibility' legitimated the 'remedying' of the patients' moral reasoning.

Morality of 'illness' and 'work'

In both sites the moral order of 'work' and of 'will', whether related to character or responsibility, legitimated judgements based on willingness to work. The main difference was that in Site One that willingness could be exhorted, and the patient's lack of show of willingness could legitimately be compensated for by the nurse ('symbiosis'). In Site Two, responsibility for showing willingness was left more to the patients. In Site One respect was accorded to patients who showed character by trying, by force of will, rather than by deliberation. In Site Two respect was due to patients who worked out problems, by deliberation: 'Well, what sort of problems?'; 'making the connections'.

The moral orders in which the patients in this study were construed can be seen as akin to the moral order which structures everyday life, that of 'work' (Schutz and Luckmann, 1974). I have put in inverted commas the concept 'work' as used by the nurses and patients, in order to emphasise that the concept was part of an ideology that reflexively structured interpretation, action and judgement.[27] However, as much as I have emphasised the symbolic character of the 'work' the patients were required to do, I am arguing that it was a form of work in that it structured interaction through which the patients participated in the production of interpretations of themselves, action on action, and legitimation. The work they participated in was 'work' of which they were the subjects and objects. Through this work they took part in the processes through which they 'passed' back to the paramount reality. The patients returned to the paramount reality of work through 'work': back to baking, mothering, washing, tending oneself, clerical work; and back to the ordinary 'emotional labour' (Hochschild, 1983) required of all in the main culture. Those ordinary forms of work and the accountability practised in planning and doing them constituted major parts of the 'therapy' of nurse-patient interaction.

The nurses' role in interaction with these patients was in part to maintain the legitimacy of the moral order of 'work' against competing moral orders: work they accomplished through being present as workers working with other patients; talking about their work; correcting illusions that the place was a hotel, holiday camp or madhouse; maintaining in 'social talk' and 'illness talk' the distinctions between those inside (including the distinction between those inside who worked and those who did not) and those outside; as well as through the more readily discernible 'work' of help with showering, discussion of problems, marital and family work, encouragement, reassurance, and so on.

The nurses and patients also participated in maintaining the moral order by enforcing the claim that entitlement to relief from obligations to work depended on judgement of illness. The articulation between the discourse of illness and problems, and relief from obligation to work, was managed through use of the concept 'responsibility'. In Site One the motto was 'we can do so much but you have to help yourself'. The ordering of work depended on maintaining the distinctions between those able to participate in maintaining the paramount reality (by taking part in work or doing work themselves) and those not able to do so. The main obligation of nurses, communicated to patients, was to maintain the site, the paramount reality of the workplace, so that the work of maintaining the paramount reality by recovering strays could proceed. Through this argument I am claiming that the main work of these nurses with the patients in this study was the legitimation of the paramount reality through the enforcement of obligations to work to restore or maintain it. This work was underpinned by an unarticulated assumption that it was right to maintain the paramount reality ('my reality' according to an experienced nurse).

Work and responsibility in Site Two

The problem of responsibility was common. The local moral orders of the two sites differed to some extent, as I have suggested. However, it was the case that in both sites the patients were held to be 'kinds of people' characterised by their problems in assuming or resuming responsibility. The commonness of the problem of responsibility could be seen in two ways. Firstly, some nurses shared their own problems with some patients; problems related, for example, to difficulty in talking about personal matters, or in coping with demands made by relatives (see Appendix 13). Patients sometimes asked nurses specifically about their relationships or problems. Secondly, the nurses generally faced problems in acting responsibly and accountably in the two sites. At times in both sites nurses complained to medical staff that the demands placed on them as the result of admission of problematic patients limited their ability to carry out their work adequately. More broadly, I have characterised Site Two as a setting in which nurses' formal responsibility for work with the patients in this study was limited.

Problems of non-responsibility of both patients and nurses had to be interpreted in light of the structure of power and knowledge in the sites. The subjectivities of patients, in particular those who could not or would not respond to the injunctions to account and talk, were liable to become the object/subjects of further 'work'. Nurses who tried to maintain alternative moral orders which sustained a discrepant view of 'the main thing' or alternative 'working relationships' did not declare their work.

Moral aspects of working relationships: resistance, symbiosis, legitimation

Both compliance and rebellion by patients reflexively maintained the moral order. In Chapter 6 I discussed nurses' perceptions of patients' resistance and 'rebellion'. The nurse did not think 'too much' about issues like rebellion. The moral order based on 'responsibility' legitimated the nurses' exercise of power in fulfilment of their responsibility to account for the patients' whereabouts. The nurse's claim that patients liked having responsibility 'taken off them' may be interpreted as a contradiction of the argument that the nurses in Site Two held the patients in this study responsible. However, the two claims are compatible, given the further argument that the nurse's claim that the nurses took responsibility was accompanied by her justification of requiring patients to tell where they were going. The price the patients paid for relief from responsibilities in the wider community was assumption of responsibilities to the nurses (and other staff, and patients) in the site. It should not be assumed that this responsibility was considered onerous at all times or by all patients. I have argued that some patients some of the time valued the nurses' asking how they were because it showed interest.

I have based the argument of this monograph on the understanding that accounts were devices for interpreting and warranting action, and that interpretation took place in and reflexively structured moral orders (see Chapter 3). Accounts were construed theoretically as devices for clarifying what was really being done, and in the course of that, legitimating, explaining, excusing or justifying what was done. My argument here is that empirically nurses justified their role in the system of accounting on the grounds of administrative or professional necessity (fulfilling the administrative requirement of accomplishing the 'main thing' of keeping the patients 'safe, fed and then happy'; or 'keeping the place anxiety free'), but more generally, on the grounds that it was legitimate to manage the accountability of patients because of what the patients were collectively or individually like: 'patients like it', 'the kind of person he was', 'patients being ordinary people'. They thus legitimated their part in the interaction and the order in which they worked, through reference to people as interpreted in the moral order. They interacted in a pre-interpreted reality in which the pre-interpretations were meaningful in the moral order.

In day to day interaction the nurses constructed the patients as kinds of people in terms of their moral character, and acted toward them on that basis. By doing so they were able to work in settings organised as moral orders, structured by systems of legitimation and the public according of reward and contempt. Like the patients, they could (and in some cases did) rebel or resist, or maintain (subordinate) alternative moral orders, but they could not work free of the moral orders in the sites. It is necessary to stress again that in establishing the relationship of power and moral order, I am not implying that the effects on patients were wholly or mainly negative. I have already presented data that demonstrate that patients often remarked on the value of nurses and what nurses enabled them to do. They legitimated the nurses' work in terms of the moral orders of the site (helping those most in need; recognising that you are ill; helping you develop responsibility) and of the wider community ('nice boy'). I have stressed the pervasiveness of moral concern and judgement in order to emphasise the necessity of interpreting the action of patients and nurses in relation to the moral orders of the sites, that is, the moral orders in which the actions were enacted and interpreted by the actors.[28]

The main critique by previous researchers was that psychiatric nurses practised on the basis of lay understandings and moral judgements. The argument of this chapter is that they operated on the basis of common, but negotiated and dynamic moral orders which articulated with those of everyday life. Far from being haphazard these were maintained in order to accomplish the work of the sites as accountable action. The meaning of common terms, for example 'responsibility', had to be interpreted through examination of their use in doing the work of the sites. The weakness of a simple dichotomy of lay versus professional understanding and judgement is that it fails to take into account the complexity of the relationship (as found empirically in this study) between ordinary and professional judgement; the extent to which ordinary understandings did and had to underpin professional judgement (cf. Cicourel, 1976; Asquith, 1977; Bennett and Feldman, 1981); and the dilemmatic character of common sense and common morality (cf. Potter and Wetherell, 1987; Billig et al, 1988). Indeed, such a dichotomy fails to take into account that it is precisely the dilemmatic nature of ordinary morality that makes it useful to professionals. The nurses depended on background understandings to do their work. I have argued here that it was because they shared concepts like 'responsibility' and 'work', 'illness' and 'problems', and because they had the power to negotiate meanings with patients, that they were able to use these terms to negotiate common and uncommon interpretations of action, reflexively interpret the moral orders in which the terms had meaning, and order interaction to ensure its accountability in the moral orders of the site and in the wider community.

Legitimation

I attended to the relationship between responsibility and legitimation because this was empirically a central concern of patients and nurses. Simply to ask a patient to tell about a conversation was to invite a legitimation (or non-legitimation) of the patient, the nurse and the site. The patients gave accounts in which they legitimated not talking to the nurses: S2P10 because she could not bring herself to, S2P5 because she was not that kind of person, S2P7 and P8 because they had no need to, S2P4 because she could not think of the reasons the nurses expected her to know, S2P6 because the nurses did not have as much time as the social worker did and because they had to help others; S1P1 and S1P4 because the nurses were busy, S1P2 because she was getting better, S1P7 because they thought her too old. In Site Two the reasons the patients gave for not talking could in most cases be interpreted as relating to their 'problems'. Accounts of not talking given by both patients and nurses may be regarded as justifications of their own availability, and attribution to the other of the blame or responsibility for not talking.

Analysis of the data indicated that the processes of legitimation and non-legitimation were complex and subtle. Thus a patient's very valuing of the nurses could form the basis of their negative evaluation of her. S2P6 valued the nurses' caring for her when she was unwell, but was criticised in a nurse's account for acting as if her symptoms were due to something like the flu. P6 valued the nurses for enabling her to recognise her moods, and S2P4 valued them for helping her to recognise her emotions; but this was countered by a nurse's critique that these patients did not take responsibility for 'work' on understanding why they had problems.[29]

It may be argued that what was common to these accounts was that the patients and nurses interpreted the same action in terms of different frames of meaning or different moral orders. Altschul (1972) noted that patients were more sure than nurses of the helpfulness of what the nurses did.[30] MacIlwaine (1980) found that the nurses and neurotic patients saw different aspects of the nurse's role as most important. The findings of this study cast new light on these earlier works, insofar as they support an argument that the differences in interpretation were themselves interpreted in the paramount moral order, generating a self-awareness and irony[31] in nurses' accounts:

> N: She (P4) may see us as being generally supportive but um, probably not seeing it from a, a planned or calculated angle, just that we're **nice people**.

My conclusion is that the data may be interpreted as indicating that, in taking the roles of the patients, the nurses in Site Two saw themselves as valued, but relatively less valued in a site in which they did not do or were not acknowledged as doing 'deep' or therapeutic work. What was implicitly not legitimated in the patient's account was the willingness of the nurses to engage the patient in work on 'it'. The patient's account, read from this perspective, could be interpreted as a form of non-legitimation of the nurse's 'potential' role; and the nurse's irony can be interpreted as countering the patient's legitimation of less valued aspects of the nurse's role (cf. May and Kelly, 1982; Kelly and May, 1982). This was not the case in Site One, where nurses' work was more often legitimated by the nurses themselves and by the consultant.

The very actions valued within the moral order structured through the working ideology of 'illness' were de-valued in the moral order structured through the working ideology of 'responsibility'. Legitimations in one order were non-legitimations in the other. In face to face contact power could be read in the capacity to command interpretation and action within one moral order. Other researchers have noted the tenuousness of nurses' power to practise this command (Chapman, 1987; May and Kelly, 1982). The data in this study indicate that a more complex explanation is needed, one not based on an assumption of uniformity of moral orders among nurses, and one capable of taking into account the varied patterns of legitimation and non-legitimation, and their dynamic character. There were differences in practises of legitimation not only between the sites and between nurses and doctors, but among more experienced nurses; between more and less experienced nurses, including students; and between males and females. Practices of legitimation and non-legitimation between individual patients and nurses changed over time, again in ways open to different interpretations. I have noted that the two sites differed in the extent to which the issue of legitimation was taken as a topic for discussion and negotiation. These different legitimations were related to different understandings of the 'kind of person' the other was and the 'right attitude'.

The finding that accounts reflected different perspectives, ideologies and moral orders and differently legitimated the interaction of nurses and patients can be related to a claim advanced throughout this monograph: namely, that nurses and patients were interdependent in 'sharing the site' and doing the 'work' of the sites. The main working ideology was shared by nurses and patients to a greater extent in Site One than in Site Two. In Chapters 5 and 6 I discussed 'forms' of knowledge and power. Here I will discuss the 'form' of accounts as interpreted in terms of the moral order; namely, 'symbiosis'.

The interdependence was represented in the analytic relationship between accounts. Patients sometimes gave accounts which emphasised how their ability to give an account of themselves depended on the nurse's having given an account to them. Nurses' accounts could be construed as 'templates' the patient could use to structure her own accounts. Patients noted that nurses gave accounts for them when the patients were unable to do so for themselves.[32] The nurses assumed responsibility for the patients. The relationship of nurse and patient and of accounts in these instances could be regarded as 'symbiotic'[33] (cf. Shotter, 1984; Harré, 1983). Thus, S2P6:

> P: See some ones'll say to (? you), 'What's wrong with you you're no looking so well?', or, 'You're maybe looking better this morning', you know, and you feel, Well, maybe I am a wee bit better, and, cos, some of the nurses here have said to me, over the last week, I have improved, and I know I have improved **myself**, over the last week.
>
> .....
>
> P: You know, sh-, the nurse sort of has the same opinions as us. Although sh-, they try to help us **explain**, and, I think they maybe get uh, to know us a wee bit better than Sally (Note: occupational therapist) does, because eh, we're **with** nurses more. And they'll say, 'Well, did you no think **this** would happen to you?'. Cos I think they get to know what kind of **person** you are...She gets to know your moods, and, what interests you, you know.

The nurses noticed her: 'And, you feel that, it is being taken notice of, you know, you're no just sitting there as a lump. And, you're being watched, but, in a, the nicest way.' Having noticed, they provided accounts of her and to her which enabled her to be understood and to understand herself as 'mentally ill'. They interpreted her as a kind of person and took the right attitude toward her: not a lump, but a person who was ill. Thus in a symbiotic account the patient was provided with an understanding of the kind of person she was, why she was 'here' and what she had to do: someone who had been mentally ill, and was recovering. The construction of her as mentally ill became subjectively real through a process of reality construction and maintenance, sustained through the system of accounts and accountability within a moral order. Symbiotic accounting was re-socialisation or 'therapy' in practise. The form of symbiotic accounting represented acknowledgement, through incorporation, of the cognitive order and the structure of power and knowledge (specifically, the power to know how one really was). The primary form of symbiotic accounting in Site One was the story with its central metaphor.

A second implication of considering accounts as symbiotic relates to the power involved in accounting. The accounts of these patients and nurses were claims in moral orders, and relationships of accounts reflected relationships in moral orders, relationships of knowledge and power. In a symbiotic relationship one member has greater power, status and knowledge. These are afforded the other until the other is able and allowed to account for himself (Harré, 1983). Thus the accounts of one member have greater authority - indeed, in the case of parent and child, they author the person of the other.

A fuller analysis must, however, interpret contradictions between the account of the patient who had given 'symbiotic' accounts and an account given by a nurse. For example, a nurse gave an account of S2P6's stay in which the patient's belief that she was 'ill' was regarded ironically, and the patient was seen as a 'hider'. The implication is that while P6 had, according to her account, developed the ability to account for herself in terms provided by the nurses, in the nurse's account she had not developed the ability to account for herself in terms which entitled her to respect in the local moral order based on 'responsibility'.

The nurse's account can be interpreted as indicating that the work of 'therapy' in Site Two was two tiered.[34] In the terms of the moral order of Site Two, the stray from the main reality ought not only to have returned to the paramount reality, in the sense of having recovered the powers that enabled her to return to the community. She ought also to have become the 'kind of person' who took the attitude toward herself that the nurse did (his ironic tone emphasising that she did not). She ought to have acknowledged the principle that sustained the moral order, ordering interaction and the production of knowledge: the principle of 'responsibility'. According to the nurse, the hazard faced by those who did not do so, was that they would, when again faced with problems, again see themselves as 'ill' and return for help. The implicit legitimation of the nurse's practise was that through taking 'responsibility' for 'looking at it' and 'working on it' the patient would not need to become again the subject and object of work in the site.[35] The stray was, in this second account, not yet returned. She had not acquired the ability to handle the tools of reality maintenance, including subjective reality maintenance. The nurse's account can be regarded as invalidating the patient's symbiotic account. The general conclusion from discussion of this case is that symbiotic accounting, in a setting in which different forms of legitimation co-existed, was complex and problematically related to the structures of power and knowledge in the sites.[36]

It should be noted that this analysis of 'symbiotic accounts' relates to the data from Site Two. The symbiotic accounts in Site One were 'mediated' by metaphors. The metaphors in Site One, enabling the nurses to treat people as kinds of people they were not but could be, may have facilitated work, as did the ideology of responsibility in Site Two. But by treating the patients as what they could be, the nurses also treated them as valued in the moral order of the site and the community (e.g. a child who could develop). They treated the patients as people with whom they could have a working relationship.[37] The symbiotic accounts in Site One, like those of Site Two, embodied contradictions. The woman who gave accounts in which the nurses were depicted as giving her more responsibility was depicted by the nurse as resisting leaving the hospital. The issues of power related to this were discussed in Chapter 6. The concept of 'symbiotic' accounts conveys that the nurses' ideologies legitimated, in different ways in the two sites, their exercise of power in accounting for or providing accounts for patients until the patients were able to do so for themselves.

Thus the concept 'symbiotic accounting' enables interpretation of some of the complex issues involved in the interaction of these nurses and patients. Juxtaposing accounts allows the development of a different perspective on the relationship between the nurse and patient. This perspective suggests that accounts in interaction between patients and nurses cannot be regarded unproblematically as devices whereby nurses enable patients to develop capacities to account for themselves, since the patient may develop capacities to account in ways which the nurse considers illegitimate.

What is at stake: person, self and community

I have juxtaposed P6's and a nurse's accounts in order to draw out some implications regarding their participation in moral orders. The process of accounting between nurses and patients was only one of a set of accounting processes regulated by the structures of knowledge and power in the sites. While the methods of this study have enabled some greater contextualisation of interaction than was the case in previous nursing research, I have not been able to account for a great deal of the interaction of the patients with other professionals, patients and families. These figures have appeared in these accounts at the 'fringes' of relevance (Schutz and Luckmann, 1974).

A similar limitation is noted with regard to the place of these conversations, and the period of admission, in the patient's life. 'Then', 'when', 'out there' - the indexical terms which located this talk in time - illustrate the limits of contextualisation. Thus the relationships of moral orders inside the site and outside has been little explored. S2P6 told of the difficulties she faced in accounting for herself in the community:

> P: (Before coming to hospital) I didna know **what** was wrong with me. I just knew I was sitting staring at blank walls. I wasna watching the television, I wasnae eating. I just didnae know **what** was wrong with me. I didnae know I had a, a problem. You know, m-, I didna know I was mentally ill.
>
> ....
>
> P: I'm going home today, but, you just canna thank them enough, for all they've done for you, you know, because, the state you come in, and the state you go out is two different, people going, out, you come in a wreck, then you're going home to face, you feel a bit nervous about going home to face, everyday reality, you know, but I **still**, know that I've got help at the Day Hospital, if I need it. And I think, **if** a-, any, o-, I **hope** it doesnae come back, but, **if**, at any time this **does** return, I can phone here, for help. Where I was sitting in the house for six or eight weeks, and I couldnae get help. I was sitting even

saying to my husband, 'Help me. G-, (? well you got to or ? will you go out to) try and help me', but, he didnae understand what kind of help I wanted, you know?

This excerpt highlights points similar to those made by other patients regarding the value of an account of what had happened to them. It highlights the stresses of inability to account for self and for the other. It also highlights common-sense understandings of agency and patienthood which, I have argued, structured interaction in accounts in the sites as well as outside. This account illustrates that, in processes of legitimation of accounts of 'illness' and patienthood, agency and responsibility, what is at stake is the person and the self of the account giver in a moral order. P6's legitimation of the site entailed future obligations (on the part of staff) to respond. I am emphasising here that the accounts of these nurses and patients may be read for their implications in relation to the broader moral orders of institutions as providers of services over time,[38] and in relation to the moral orders which structure life in the community.

I have used the concept 'therapy' and the notion of recovering strays from the paramount reality, in order to convey some of the key conclusions regarding the interaction of these nurses and patients. While the concept 'community' has had to play various functions in this discussion, it is important to emphasise that the work of nurses and patients was the actual practical work of sharing the site and helping to get the patients 'out the door'. Patients came to the site from positions in moral orders and had to return to the community.

The patients who gave the accounts in this study were people whose status in the predominant moral order of the society outside could be considered low. Among them were people who were unemployed, old, out of work, women, lonely, eccentric or bizarre, homeless and unhousable, deaf, lame, recovering from severe psychotic illness, grieving, in difficulties in marriage, abandoned by children, displaced.[39] The nurses, in working to return them to the community, worked to return them to the moral orders structured to accord them those statuses. In the sense that 'a person is 95 per cent juror before he comes near a court' (Garfinkel, 1967, p. 110), so much of the participation of nurses and patients in the moral orders of face to face interaction and the sites was structured by their understanding of and participation in the moral orders of everyday life. This was explicitly the case for some student nurses, in ways that I have recounted. They accorded respect to people they recognised in terms of the ordinary morality of everyday life: the football fan, the father, the mother, the middle aged woman with demanding relatives, the lonely. In doing so, they sometimes supplemented what they saw as a deficient system; one that left people to 'ditter away'. They structured their work on the moral principles they brought to the work, in contradiction to those they found in the site.

Hazards to the person

I discussed in Chapter 6 the politeness and circumspection with which nurses approached patients. Their accounts emphasised the status of the person in the moral order and her entitlement to shows of respect. However, to do their work the nurses had to violate these moral rules. Not only had they to talk to and share places with strangers, they also had to violate the rules of normal social interaction - asking relative strangers to talk about personal things. Moreover, in many cases they had to violate a basic rule (respect the other as best authority on her action) to suggest that the patient's way of seeing the world and accounting for action ('it') might be problematic.

The patients faced the problem of having to respond to the expectation not only that they regard their way of life and view of themselves as problematic, but that they discuss this with relative strangers. Interaction in the sites thus posed 'hazards' (Harré, 1979) to the patient as a person. At stake was the patient's view of herself. Most of the patients valued the nurses' help in managing losses of self-control. However, they faced a hazard in becoming subject to work on locating and working on the 'it' held to be responsible for the loss of control. The data suggest that patients coped with this threat to self in different ways. A patient could cast the nurses in roles which enabled her to relate to them: not a friend, not one of my circle, not family; someone who cares and understands; someone with training who recognises signs of illness (cf. Altschul, 1972; MacIlwaine, 1980).[40]

Nurses faced a similar problem. In interviews they noted that they had difficulties in talking with neurotic patients because these patients were like the nurses, they were 'on the same level', 'they could challenge' the nurse. The ideology of 'responsibility' can be construed as enabling the nurses to structure a relationship through interaction with the patient seen as 'not ill' (cf. MacIlwaine, 1980;

Towell, 1975). The data of this study do not illuminate how the nurses structured their interaction with patients considered 'ill'.

Self protection by nurses and patients

Both nurses and patients developed strategies for defending themselves from observation and interaction in moral orders structured reflexively through the ideologies of responsibility and honour. I have discussed the charge by nurses in Site Two that patients 'hid'. I have also discussed (Chapter 6) the nurses' practise of screening out their subjectivity(ies) in formal accounts recorded in nursing records (the Kardex). The strategies of self-protection had consequences not only for the person herself, patient or nurse, but for the other as well.

In their written accounts the nurses practised a form of objectivation which emphasised the 'objectivity' of their observation. In their Kardex entries the nurses participated in the 'management out' (Munro, personal communication) of their contribution to the work of interpretation and action in the sites (cf. May and Kelly, 1982; Towell, 1975). In presenting the patient as if she were represented 'objectively' they participated in reification of the patient's socially constructed being. By screening themselves out of their reports, the nurses implicitly constructed the patient as responsible for the interaction. The nurses' reporting practises could be seen as legitimating the institutions of observation and sustaining the ideology that the patient was responsible for the picture of her (cf. Raffel, 1979), thus legitimating the staff in their work of 'assessment and treatment'. Their 'management out' could also be seen as legitimating the nurses' role of reporting rather than determining policy for patients (especially in Site Two). The system of recording may have served to protect the nurses from further accountability in a system in which accounting constituted a moral hazard.[41]

What was managed (out) through participation in the institution structured reflexively through discourse based on the ideologies of illness and responsibility was the conflict of world views of nurse and patient. The experiences and views of the world of patients and nurses were honoured or not within the moral orders of the sites. By managing their selves out of accounts of work the nurses set limits to the development of understanding of their interaction with patients. I will address some implications of this in Chapter 8, arguing that in privileging and participating in institutions which privileged the appearance of the patient as responsible for interaction, and which protected the subjectivity of the nurse at the expense of objectification of the patient, the nurses participated in processes which were personal, interpersonal, social and political.[42]

The location of tension, mixed messages and contradiction in the moral orders

I have argued at various points that patients participated in different discourses in the sites: 'ordinary talk' and 'illness or problem talk'. The distinction may be recast in order to explain some of the tensions and contradictions in accounts. I am arguing here that the patients and nurses participated in, not a single discourse, but discourses of illness and discourses of problems. There were contradictions not only between the nurses and patients, but between the discourses, and also within the discourses. I am arguing that nurses used the concepts in the ideology of responsibility to manage the contradictions.[43] The contradictions in discourse in this study centred on the rights and obligations to give accounts and on whether talk was legitimated as 'work', entitling the actors to respect.

The nurses' and patients' moral reasoning in face to face interaction and in accounts reflexively reproduced the contradictions in discourse (Potter and Wetherell, 1987). Among the contradictions in Site Two were: you don't have to talk, but you do, really; we don't mind your going out without telling us but we do, really; we can't tell you what to do, but we have to; we are the authorities but you shouldn't treat us as the authorities; be responsible for yourself but be responsible to us. Among the contradictions in Site One were: we can help but you have to do it yourself; you are like a child but you have to go into the community; you are not being put out but you do have to move.

This analysis has not resolved the question of the location of the contradictions.[44] Are they in the individual patient or nurse, between them, in wider social structures, in reality? In different moral orders the contradictions were located differently. Where the contradictions lay was part of the knowledge legitimated in the moral order. Remedies for contradictions were legitimated in the moral order. The conclusion of this argument is that empirically the appearance of the contradictions was mediated by the actor's place in the moral order and his command of the facilities of knowledge and power, in particular the locally legitimated discourse, to structure the appearance of himself and the others as agents or patients, as actors worthy or respect or contempt in the moral order.

The meaning of conflict

I have emphasised throughout this monograph the empirical links between knowledge, power and moral order. In arguing that the nurses could not oblige patients to talk with them about problems, I have highlighted the limits of their power, and their relations in moral orders organised for knowledge production.

The findings of this research may be interpreted in light of the work of various writers whose comments on the limits of nurses' power in relation to limits on control of discourse are relevant to discussion of nurses' and patients' relationships in moral orders (Strauss et al, 1964; Belknap, 1956; John, 1961; Altschul, 1972; Sladden, 1979; Towell, 1975; May and Kelly, 1982; Chapman, 1987; Robinson, 1985). The conclusions cannot, however, be reduced to a claim that the nurses construed patients in lay terms, nor to a claim that their discourse was peripheral to that of other professionals. The nurses used concepts including 'illness', 'problems' and 'responsibility' to manage their own, other nurses' and the patients' 'work' in the moral orders of the sites.

No monologic account can resolve the contradictions in the discourses produced through that work. The contradictions lay in the meanings in use of the terms of the discourse. Nurses and patients both had to manage the concept 'responsibility' in settings characterised by contradiction and conflict related to the functions of the sites; relations between professionals; and protection of and revelation of self. To manage 'responsibility' they had to manage the concepts 'illness' and 'problems'; and vice versa. Their facility in and rights to use of the terms reflected their positions in the moral order, their rights, obligations and power to claim legitimacy for their own and/or the other's interpretations. The claims they made using these concepts were heard and responded to in the moral orders of the sites, occasioning further claims regarding 'illness', 'problems', 'responsibility'. The use of the terms occasioned contradictions and location of responsibility for contradictions. They thus enabled ongoing accomplishment of the work of determining 'responsibility'.

Summary

In entering the sites the patients entered conversations. In entering conversations they entered worlds structured as moral orders, mediated by discourses. Among the discourses were those of everyday social life, and those in which they could be constructed as, acted towards and legitimated as 'ill' or as having 'problems'; as 'responsible' or not. They were constructed as subjects in the discourse in talk and in the nurses' talk about their talk.

They came to occupy places in the moral orders of the sites reflexively shaped by the discourse: rights and obligations to be acknowledged best authority on their own reasons; to be regarded as agents or patients, responsible for playing the part of the characters they were held to be (Site One) or responsible for or subject to 'it' (Site Two). Who they 'really' were was ongoingly negotiated through processes of externalisation (or interpretable failure of externalisation), objectivation (subject to dispute) and internalisation (sometimes problematic) (Berger and Luckmann, 1967). The problems in interpreting their appearance in the moral orders of the sites reflected real contradictions and problems in their interaction and talk about it, that is, in their 'work' or 'therapy'.

I have described how in Site One nurses ordered and legitimated interaction to maintain the patient as responsible through exhortation, appeals to 'will', and stories and metaphors which constructed them as 'characters' actually or possibly responsible for themselves.

I have described how in Site Two the nurses organised their work to sustain the patient in the moral order as a (potential) moral agent (potentially) responsible for her action. The conditions for maintenance of the moral order included: the construction of 'responsibility' through obligation to talk, unforced (a condition of agency); promulgation of norms, e.g. 'it's good to share your problems'; definition by the nurse of the patient's role, the patient being responsible for working with the nurses and for finally accepting readiness to help herself; knowledge of typical moral careers ('if you leave the ward in these circumstances you will find it difficult to get readmitted'); construction of reputations (recounting the GP's story of the patient who 'wasted time'); and construction of responsibility.

The moral orders in both sites were based on accounting for the presence and the location of accountable subjects, subjected to the discourse. The nurses managed the concepts 'illness', 'problems' and 'responsibility' to manage their accountability - their ability to account for all patients - within the terms of the moral order structured through the discourses on 'illness' and 'problems'. The concept 'responsibility', as a 'working word', can be construed as a device enabling them to account for people who had to be judged 'present' or 'absent' as accountable subjects (subjects ready for work) but not 'ill', not psychotic. The concept enabled them to subject the 'absent' person (in talk with them and about them) and to require the person to subject herself to search for her accountable self. The concept 'responsibility' was used by nurses to maintain the (potential) working relationship with patients whom they claimed were not working or who were not working with them. Through command of the discourse, nurses in both sites managed treatment of the patient as the kind of person she was, and legitimated taking the right attitude toward her. Management of 'responsibility' reflexively constituted 'the main thing' with these patients.

I have in this chapter tried to convey how nurses and patients managed to order their interaction and legitimate it. I have explored the fine grain of interaction: the 'microphysics' (Foucault, 1979, p. 149) of the acts of excuse and justification; the points where people were pinned down or released from obligation, shown or denied respect. I explored how nurses negotiated their rights and obligations in order to share the sites and play their parts in complex processes of what appeared, through this analysis, as essentially moral work. They had to manage interaction in worlds already structured as moral realms. I have argued that they did so by negotiating understandings of 'work' related to 'illness' or 'problems', understandings entailing commitments in moral orders. In the negotiation nurses had the greater power to interpret interaction and require accounts, and the order reflected the legitimacy of their interpretations. Their practises of knowledge and power were legitimated through their places in and command of the discourses which structured the moral orders.

In nurses' and patients' conversations the moral order was reflexively realised: through the hazard of talk patients and nurses could win respect and avoid contempt (Harré, 1979). The kinds of person they came to be known as through the conversations depended on their abilities to interpret and impose moral orders; their facility for taking their part in the moral order as defined; perhaps their gender; and their rights to display knowledge, exercise power, and judge. The accounts of patients indicated that they changed, in some cases, through talk with the nurses. I stressed that different and competing moral orders were available to or imposed on patients in the sites. How they came to appear to others and to themselves depended, to an indeterminate extent, on which nurse they talked to and how they were able to negotiate maintenance and repair of moral orders through their talk.

Notes

1 Foucault's (1979, p. 250) analysis of 'moral accounting' by warders in prisons is relevant to this analysis.
2 The logic that the nurse is responsible for judgements of the patient's responsibility is central to the problem of this monograph. What is required is another judgement - of the basis on which the nurse is judged. That issue was addressed in the review of literature, in particular MacIlwaine (1980) and Altschul (1972).
3 Any 'dirty work' in Site One 'showed' more, because action was packed into a space shared by patients and nurses, especially at times of staff shortage. The moral context was realised in the empirical settings of space and time in the sites.
4 An exception was an occasion when a man who had tried to commit suicide returned to the ward.
5 Throughout this period a debate went on about whether P6 'should be here'. This was tied up with questions of diagnosis. In a previous footnote I told how the nurses devised a 'game' to 'let P6 know' that she was acting as if she did not want to 'be here'. Nurses were not entitled to claim the authority explicitly to determine grounds for admission or discharge.
6 A method which would have focused only on the individual nurse or patient could not have captured important aspects of this process.
7 See Appendix 4.
8 Previous nursing researchers (John, 1961; Altschul, 1972; MacIlwaine, 1980) do not acknowledge that their claims about patients' emotional states (claims which contradict those made by the nurses) are based on interpretation of the patients' personal states in a moral order different from the moral order constituted in face to face interaction. The legitimacy of the researcher's moral order is problematic from the reader's point of view. The problem is not resolved by use of 'objective' instruments because these cannot establish the basis of moral judgement.

9 This was the common-sense notion of 'neurotic' used by medical and nursing staff.

10 The 'common sense' here is that weddings are 'happy occasions', etc. Opposite constructions of weddings are, of course, available in 'common sense'.

11 Harré (1983) and Shotter (1984) discuss the social psychological proposition that 'internal' talk and conversations - interaction with self - is an importation of the conversations, dialogues, debates available in the social sphere (cf. Billig et al, 1988).

12 See Smail (1987).

13 For example, a doctor was irritated when told that he could not charge a patient for damage to property because the man was in hospital under a Mental Health Act order which legitimated his involuntary hospitalisation on the grounds that he could not be held responsible for his behaviour. Judgments of illness had administrative consequences and moral consequences. To say, as a doctor in Site Two did of P2, that she was not taking her stay seriously, was to preface her discharge and to criticise her as a deviant patient (cf. Turner, 1987).

14 Because 'because' and 'in order to' motives are so closely related to judgements of agency and patienthood, they are important in interpretation of accounts.

15 For P4, being required to account to the nurses constituted a 'hazard' (Harré, 1979). She thought that she might have been construed as 'acting young'. The concept 'young' occurred in both P4's and the first nurse's accounts of this episode of interaction. The nurse thought that P4 like other patients might have rebelled at being asked to account to someone younger than herself. P4 construed the nurses in terms of age (see Chapter 6).

16 See Sacks (1984) on the accomplishment of 'being ordinary' through story-telling practices.

17 Students sometimes revealed severe doubts about their practice.

18 There were thus two levels to the discourse and of accountability: first, in face to face interaction; and secondly, in talk about the interaction. The rights and obligations in each were different.

19 The capacity to plan is related to reflexivity and agency (Harré and Secord, 1972).

20 See also argument in Chapter 6 on 'time' and management of the 'working relationship'.

21 Time and type of support were related - exploration taking more time than 'just support'.

22 In symbiotic accounting (see Shotter, 1984), legitimation of one's action and the representation of one as a person (or a 'kind of person') is accomplished by another. The primary example is that of mother and child. Symbiotic accounting is necessary when the requirements of autonomous accounting are not fulfilled. In particular, since accounting is dependent on and springs from reflexivity (see Mead, 1934), symbiotic accounting may be required when reflexivity is impaired. That is, when one is unable to take the role of the other and direct oneself to participate in the social acts which comprise ordinary life, one may require or have imposed on one a form of symbiotic accounting. Harré (1983) argued that there are three aspects of personal being which are dependent on reflexivity: self-consciousness, autobiography and agency. The accounts one gives of another will depend on the local theories of persons and selves (Harré, 1983). People are 'grown' as personal beings by having provided for them reasons for and interpretations of action which interpret it as meaningful in the local moral order. Among these are theories of what a person is. In Harré's (1983) view, the self is an appropriation of the local theory of persons.

23 Recall S2P10's account of herself as someone whose anxiety was 'exaggerated'.

24 See Chapter 6.

25 I am not questioning the legitimacy of this management, or the care given to ensuring her participation in decisions about the move.

26 Mead's (1934) conception of 'reason' was useful in understanding the relationship between social conduct, responsibility, discourse and reason.

27 It could be argued that in any form of practice involving prolonged day to day contact, the moral orders of work and of everyday life will (must and ought to) articulate.

28 The analysis here can be compared to that in Towell (1975). Other nursing researchers, for example, Altschul (1972) and MacIlwaine (1980), have not addressed as directly the question of the constitution of moral orders.

29 Giving reasons why she should be in hospital laid S2P2 open to blame by a student: N: 'I had it mind that because of, em, her, sort of, her unwillingness to stay **away** from the hospital while she was, actually a patient at a different hospital, i.e. the Epton

Downs, she still kept coming back here. And at every given opportunity gave reasons why she should still be in hospital, as in-patient. That's why I presumed that, you know, this was another ploy of, of needing to stay in.'

30 However, this finding is open to an interpretation that the nurses, accounting in a context in which they knew that patients would also provide an account, might have made weaker claims of helpfulness to avoid being seen as boastful or presumptuous.

31 The reflexivity of the social sciences has been noted by Schutz and Luckmann (1974), Giddens (1976) and others. This nurse can be heard as echoing the interpretation of nurses common in the nursing literature (e.g. Altschul, 1972; MacIlwaine, 1980; Shanley, 1988).

32 I observed this in the case of accounts given to excuse patients who were psychotic.

33 Symbiotic relationships are essential to development of persons. In a symbiotic relationship, one learns what one is doing through the accounts given by another of what one is doing (Shotter, 1984, Harré, 1983).

34 This 'two-tier' interpretation relates to this nurse's accounts. Other nurses interpreted patients in terms of whether they were likely to 'come back' if problems were not resolved.

35 The implications of being unable to negotiate accounts spoken from different places in the moral order or different moral orders will be discussed in Chapter 8.

36 The differences in accounts are theoretically salient from a sociological perspective and from a nursing perspective, not because they ironically cast into doubt the interpretations of either nurse or patient, but because they indicate that both the nurse and the patient - whose 'strength, will or knowledge' (Henderson, 1966, p. 15) are the focal point in definition of nursing - may be defining each other and their relationship is substantially different ways. The theoretical problem then is how to define a relationship the existence of which is subject to competing 'first order' interpretations.

37 It was notably the case that nurses in Site Two could, in their accounts, re-cast 'work' and with it the legitimacy of the working relationship.

38 That is, the sites were the places to which the patient would return if she did not 'get better'. She could become 'repeat business'. The nurses, in particular the permanent staff,

therefore saw patients in relation to a backdrop of 'out there', and in terms of potential psychiatric careers (see Goffman, 1962, 1967).

39 The list of characteristics of the patients could be matched with a list of antonyms: in work, men, having company, normal, having a home, fit, mentally well, married, happy, having a place in society, young. These antonymic characteristics correspond to characteristics of some of the male nurses in the sites.

40 Another way of managing the threat to self was to sustain a notion of 'someone like me who doesnae talk about problems' while talking about problems in groups (S2P6).

41 See Pollock (1989) and Menzies (1970) on nurses' strategies for managing their participation in systems of accountability. Pollock documents CPNs' strategies for dealing with work which could impose administrative/legal accountability. Menzies discusses the role of the institution in structuring work to defend nurses against anxiety.

42 This may be read in conjunction with Peplau's (1978) argument that the work of the patient could be construed in terms of interpersonal, intrapersonal, or systems models.

43 The contradictions included: in the discourse of 'illness', patients were held to be non-responsible but still obliged to participate in treatment (Parsons, 1951; cf. Freidson, 1970; Turner, 1987; and Towell, 1975). This occasioned the distinction between 'ill' ('oh aye, they're definitely sick or they wouldna be here') and 'really ill' (non-responsible).

44 See Peplau (1978) on where the work of treatment of mental illness is to be done.

8 Conclusions

Introduction

In Chapters 5, 6 and 7 I presented arguments based on analysis of the data on knowledge, power and the moral order in interaction between nurses and neurotic patients. I will summarise the main conclusions and discuss the implications for theory development, methodology and nursing practice.

I set this monograph in the contexts of my questions in practice and issues in the nursing literature concerning the practice of nurses with neurotic patients. To answer the questions I adopted a theoretical perspective which enabled me to interpret interaction through the interpretations of those involved in it: views 'from the inside' of social practices (Shotter, 1984, p. 184). I have conveyed the theme of 'developing understandings' by regarding these nurses' work as responses to the questions 'Why is she here now?' and 'What do we have to do for her?'. I found that the question 'Can you tell me about your conversation?' provided access to varied, situated and contradictory understandings. Nurses and patients in their interaction depended on shared background understandings and common sense to engage in and order their talk with each other. In talk they interpreted common sense and deviations from it. The dilemmas and complexities of common sense (Billig et al, 1988) afforded them the topics and resources for the work of understanding each other.

Conclusions on knowledge, power and moral order

The main conclusion regarding knowledge is that nurses depended on common sense to recognise each other as kinds of people, to place each other in the world and to work to mend realities. They depended on it to sustain through their interaction the paramount reality of everyday life in the institutions in which they worked as sense makers making sense of sense makers. I identified the working ideologies in the two sites and suggested that nurses drew on both common sense and specialist knowledge to manage their parts in interaction in complex social institutions, institutions reproduced in part through their interaction.[1] In analysing the patients' knowledge in terms of 'ordinary talk' and 'illness/problem talk' I have provided an empirical guide to understanding talk from the patients' and nurses' points of view, a guide of potential use to nurses and patients. In analysing the nurses' knowledge in terms of site, stay, patient, illness/problem, remedy and personal knowledge, I have provided an empirical description of psychiatric nurses' knowledge in practice. In analysing the centrality and significance of story as a foundation of nursing knowledge I have contributed a conception of how nurses actually interpret and shape their practice. I have also argued that nurses' knowledge was diverse, divergent, possibly gender-related, related to context, and dynamic.

I drew on the nurses' interpretations of their practice to discuss the issue of the knowledge base of psychiatric nursing practice with neurotic patients in admission wards. The nursing literature interpreted psychiatric nursing in terms of a dichotomy between, on the one hand, 'lay' understanding or common sense; and on the other hand, 'deliberate, purposeful' talk or talk based on an identifiable perspective and theoretical knowledge. I have concluded that the nurses in this study drew on a wide variety of kinds of knowledge, some specialist, some grounded in the practical knowledge of the site. 'Worldly knowledge' was vitally important in interpreting, maintaining and repairing the 'world' of the site interpenetrated by the world of everyday life. Nurses and patients as sense makers making sense of sense makers 'worked' against the background of 'worldly knowledge'.

Nurses' second level accounts provided an insight into their second level concepts. The nurses' knowledge was mainly oral and intersubjective, and interpretations were screened out of written documents. The knowledge was knowledge in practice, knowing the main thing at the time for the practical purpose of accomplishing the practical aims of managing the site and moving people on in their stays. It was 'working knowledge' (Harper, 1987). The forms of knowledge were the forms of practice. Among the forms I found were the circle of interpretation, the cycle of interaction, the symbiotic account, and the story of the main thing. I will suggest below further research on understanding and developing forms of nursing practice.

I reviewed the theme of knowledge in the psychiatric nursing literature by teasing out the oppositions which structured the literature as discourse. In doing so I indicated how the nursing researchers' search for 'rational, deliberate' knowledge related to the aim of identifying a body of knowledge adequate for justification of claims to professional identity. I concluded from the present study that the rationality of the nurses' practice did not depend on deliberation or reference to a set of principles, if by that is implied a set of decontextualised elements. Rather, the rationality was always underpinned by reference to indexical, reflexively accountable features of the reality of the work settings; to the resources of common sense; and to the terms of 'working ideologies'. On the basis of this study I can offer no conclusion on the value of theoretical knowledge in psychiatric nursing practice. However, I argue that decontextualisation would have stripped the knowledge of its practical force. Theories in use in practice should be interpreted in relation to the contexts in which they are used.[2]

The main conclusions regarding power related to the analysis of nurses' and patients' interaction in terms of their powers in relation to each other; in particular, analysis of 'work' on the patients' 'powers' to act as accountable agents. I provided an original analysis of the form and process of psychiatric nursing with these patients. I emphasised that the nurses practised a form of rhetoric, or 'persuasive speech' (Aristotle, cited in Szasz, 1979, p. 13) in which 'each tries to move the other to see or do things in a certain way' (p. 11).[3] According to this analysis, both nurses and patients could be construed as rhetoricians. To construe them thus is to construe them as moral agents pursuing aims (cf. Szasz, 1979, p. 15). Empirically, the question of the patient's status - as patient or as moral agent pursuing aims - was often the matter under dispute. This study did not intend to resolve the issue of the agency of patients. However, the description of nursing practice with the patients in this study has included a claim that, in their accounts in interaction, the nurses and patients can be seen as rhetoricians disputing issues of agency, will, and aims; using the resources of a dilemmatic common sense (Billig et al, 1988).

I stressed the reflexive relationship between knowledge and power, mediated by practices of knowing. In particular I noted the organisation of observation, including observation through accounting, which constituted assessment. These practices can be construed as a form of 'discipline', through which the subject is constituted through talk (Foucault, 1979; Dreyfus and Rabinow, 1986, p. 175). (See also below.) I explored aspects of the patients' power, including resistance and 'rebellion'.[4] The main practical problem of power which nurses and patients had to solve in their interaction derived from questions of 'can't do or won't do?'[5], the ordinary equivalent of questions of agency.

I explored the role of metaphor in enabling 'working relationships', and focused on the complexities of analysis in which nurses' action on patients' action was interpreted through their accounts. I argued that the complexity and problems of analysis reflected features of the nurses' and patients' work together: problems of interpretation; having to 'see her through her words...what she is doing'. This, however, entailed some difficulties in discriminating between, on the one hand, the rhetoric involved in constructing a picture of interaction and of the nurse and patient as agent/agency in it; and, on the other hand, the power in interaction. This reproduced the 'problem' noted in discussion of knowledge, namely that of interpreting a pre-interpreted reality on the basis of accounts. The problem of the analysis reflected the problem of interaction: it was essentially the problem of interpretation itself, and of the power involved in negotiating and making interpretations 'stick'. What made the 'work' of the nurses and patients, the 'dramas of push and pull' (Peplau, 1952) problematic was that it was interaction between people, each of whom could relate to the other(s) as both agent and agency, and interpreting being(s). The moves in the 'games' of interaction (Mead, 1934) were related to issues of power in struggles to command the definition of the game, the rules, and the players' rights and obligations. I interpreted these as issues of power, will and agency.

'Actors acting on actors', the nurses acted on the basis of their interpretations of the patient as agent, taking account of the possibility of the 'con'[6]. Thus issues of knowledge and power were utterly intertwined. The complexity inheres in the social construction of the power of nurses or patients. The appearance of powers depended on the power, the account giver's command or facility in persuasion to a view from his or her position. Thus rhetoric and power in nurse patient interaction were so closely interlinked that study of one entailed study of the other. The confluence of power and rhetoric was conveyed in the centrality of metaphor[7] in structuring the common understandings which shaped interaction.

This monograph has focused on the 'appearance of power' and on the rhetoric which commanded the appearance of action on action, rather than on 'examination' of the practices of power in interaction. This was justified by an argument that the capacity to 'command' the appearance of powers was a practice of power; and that the patient had the power to resist 'commands' to participate in processes through which she would be defined. However, there is clearly a danger of a regression, in which the analysis of the 'reality' of power is forever deferred, with analysis of the representation of power privileged. (See the argument below on the potential for a Foucaultian analysis of the data.)

I noted that the practices of power were always contextualised. Criticism of nurses' 'missed opportunities' which does not take into account the social construction of 'opportunity' is inadequately grounded. Nurses' references to indexical features of interaction, in their accounts of 'opportunities' they saw and took or did not take, should be read in light of Dreyfus' (1983, p. 14) argument that:

> The pragmatic background and its practical kind of understanding is the source of the problems confronting a theory of everyday capacities.

In the psychiatric nursing literature, 'missed opportunities' have been constituted by the observer/researcher, on the basis of decontextualisation; rather than by the actor in the situation of pragmatic, involved action. In this monograph, the perspective of the latter has been taken as the basis for understanding practice.

As I related the analysis of knowledge to nursing researchers' interest in knowledge, so I want to highlight the power involved in nursing research. Because nursing researchers produce knowledge of practice which is used to shape policy, they are in unusual positions of power in relation to those with whom they engage in research. The analysis in this monograph revealed the complex relations of power, and the different perceptions of relations of power among various staff and patients. Nurses worked in webs of power. I investigated one group of patients in the context of the main work of the sites; saw fragments of action, phases of episodes; and saw the nurses struggle at times in situations which to me seemed exceedingly stressful. The account of power, like the account of knowledge in this monograph, should be taken as a partial account, but one that conveys some clear implications about power in practice. Among the implications are these: because nurses' practice is situated in relation to the working practices of other professionals, the political context of the institutions has to be taken into account in discussions of nurses' accountability; and because nurses manage themselves as scarce resources they are vulnerable to stresses generated by a 'flow of work' (admission and discharge) they can control only indirectly. The 'site' and all 'work' in the site were always subject to sudden and dramatic redefinition through admission or discharge.

The main conclusion with regard to moral order was that the nurses' and patients' interaction was essentially a moral order. The accomplishment of everyday life, of sharing the sites, could be interpreted as a legitimation (and a reification) of the moral order of the everyday world. I interpreted the sites as systems of excuse and legitimation. The moral order in which action was interpreted at a given time depended on the people in interaction who sustained and challenged it, always against the backdrop of the moral order of the paramount reality of the wider community, which interpenetrated the sites. The relevance of concepts of moral orders based on honour and deliberation was explored. However, I stressed that these concepts were inadequate to account for the complexity of interaction. I also described some of the tensions in 'symbiotic accounts', in order to investigate contradictions in relationships between nurses and patients as understood through accounts. The analysis of the main orders of the two sites may have understated the diversity of interaction, sustenance of other orders, subversion.

Nursing researchers have appraised nurse-neurotic patient interaction in terms of the inappropriateness of 'lay' moral judgements. While I have emphasised the dependence of nurses' and doctors' judgements on common-sense categories of moral judgement, I have tried to advance the understanding of this aspect of nurse-patient interaction by interpreting the meaning of the maintenance of the moral order of everyday life in these settings (cf. Chapman, 1987, for a related analysis in a different setting). The nurses' moral judgements were mediated by the conception of the patient as a person, based on interaction in the moral orders of the sites structured as places of work. A simple dichotomy of 'ill'/'not ill' as the foundation of moral deliberation did not account for the complexity of the nurses' and patients' moral reasoning. Rather, occasions of excuse and justification were negotiated against a backdrop of shared understandings of the obligations of everyday life, and of 'work' as structured by the rights and obligations of nurses and patients. By maintaining the moral order, the nurses enabled people from various and at times unknown positions in the moral orders of the main community to share the site and take part in the 'work'.

Nursing researchers have interpreted nurses' practice within the moral order of professional discipline. Nursing research is construed as part of nursing, and nursing is structured through lines of accountability.[8] It is therefore important to emphasise that it was not the intention of the present study to provide a basis for evaluation of the work of nurses in the two wards, nor to provide a basis for generalisation to other settings. Rather, the intention was to interpret interaction as construed by the actors who both structured it and provided moral commentary on it. In this I, like previous researchers (Altschul, 1972; MacIlwaine, 1980), have been only partly successful.[9]

The analysis summarised above was based on understandings from an interpretive perspective. Adopting this perspective involved treating people as the centres of their worlds, as managing interaction and maintaining subjective identity. Attention to language was a central feature of the methodology. Viewed from an interpretive perspective, psychiatric nursing involved reality definition, maintenance and repair, based on use of facilities afforded by language for creating and inhabiting social worlds (Berger and Luckmann, 1967). The nurses' discourse comprised working words and working usages. It was a set of variations on the discourses of everyday life, on grounding in which it depended. The *parole* of psychiatric nurses and patients shaped the worlds of their day to day life.[10]

Implications

These considerations lead to a discussion of some implications of this study for theory, methodology and nursing practice. The study was grounded in a tradition which emphasises the ontological priority of first order constructs in ordering the socially constructed reality investigated by the researcher (Schuetz, 1943; Harré and Secord, 1972). The problem of actors' and researcher's knowledge, discussed in Chapter 3, is thus a central theoretical concern. A theoretical problem at the heart of this monograph concerns accounting for 'contradictions' between accounts when questions might be raised about the ability of one of the sources of the accounts to give 'valid' accounts. Harré and Secord (1972, p. 235) cite Freud's concern with the 'authenticity of an account which supplied the reasons for a hitherto inexplicable action'; and claim (p. 256) that a person who is chronically anxious may be 'assigned' by doctors 'to a certain category of human being, namely, the neurotic'; by implication a category of persons the authority of whose accounts may be suspect. This suggests that Harré and Secord might support the privileging of another's account (for example the Freudian account) over that of the 'neurotic'.[11] Habermas (cited in McCarthy, 1976) likened neurosis in the individual to ideology in society. The term 'neurotic' in his account refers to people who have unconscious motives which they cannot make available to themselves or to another in accounting for their action (Habermas, 1970). Harré and Secord's (1972) analysis of the 'assignment' of the 'neurotic' may refer to the social construction of the neurotic.[12] However, it remains unclear whether in these writers' views, 'neurotic' may refer to a class of people whose accounting practices are considered especially problematic in a theoretically significant way.

A further conclusion on the relationship of theory, method and substantive topic relates to the first. I noted in Chapter 4 that issues of validity and reliability in this study were in part addressed by checking out my understandings with those who had given the accounts or been present during my periods of fieldwork. In this, however, I was only partly successful, due to the assurance of confidentiality. I could not identify specific differences between a patient's account and a nurse's account and ask for clarification. Therefore, some of the findings, specifically those related to differences of view, may be regarded as having been differently validated. These issues relate directly to my discussion of implications for practice.

One of the main conclusions I reached through doing this research is that the nurses in their practice faced counterparts to the theoretical and methodological problems I faced. Thus I highlighted in Chapter 5 how the nurses construed issues of reliability and validity for practical purposes. In feedback sessions the nurses grasped the relevance to their work of the notions of social construction of reality, defence of the paramount reality, and therapy. The problems faced in practice and in this form of research centred on issues of knowledge, power and moral order. These problems were essentially related to the basic problem of intersubjectivity; the problem of constructing and making sense of a social world, given that all that is known is interpreted from the different perspectives of individual actors.

An implication of the conclusion that 'practically methodologically' the nurses faced variations on problems faced by social scientists - problems of knowing, knowing better and demonstrating the grounds of knowledge - is that further research is needed on nurses' methods of managing issues of reliability and validity for practical purposes (cf. Garfinkel, 1967).

I placed this study in the context of the body of knowledge of psychiatric nursing by arguing that each work in the field has to define the field[13], because there is no paradigm of psychiatric nursing. In this monograph I have defined the literature on psychiatric nursing as a discourse, and related the discourse of the nurses in the study to that in the literature. In doing so I have tried to advance the debate, the 'conversation' or argument about and in psychiatric nursing construed as a set of practices and as an object of social scientific study.

As an object of social scientific study, what characterises psychiatric nursing is that, both in the sphere of practice, and in the sphere of theoretical, educational or professional development, psychiatric nursing is concerned with practical and theoretical issues of 'who knows better?' and 'who will command the definition of the situation?'. Two main implications concerning the relationship of nursing theory and practice and the definition of psychiatric nursing follow from this research.

The first implication relates to issues raised by Peplau (1952). I have discussed Peplau's (1978) understanding of the relationship between the work of the patient and the work of the psychiatric nurse. I have argued from empirical evidence that the nurses and patients in this study were, and saw themselves as, interdependent in doing the work of the sites. The methods of the study enabled nurses to recognise and reflect on aspects of their practice which are of theoretical significance in nursing. Having adopted the role of participant observer, I asked nurses to produce accounts in which they took their own work as a topic for further explanation. This study indicates the potential usefulness, for British psychiatric nurses, of Peplau's (1952) understanding that the nurse in practice is a participant observer.[14] I am arguing that the definition of the 'work' of these nurses and patients, and the 'parts' they play, could be further developed by legitimating the nurses' 'participant observer' role as a form of practice and education, and as a device for defining practice for the purposes of quality assurance.[15]

The conclusions of Chapters 6 and 7 suggest the possible fruitfulness of further work based on Peplau's (1952) understanding that the person that the patient becomes depends to some extent on the person that the nurse becomes. My experience throughout the research was that, given the right conditions, nurses wanted mirrors held up to their practice. Their opportunities to develop understanding of their practice, and their own involvement in the processes of interaction, were few.[16] The present study suggests a potential remedy for this 'lack of opportunity'. Nurses' narrative practices - including accounting and telling of stories about practice - could be legitimated as developmental practices whereby nurses might increase their command of social resources for telling what they do.

It may be countered that my finding that nurses 'screened out' their interpretations in writing formal records indicates their unwillingness to bring 'self' more into practice. However, I am suggesting that this process of interpretation should be based on talk; and that, in the first instance, it might be conducted outside the current framework of accountability.[17, 18]

It could be further countered that this proposal is a form of research-based imperialism, and that it contradicts the conclusion of this monograph that nurses know, for practical purposes, what to do. Both objections are somewhat valid; though I have outlined some of the problems nurses faced in their work with these patients, and the limits of their ability to help. Nonetheless, the context of practice is changing with increased demands for accountability. What I propose is a set of methods which nurses in practice could command in inevitable struggles over definition of 'work'. The present study suggests that struggles over definition of 'work' will entail (for both patients and nurses) struggles over definitions of self, other and community.

The second main implication for nursing theory and practice concerns Henderson's (1966, p. 15) definition of nursing. The empirical data of this study may be used to illuminate problematic aspects of that definition:

> The unique function of the nurse is to assist the individual, sick or well, in the performance of those activities contributing to health or its recovery (or to peaceful death) that he would

> perform unaided if he had the necessary strength, will or knowledge. And to do this in such a way as to help him gain independence as soon as possible.

Firstly, it is important to note that the work of the nurses in this study may be interpreted as a form of nursing in terms of the above definition (granted that the definition of 'health' requires some mediation through Peplau's concepts (Peplau, 1978). Secondly, it may be noted that the conclusions of this monograph indicate that the phrase 'that he would perform unaided if he had the necessary strength, will or knowledge' pinpoints problematic matters of central importance in defining the work of these psychiatric nurses and patients.

These conclusions regarding the relationship of practice and theory centre on the nurses' practices of responsibility ascription: interpreting the patient as agent or patient, and making ascriptions 'stick'. The nurses' knowledge, power and interaction in the moral order were based on interpretations of the patient's (and other nurses') action. I have stressed that accounts were crucially important in this process. The method I chose, and the one that I recommend for nurses in practice, is based on construing accounts as occasions for interpretation and responsibility ascription.

The argument of this study indicates that the definition of what is to count as knowledge, of whether or not the patient possesses necessary strength (powers), and of whether or not the patient is acting willfully in not doing, are practical issues which reflexively affect the definition of nursing (cf. May and Kelly, 1982; and Kelly and May, 1982, on mutual legitimation). On the basis of this study I suggest that the definition of nursing in any setting or situation will involve a social process involving interpretation, definition and negotiation of what constitutes knowledge, power and will. An implication is, therefore, that nurses would benefit from interpreting the empirical social processes through which 'nursing' is defined. The ways in which nurses accomplish those definitions for practical purposes can usefully be construed from the perspective of the social construction of reality. This study indicated the importance of recognising that the definition of psychiatric nursing is always occasioned. It takes place and is commanded in settings structured by relations of knowledge and power; that is, it takes place in a political context (cf. Pollock, 1989). The definition of 'necessary' knowledge, strength and will is negotiated daily in face to face interaction between neurotic patients and nurses; and thereby the definition of nursing is accomplished for practical purposes.

These arguments based on the findings of the study suggest further implications for practice. In this monograph I have explored issues related to the nurses' practices of responsibility ascription. The relationship between story analysis and responsibility ascription can be fed back into nursing theory development. Any account of doing for the other what she would do for herself if she had the necessary 'strength, power and will' implies complex reasoning which can be articulated in story: the nurse as agent in helping the patient, and as agency in doing what the patient (as agent) would do for self.[19] The theoretical significance of the analysis of story, from the point of view of psychiatric nursing, is that the dramatist pentad may be used to explicate matters of motive. Story analysis in clinical practice could form a basis for interpretations not only of motives, but also of the processes of motive ascription and of definition of nurse and patient roles.

I have described in the text the inadequacies of conceptions of nursing (e.g. MacIlwaine, 1980) which assume that problems of responsibility ascription and legitimation of practice can be solved through 'recognition' of the implications of diagnosis. Further research is needed not only on the conceptual and empirical links between diagnosis, formulation and common-sense reasoning but also on how diagnoses and common-sense terms are used to accomplish nursing as warrantable conduct.[20]

Implications for nursing education and practice

I will now consider some of the implications of this study for nursing education and practice. The methods used for developing understandings were innovative in the field of nursing studies. This study suggests that accounts of conversations from both patients and nurses, series of accounts by the same patients, and second level accounts are all potentially available as data bases for interpreting nursing practice.

There are at least three ways in which the interpretive methods used in this study could be used in nursing practice, education and research. Firstly, because they enable nurses to define what they consider qualitatively meaningful aspects of their work, they should be incorporated into quality assurance programmes.[21] With regard to quality assurance, an implication of this study is that the patient's view of interaction and the patient's role in definition of nursing practice must be taken into account.

A second use for the methods in practice lies in their potential as a form of nursing practice. The method of accounting might be used by nurse and patient to facilitate discussion and negotiation of their roles; within the framework provided by use of the analytic categories developed in this study - 'knowledge', 'power' and 'moral order' - or within a framework generated locally. Other possibilities for nursing practice development include joint analyses of stories and accounts, and the elaboration of symbiotic accounts and shared stories (cf. Mair, 1987; and Hobson, 1985). Psychiatric nursing may thus develop as local practices.The methods of developing nursing practice as understanding, used in this study, could inform nursing practice based on a 'social behaviourist' (Mead, 1934) stance.[22]

I noted certain limits imposed by the use of the methods in research. I could not 'negotiate' views between nurses and patients. This could, however, be done in practice. A second limitation was that, in order to tell me about their talk with nurses, in particular 'illness and problem talk', patients would have had to have recapitulated the talk and associated feelings. I sometimes sensed that this set limits to what they could or would tell me and to what I was willing to explore in the research context (Appendix 2). It is possible that nurses using these methods in practice would generate kinds of data different from those reported in this monograph. One finding of this study is that processes of telling and being told about are so infused with power and so closely related to the implications of the moral order that the uses of telling would depend on the roles and relationships of the teller and hearer, and these in turn would depend on the wider contexts of the settings in which nurses and patients talk.

I will now discuss implications for education of nursing students. I noted that student nurses gave accounts of some of the most stressful interaction, and that on some occasions they made (and felt that they had to make) decisions regarding interventions, on the basis of inadequate training and support. In some cases the consequences of such interventions, and the associated distress, were unknown to the ward staff. Students structured their work on the basis of their places in the moral orders and the structures of power in the sites. Melia (1981) found that student nurses felt they were 'working in the dark'. Some students in this study felt that they worked in the dark, and on occasions deliberately kept trained staff in the dark about their work (cf. Altschul, 1972, on 'involvement').

I suggest that some of these issues could be addressed by using the categories 'knowledge', 'power' and 'moral order' as guides in accounting and negotiation of accounts between student nurses and patients, and between student nurses and staff responsible for their clinical education. Use of these categories would enable articulation of interpretations of nursing practice with understandings in related social sciences. Alternatively, student nurses like other nurses could develop skills of qualitative data production and analysis to devise categories relevant to their own, patients' and more senior nurses' understandings of interaction. In doing so they would take a lead in developing systems of accountability shaped by their understandings and used to shape their further action in clinical work.

I have highlighted the role of language in psychiatric nursing practice. I recommend that student nurses be given opportunities to participate in development of practices of accounting and story telling. An implication of the theoretical perspective adopted in this study, in particular work by Mair (1987, 1989), Shotter (1984) and Harré (1979, 1983), is that development of 'powers' of accounting is a form of development of self and of social accountability.

An implication of this analysis is that the process of nurse-patient interaction in psychiatric nursing is potentially a process of self-development for the nurse as well as for the patient (cf. Peplau, 1952). Cultivation of accounting as a form of development, and reflection on self in interaction with others, would be valuable for nurses being educated, not simply trained, to relate to and work with patients. I have highlighted that the nurses' case management was mediated by an oral culture. Students in settings where this is the case should be enabled to 'read', deconstruct and interpret the knowledge in talk; and also be enabled to develop written records suitable for nursing development and communication with other professionals.[23]

In arguing that forms of practice and education based on dialogue among nurses and between nurses and patients are 'suitable for nursing development' I am claiming that knowledge of the practice of psychiatric nursing is not fixed, and is not owned by individual nurses, or by nurses alone (it is to some extent shared with patients). It is a form of social knowledge, shared and articulated collectively, and dynamically produced and reproduced. The function of the methods I have outlined above would therefore be to enable nurses' development as practitioners able to articulate in appropriate forms the knowledge that guides their work, to recognise the practices of power in which they are engaged, and to articulate and argue the moral dilemmas of their work. It would be a form of praxis (Clark with Asquith, 1985).

In this monograph I have focused on responsibility as a central issue in the psychiatric nursing of neurotic patients. As a researcher I participated in the sites in a role of relative non-responsibility. A main contradiction[24] in this monograph consists of saying, from outside practice, that knowledge is in practice but ought to be developed; that nursing practices as forms of power ought to be critically interpreted, developed and directed; that moral reasoning is essential to psychiatric nursing and ought to be developed. In Chapter 2 I criticised researchers and theorists who sought to impose 'remedies' for psychiatric nursing on the basis of judgements based on standards of rationality or ethical standards derived from outside the settings of practice. Because it may appear that my argument, based on the conclusions of the study, proposes precisely such a 'remedy', it is important to stress the central recommendation that I am making, and the grounds for it. The contradiction necessitates a further conclusion.

I am arguing for the development of methods and practices of 'developing understandings' in psychiatric nursing, not because the good of psychiatric nursing is known, in the form of a theory, but because I believe that the development of understandings is itself a good. This is not a conclusion of the study, but one based on the acceptance of moral reasoning articulated by various authors (Harré, 1983; Shotter, 1984; Habermas, 1963, 1971a, 1971b). In proposing use of the above methods by psychiatric nurses in their work with neurotic patients, and in psychiatric nursing education and practice more generally, I am proposing methods which would involve political change (on the personal and social levels) based on attempts to create the conditions for unconstrained communication. That proposal, however, follows from the argument of this monograph. In their work with patients nurses were already involved in forms of 'therapy', work to restore the 'strays' from the paramount reality and to legitimate that work. In that work the nurses and patients participated (as I did in a different role) in daily struggles to define reality and to shape the world to human ends. In that work they defined common sense and uncommon sense, playing their (structured) parts in structuring the shared world.

In arguing for methods of 'developing understandings' I am arguing for methods that would enable nurses and patients to explore more fully and freely how they make common and uncommon senses and use them to shape the world. Previous nursing researchers have critiqued the nurses' common sense on the grounds of its inadequacy for (professional) practice. My claim is not that theory is not necessary for practice - I have noted that nurses drew on theoretical and other knowledge in doing their work. My claim is that the common sense of psychiatric nursing is always being made. Investigation of psychiatric nursing is therefore investigation of a form of social reality in which the paramount reality is produced and reproduced. Critique of this process by practitioners may enable them to understand the ways in which the practices of psychiatric nursing may reify the social processes of the paramount reality. The role of research in this process may be to facilitate practitioners' interpretation and critique of their practices.

I have highlighted the contradictions in my discourse, as well as in the discourse of other researchers, and of nurses and patients. The contradictions in practice and the contradictions in the nursing literature are contradictions in different discourses. My conclusion is that the contradictions in practice can only be resolved by those involved in practice. The form of theory that would help them would be, not theory based on decontextualised knowledge, but critical theory. The claim for the good of accounting is in part based on a claim of the good of personhood related to ability to account for actions in terms recognised in the locally valued discourse (Harré, 1983; Shotter, 1984).[25] The potential conservatism of practice on these terms is balanced by the prospect that in every interaction one may choose to reproduce, or not to reproduce, the locally valued discourse (see Harré, 1979). The claim for the good of accounting is also based on Habermas' (1963, 1971b) argument that discussion intended to define the good life depends on the linguistic competence of speakers, and on unconstrained speech. Among limits to freedom Habermas includes the constraints of communication imposed by neurosis in the individual, and by ideology in the society (Habermas, cited in McCarthy, 1976, p. xv). I am arguing for the development, in practice, of better common-sense ways of revealing and resolving contradictions, on the grounds that common sense provides the 'seeds of arguments' (Bacon, cited in Billig et al, 1988, p. 16) used by nurses and patients in their struggles to share and to shape a common world, and to develop their own and each other's 'powers' of argument.

The limitations of the present study must be understood in terms of limitations of the theoretical perspective, of the method, and of the analysis. Some of the problems inhere in trying to relate interpretations of the microcosms of interaction to interpretations of the macrocosms of the sites and the wider social order. One of the weaknesses of this study is the inadequacy of articulation between, on the one hand, the second order concept 'ideology' at the level of sites, and the first order concept 'savvy' which may be seen as its correlate; and, on the other hand, the second order concepts ('agency', for example), and individual nurses' and patients' first order understandings (for example 'the kind of person'). Another weakness lies in the limits of articulation of the macro-processes of the wider community and the site, with the micro-processes of interaction. The analysis of 'working knowledge' (Chapter 5) is only partially successful. Some of the limitations reflect limits of the theoretical perspective. Giddens (1976, p. 171) criticises Berger and Luckmann (1967) for their failure to 'reconcile a theory of action with one of institutional organization'. Researchers in the ethogenic tradition (Marsh et al, 1978) have been criticised for similar failures (Totman, 1980). My attempts to articulate the macroprocesses and microprocesses have to an extent been driven by interpretations of links at a theoretical level between concepts of agency, theories of action, and understandings of moral orders based on conceptions of the person. While I argue that the interpretations of the first order constructs in the data support the weight of inference from them, they have in some instances greatly oversimplified the world the actors sustained in interaction. I have to some extent relied on a notion of 'ideology' which glosses the complexities of interpretation and interaction. Likewise, my analysis of metaphor glosses the problems of articulating the relationship between the nurses' discourse, based on interpretations, and the organisation of work in the sites.

Despite these limitations I argue that conclusions from my analysis of empirical data support a claim that what is of sociological significance in nurse-patient interaction in institutions such as the two psychiatric admission wards is how nurses and patients solve the problem of interpretation, practically, by negotiation of common sense. What is of particular theoretical significance, from the phenomenological perspective, is that they coordinated interaction ('shared the site') by organising it in terms of the paramount reality of 'work' (Schutz, 1968). The phenomenological perspective is thus relevant to the central concern of the nurses in the two sites as interpreted in this study: the work entailed in responses to the questions 'Why is she (am I) here now?' and 'What do we have to do for her (I have to do)?'.

In indicating the potential fruitfulness of these theoretical understandings it is necessary to indicate some tensions and problems associated with them. The main tension[26] has come through the text of this monograph at various points. It is the tension generated by considering that each person is the centre of a world, and a world maker; while also depicting one social world that all inhabit. The problem can be construed as a problem in the sociology of knowledge (Berger and Luckmann, 1967).[27] No conceptual machinery for universe maintenance adequately explains how the social world is sustained.[28]

Ending and unfinished work

I began this monograph with a story of how questions in practice led me into a conversation with nursing literature and theoretical literature, and then into conversations with patients and nurses in practice. The question was 'What am I doing?', spoken within the context of practice as a psychiatric nurse. My way of answering was to ask others to tell me what they were doing. The problems of knowledge, subjectivity and intersubjectivity have thus been present in each dialogue of this research. Through the research I opened and closed dialogues with nurses and patients in the practice settings. In the monograph I have opened and closed dialogues between others' talk and texts and my own text. I have recommended to nurses the theoretical pespective and the methods of interpretive, interactive investigation as the basis for further dialogues about reasons in practice and the practices of reason.

The conclusion of this monograph is thus that the work of finding the common sense of psychiatric nursing in practice remains to be done. The struggle to find truly plurivocal (Bakhtin, 1984) forms of expression is a political struggle to be undertaken in practice. Research in practice, action research (Webb, 1989) in which the researcher's voice is committed to the development of discussion in the sites of practice, may be one form of that struggle.

Psychiatric nursing, portrayed in the monograph as a form of 'social argumentation (which) can be seen as providing the model for social thinking ...(and) the arguments which arise within a particular common sense, as people debate about the common sense they share' (Billig et al, 1988) awaits further realisation and definition. This monograph has been a form of interpretation of an aspect of psychiatric nursing. The conversations that sustained it are over, but echoes of them, and of 'voices' in the literature, persist.

Notes

1 I argued that the institutions were structured to produce knowledge of patients, to remedy deviations from the paramount reality.
2 See for example, the note on the 'vestigial' knowledge of responsibility in Site Two.
3 I noted in Chapter 3 that Szasz construed rhetoric as 'a certain kind of conversation' by means of which one could heal or harm depending on the speaker's intention, and 'concerned with what comes within the ken of all men and belongs to no definite science' (Aristotle, in Szasz, 1979, p. 13). The concept of rhetoric was drawn on to relate the nurses' accounts to a conception of speech as action intended to persuade others to a view of the world. Specifically, Szasz notes the distinction between the noble and the base rhetorician, the former misportraying the world by depicting 'cause without consequence or consequence without cause, acts without agents and agents without agency (thus blocking) definition and cause-and-effect reasoning' (Weaver, in Szasz, 1979, p. 20).
4 The sites could be construed as 'provinces of knowledge' (Schutz and Luckmann, 1974) 'commanded' by nurses, most of the time.
5 This argument about power/powers can be read in terms of discretionary powers (cf. Adler and Asquith, 1981). The argument would be that, from the nurses' points of view, several of these patients had and exercised discretionary powers - they were agents and strategists, they could subject themselves to their wills or choose not to. Nurses had discretionary powers to help patients, depending on their recognition of or interpretation of the patient's discretionary powers. The practices of power were thus based in a system of knowledge of what kind of person the patient was - agent or patient. However, the thrust of the argument is that the analysis of powers could be more complex (for example, see the discussion above on 'opportunities'). The ideology of discretionary powers is closely related to the question of professional judgement - should nurses recognise that patients do not really have discretionary

powers? It is therefore related to professional ethics and practical ethics. What kinds of person are entitled to help provided by the nurse on the basis of her discretionary exercise of power? These questions relate to larger issues of use of nurses' power in the community (Wooff and Goldberg, 1988). The analysis of discretionary powers in this monograph shows that the problem should be examined at the microprocess level and also in relation to the macroprocesses of practices of discretionary power in the sites - what discretion do nurses practice in the exercise of their powers? How does the patient get to be defined as someone with discretionary power? The social processes by which this is accomplished are complex. The question concerns what is involved in diagnosis or clinical decision-making based on recognition of discretionary power. Some nurses regarded some neurotic patients as people with sufficient discretionary powers to have worked had they wanted to. The management of the nurses' work in a system in which they were recognised as having discretionary power was closely tied to their management of the definition of the patient's discretionary power.

Put simply, the definition of the nurses' work, and more generally of the nurses as workers, was reflexively related to the definition of the patient's work and of the patient (cf. Peplau, 1978)

6 The possibilities included the patient as agent acting as if she were a patient; and as patient acting as agent.

7 Sackmann (1989) noted the usefulness of 'adaptive' metaphors in organisations when 'a different reality is being developed' (p. 482). See her discussion of the metaphor of 'gardening' in the context of the discussion in this monograph (cf. Barker, 1989).

8 I noted that calls to get nurses to account for their practice could entail reproduction and reification of the moral order of professional relations (Altschul, 1972). In recent literature (Clark, 1988) nursing research has been directly linked with accountability. The implication is that nurses' accountability may be judged in terms of the fit between the knowledge base of their practice and current research-based evidence (Swaffield, 1990).

9 The submerged voices in the moral orders of the sites remain largely submerged in this monograph: the quiet and the difficult patients, the student nurses. I reproduced and to an extent reified the feature of the moral order whereby the most

privileged members had the last word. For example, when I asked for accounts of 'what the patient's stay has been about' in Site Two, I sometimes asked more senior nurses to supplement accounts given by student nurses. Also, when a patient left hospital, her or his 'file self' (Harré, 1983) remained, mainly articulating the medical voice. To some extent less valued and privileged voices have been 'managed out', simply by use of documents and occasions for interview structured by the 'hierarchy of credibility' (Becker, 1967).

10 Nursing researchers have argued that nursing is an art, and that the skills of the dramatist or novelist are needed to capture aspects of it (e.g. Peplau, 1988). In this study I found some nurses who practised their use of language to guide their practice: for rhetorical purposes, and to grasp and convey through speech something of the richness and significance of what they did in sharing and shaping worlds through talk with patients.

11 Smail (1984, 1987) argues that it is generally the case that others can know what we do better than we ourselves can.

12 See Lemert's (1962) analysis of paranoia.

13 'The field cannot be well seen from within the field': Emerson (1982, p. 232).

14 One nurse commented that giving a second level account was like being involved in an interview with a patient, in which he had to think while trying to 'steer' the conversation in therapeutic directions, to respond to his own feelings while attending to what the patient was saying. The same nurse, who had recently completed training, said that in giving accounts to me, in the course of the working day, about apparently insignificant actions (a patient knocking before coming into a room, rather than barging in), he understood through telling what it was that he was doing. Thus, accounting in the course of nursing practice enabled development of the nurse's understanding of how his own practice was developing (through noticing small differences and understanding their significance with regard to that patient).
Nurses in both sites recognised the broad pictures of their working practices as I fed them back, but said that they had never considered their work from the perspective I provided. A charge nurse said that he would often have liked to have been able to be a 'fly on the wall' in his own ward.

15 This qualitative study has indicated the nurses' ability to define qualitative aspects of their work.

16 In this they might be said to have 'mirrored' the patients.

17 The plans for continuing education in nursing offer one set of opportunities.

18 The latter suggestion is balanced by an awareness, based on the conclusions of this study, that nurses' interpretations are part of the socially constructed reality of the wards and interaction in the wards. Nurses need to attend to the implications of their participation in systems of work in which they and others 'excise' their interpretations from documents that form the basis for evaluation of services (cf. Campbell, 1984). A realistic quality assurance programme would take account of the social construction of the reality of psychiatric nursing.

19 This monograph can therefore be read in relation to Barker's (1989) exploration of issues related to the self of the nurse in relation to the patient, and the elision of distinctions of patient and nurse in caring interactions; and to Faugier's (1990) use of psychotherapeutic understandings in psychiatric nursing practice.

20 See Kelly and May (1982) for an argument on the need for an interactionist perspective.

21 Barkus (personal communication) has observed that present quality assurance systems do not accommodate qualitative evaluation.

22 Behaviour therapy has provided one model for nursing practice and case management (Marks, 1977; Barker, 1982). Behaviour therapy practice is undergoing radical changes with the incorporation of 'cognitive' perspectives.

23 With hindsight I have concluded that a benefit conferred by a specialist training in behaviour therapy was the practice of developing forms of accounts (stories) of practice with patients, and translating those accounts (stories) into forms of communication which other professionals recognised as accountable knowledge.

24 I have at various points in this monograph referred to the tensions and dilemmas in discourse. I located them in the nursing literature and in the discourses of nurses and patients. This monograph is also a discourse characterised by tensions. I have not been able to resolve these, and have concluded that they reflect tensions in the theoretical positions I have used, methodological tensions, and tensions in the work of psychiatric nurses with neurotic patients. In order to conclude

this monograph and suggest further work, I will summarise some of these points.

There are two tensions related to the theoretical perspectives I have adopted. Firstly, at various points I used different theoretical sources which have different if not antithetical foundations. The phenomenological perspective centres on the experience and world view of the individual person or subject. However, I also adopted at various points a Foucauldian or discourse-analysis perspective, in which the individual could be seen as constituted as a subject through discourse and practices of power (Foucault, 1979). These tensions characterise some of the theoretical sources of this study. Harré (1979, 1983) can be seen as arguing for a view of subjectivity as highly structured by the forms of subjectivity made available in a society. Smail (1984, 1987) and Mair (1987) examine some of the tensions in a view of people as beings subjected to objectifying discourses, but able to resist the privileged forms of subjectification and objectification. The 'social construction of reality' thesis (Berger and Luckmann, 1967) is based on the notion of the individual subject created through socialisation. Implicitly, socialisation in a 'disciplinary society' might yield the sort of processes of subjectification and objectification described by Foucault (1979). Indeed, Schutz and Luckmann (1974, p. 245) note that '"responsibility"' for one's own acts...is imposed on the individual by means of the other'.

Methodologically, the tensions were present in the process of 'gaining access' through the Ethical Committee, intersection of the structures of power and knowledge which control the production of research-based knowledge. The tensions were present at every phase of the research as I tried to find out what nurses and patients were doing in their talk. A merit of the methodology of this study is that it led me to share the places in which talk took place, and thus to be aware, through my own senses of subjectification and objectification, of some of the processes of power in the sites. Foucault (1979, the source of the references below except where otherwise indicated) claimed that disciplinary practices were characterised by: 'hierarchical observation, normalising judgement and...their combination in a procedure that is specific to it, the examination' (p. 170). I 'passed' through the examinations of the Ethical Committee and the structures of the sites and entered new forms of examination. The whole process of my research can be viewed from a Foucauldian perspective, in the sense that I 'examined' the nurses and patients to produce the knowledge of this monograph. In doing so I took my place in systems of observation and judgement. In speaking to patients I spoke to people who knew that their talk and action, they themselves, were being 'watched' in the sites. I often knew, having had access to other talk, how they were 'known'. In talking to nurses I examined part of their practice not normally 'seen'. My analysis in Chapter 6 can be read as an analysis of the nurses' practice of discipline through talk: anything could be observed through talk, anything could be normalised ('normal grief', 'normal marital problems', 'ongoing things'). The distinctions 'ordinary talk', 'illness/problem talk' can be seen as resting on processes of normalisation and as producing new forms of normalisation. In short, my methods of knowledge production depended on the methods in use in the sites. The analysis of moral order in Chapter 7, and more broadly the analysis of the 'work' as a form of 'therapy' can be interpreted in terms of Foucault's 'techniques for making useful individuals' (p. 211). In the context of my analysis of 'social talk' and 'illness talk' (the concern with 'the things of every moment', p. 213), and of 'the visibility and unverifiability' (p. 201) of nurses' power in 'observation' (the second order construct or the view of interaction 'screened' through the Kardex), psychiatric nursing with these patients appears as one of 'those systems of micro-power that are essentially non-egalitarian and asymmetrical that we call the disciplines' (p. 222). My analysis of the nurses' work can be read that way.

The analysis which yielded metaphors of 'person growing' (Shotter, 1984) and 'symbiotic accounting' can be analysed from the above perspective. The discourses on 'discipline' and 'person growing' both concern the production of individuals. (See also Barker, 1989.) In Foucault's terms this is accomplished through 'the technology...of individuals' (Foucault, 1979, p. 225); in Shotter's (based on Vygotsky) through 'development'. The shared ground would be some concept of the 'development of powers' including the power of the self-as-introjected-other to observe, monitor and direct one's own action. Harré's (1983) account of personal development based on exercise of the will can be read this way. The organic and technological metaphors make claims on the same territory, the individual. Particular others, especially mothers, the 'generalised other' (Mead, 1934, whose work underpins that of Shotter, 1984; Harré, 1979, 1983; and Berger and Luckmann, 1967) and the 'panopticon' (Foucault, 1979), constitute gazes that subject the individual and constitute the self, subjectivity. The creation, repair and maintenance of reality (including the person) and of subjective identity through talk are interpretable as forms of discipline; the recovery of 'strays' a form of the 'pastoral' power which Foucault (1982) saw as characteristic of contemporary society. I have noted that in coming to the sites patients came 'from one disciplinary authority to another' (p. 227-8).

In this analysis, nurses too appear as constituted. I noted that in Site One nurses came to be known as the 'kinds of people' they were. The gaze of the 'community' fell on nurses too: in Site One a nurse said that because they saw the patients or relatives outside the hospital, they (the nurses) could not pretend to be other than themselves inside. The new staff nurse moved from the discipline of a school of nursing to that of the site. A consultant reprimanded a nurse for being over-zealous in reporting that a patient had been seen consuming six drinks, by claiming that the nurse might have been drinking more. I have stressed throughout that power, while asymmetrical, was not one-way. There is potential for further research on the relationship between the nurses' practices of 'examination' of patients and the knowledge produced - knowledge of 'resistance', 'rebellion', 'hiding', 'not working'.

This monograph could be read as a legitimation of the forms of nurses' 'power/knowledge' (Foucault, 1979), their practice of the disciplines of 'observation' which constituted them as 'experts in normality' (p. 228). This critique of the monograph, that submerged in it is the basis of a Foucauldian analysis of power, is sustainable. The turn toward the power/powers analysis in Chapter 6 reified, to some extent, the practices of power. The logical conclusion to that reification can be seen in the focus on the 'metaphors of power', construed as practices; and in the notion that it might have been as valid to have interrogated the patient's resistance to power for what it might 'tell' about the patient (and what it might provide, therefore, as 'fuel' for further investigation of the nurse-patient relationship), as to have interpreted it as a product of the practices of power. The 'gaze' I trained on the discourse of earlier nursing researchers, which revealed them as objectifying the nurse and constructing a 'super-observation' of the patient (seeing 'missed opportunities') through interpretation of nurses' accounts of the interaction - all in the interests of discipline in the profession - could be turned on this monograph. Under that gaze this study may appear to have submitted the nurses to scrutiny without fully examining the processes and structures of discipline in which they participated, and as having done so in order to develop better methods of 'examination', an accounting system which would subject the nurses' subjectivities to scrutiny. In the 'inverted hierarchy' in which 'individualization is "descending"' (p. 193), the nurse could be subordinated to the enquiring gaze of the researcher or peers not only in the interest of getting at the 'reality' of psychiatric nursing (by including in the picture the nurse as a person, an individual, the person he becomes through interaction - cf. Peplau, 1952), but also in the interest of 'developing' practice. In short, the study could be seen, in this analysis, as a step toward a new form of discipline.

The force of this critique of the monograph and of the limits of its analysis indicates that the tension that has been carried throughout this text (and was carried throughout the study) is a tension in psychiatric nursing. The tension reflects the power that is exercised in nurse-patient interaction and in research by nurses on nurses. The very interdependence that I found symbolised in the metaphors can be seen as the tie that binds the seer and the seen, the knower and the known (the master in the panopticon, p. 204). Indeed, the metaphors of power can be seen as precisely that: metaphors, which collectively were a metaphor for the discipline which enforced a screening of the practices and effects of power. Thus I acknowledge the force of a deeper analysis of power. My argument is that it remains unknown whether such an analysis can be carried on in practice through the analysis and critique (in practice) of the practices of power, the forms of discipline which constitute psychiatric nursing with neurotic patients as interpreted through this monograph, and which according to this analysis are implicit in each act of definition of self and other in which nurses engage with patients. The forms of resistance currently practised by patients and nurses are part of larger struggles over identity, dependence, interdependence (Foucault, 1982). Critical theory (Habermas, 1963, 1971a, 1971b, 1976) appears a candidate for use in directing the analysis in practice. However, the argument of this monograph is that the struggle over definitions of reality and subjectivity which characterised nurse-neurotic patient interaction requires theory free from the contradiction of requiring further subjectification (of the 'neurotic') as a condition of argument about the good.

This monograph stemmed from my attempt to account to myself and to others for what I was doing in practice. That attempt led me into the practices of power which produced the knowledge of this monograph. Nurses will be called upon increasingly to account for their practices in various systems of knowledge and power. Knowledge of the issues involved in participation in systems of accountability, constituted in processes of accounting, may enable them to recognise the part they play, how they are constituted, and how they constitute themselves and others in those systems.

25 An implication of this study is that as well as considering 'locally valued discourses' we must consider locally devalued discourses; and the 'provinces' of knowledge and power maintained to devalue those discourses.

26 While the tension between the view of interaction as structured by discourse and as structured by interpretation is a tension between theoretical perspectives and cannot be resolved on the basis of this empirical study, I will suggest the implications of the tension for the conclusions of this monograph and for future psychiatric nursing research.

The tensions centred on those not resolved in Chapter 6, on 'power'. I will explore a few ideas developed there on the basis of the empirical data. I provided a basis for an argument that what was at stake in interaction was subjectivity. I followed some of Foucault's (1980, 1982) ideas to suggest that in interaction the person is subjected to the truth of her being, that is, of being as subject ('I') and object ('you'). In saying 'truth', however, I am begging the question of how that truth is established. It is a foundation of the theoretical perspective of this study that the 'truths' constituting knowledge of the other are social constructions, interpretations. What is at issue in the interaction is whose interpretation is acted on to structure further interaction. I suggested that one of the forms of power in the sites was the power to make the staff members' interpretations 'stick'. Those views were legitimated through a discourse which privileged the interpretations based on command of the concepts 'illness' or 'responsibility', 'it' or 'the kind of person'. In that way knowledge and power were interconnected. The patients in Site Two were non-privileged in that they were regarded as people who defended their views through avoidance of tests ('not wanting to look terribly deeply at that') which might confirm the view others hold of them and their 'problems'. The very acts of denial and avoidance confirmed the picture of them, their objectivity as a 'kind of person', and the privilege of the view that held them in that gaze. The patients in this study were construed (by some nurses in Site Two) as defended, as strategically maintaining self by thwarting the therapeutic efforts of nurses and others. The 'truth' of this view is pragmatic, if nothing else, in that the social processes of 'resistance' and 'rebellion' confirmed the privileged view. 'If two of you say so, it must be true' (S2P8), even when the 'truth' is one's subjectivity, one's 'privateness'.

It is here that the patient diagnosed as 'neurotic' confronts an 'ideology'. The maintenance of the collective view against that of the patient is based on numerous small acts of power, in gaze and in talk, founded on an interpretation of her as a kind of person blind to herself. As I noted, this 'ideology' was never fully realised, and varied and competing strategies based on different views were sustained. The 'ideologies' were drawn on to render action accountable.

The power of others in sustaining a collective view can also be interpreted from the interpretive, story-telling perspective. If others share a story about one and act in relation to it, it becomes reality insofar as one lives in the world structured in part by the story others tell about one (Scheff, 1966; Smith, 1978; Erikson, 1968; Mair, 1987). The nurses' view, based on common sense, was dilemmatic and plurivocal, and may have offered the patient more stories, more views of self than a monologic, theoretical text might have done. What was sacrificed, the 'truth', the monologic, privileged view, may have been compensated for by the variety of interpretations. While this study makes no claim to being an outcome study, I am arguing a *prima facie* case for the possible good of the nurses' conflicting, 'haphazard' (see Chapter 2) views.

The problem patients faced was 'being here'. They entered a place governed by an assumption that there must be a 'reason' for their having 'come to the door' (see Appendix 11 for an account by a student nurse about a patient said by a trained nurse to have been 'unwilling to move' from an 'entrenched position', frustrating the nurses so that they had to 'withdraw').

In 'being here', in the institution, the politics of self and of the larger society were linked. The link was through the ideologies and practices of power in institutions sustained for management of 'illness' and 'problems', including 'personal states' dealt with in the public places of psychiatric admission wards (cf. Goffman, 1967). In these institutions the definition of the person was accomplished and sustained, negotiated, disputed, accommodated. The view of the person sustained by others through the 'programme', the view sustained through the gaze of the 'generalised other' became, in time, the view of self (S2P4) or it was negated (S1P7). This was the process of re-socialisation, of 'therapy' (Berger and Luckmann, 1967). As I have emphasised throughout, this analysis does not account for the diversity of approaches, interactions, alliances, strategies that were worked out 'below' the ideology, at the level of 'I think it's loneliness'. The nurses in their interaction with patients were less monological than plurivocal, less a single gaze, more a set of glances and further looks.

The politics of self appeared, in the microcosm of discourse, in the politics of the speaking self, the 'I' who spoke and the 'I' who was spoken (Lacan, cited in Selden, 1985). In speech, in day to day life, the politics of self (being objectified by others and by self) were played out, the definition of self and world played out in the mundane conversations of daily life ('not the drugs, you', 'another reason', 'I was bad'). Viewed from this perspective, accounts were political acts, acts of power in systems of power. They were bids to relieve self of the responsibility imposed by others or self on the one the others took self to be. They were claims for relief from the forms of objectification imposed by others on oneself, and hence challenges to the other's view of the world, the other's 'reality'. Accounts were the points where 'the world' was rendered versions of the world to be agreed, negotiated, fought out. Viewed from this perspective, the nurses were engaged in political acts, not only in interpreting the other and acting towards her - 'it's loneliness' - but in playing a part in the wider society in which the hermeneutic tasks of mediating 'loneliness' and 'depression', and of distributing 'company', were negotiated in admission wards of psychiatric hospitals. Versions of 'why she is here (I am here) now' and 'what we have to do for her (I have to do)' were negotiated. Accounts relieved self of responsibility 'outside', but at a cost -

participation in the 'discipline' of the sites ('the programme', 'deep work').

One of the tensions of this monograph can be located in the emphasis on the role of metaphors in the systems of power in the site. Metaphors were ways of discovering or recognising one's being in the common story or view. They were ways of getting the common view inside one, so that one was inside the common view, as a child, a business partner, and so on. These metaphors highlight that what was at stake in the practices of power in the sites was being, mediated by discourse. One implication of these comments is that nurses' education should focus not on 'social skills', but on what underlies the practice of social skills, the ways in which we live in discourse and talk, and are constituted as and constitute ourselves as who we are, under the gaze of others and self. We need a realistic, that is, symbolic, interpretation of nursing practice.

27 The nurses and patients could be construed as practical sociologists of knowledge. In Chapter 5 I indicated their knowledge of knowledge and its social distribution and ordering. They practised common-sense ways of sustaining the articulation between the macroprocess of the site and the microprocesses of interaction: keeping the programme going, trying really hard, doing so much for yourself, sustaining the definition of the hospital. The standard nurses' phrase when things were hectic was 'it's no (Note: Scots 'not') real'. It is important to indicate some of the implications for personhood of adopting the theoretical perspective and methods used in this study. One effect of adopting a phenomenological perspective may be to render the paramount reality problematic (cf. Bennett and Feldman, 1981). Insofar as my analysis is apt, psychiatric nurses in their ordinary practice worked to sustain 'my (Note: their, especially the charge nurse's) reality'. I have argued that they maintained and may have needed to maintain their definition of the world, in order to order other realities which may have threatened the legitimacy of the world of common sense (Berger and Luckmann, 1967). While potentially problematic, the phenomenological perspective could illuminate the role of common sense in nursing, and illuminate the nature of disturbances in reality and the processes of reality maintenance and repair needed to counter them.

28 See Giddens (1976) on the problem of intersubjectivity in the phenomenological tradition. This may be compared to Harré's (1983) description of Schutz' solution to the problem of intersubjectivity - the assumption of intersubjectivity, the assumption that the other is a 'man like myself' - as 'heroic'.

Bibliography

Adler M and Asquith S (1981) Discretion and power, in Adler and Asquith (eds.) *Discretion and welfare*, Heinemann, London.

Allport G (1942) *Use of personal documents in psychological science*, Social Science Research Council, New York.

Allen H (1981) Voices of concern: a study of verbal communication about patients in a psychiatric day unit, *Journal of Advanced Nursing*, *6*, pp. 355-362.

Altschul A (1972) *Patient-nurse interaction*, Churchill Livingstone, Edinburgh.

Altschul A (1978) A systems approach to the nursing process, *Journal of Advanced Nursing*, *3*, (4), pp. 333-340.

Altschul A (1980) Hints on maintaining patient-nurse interaction, *Nursing Times*, *76*, (15), pp. 650-652.

Altschul A (1984a) Do good practices need good principles?, part 1, *Nursing Times*, *80*, (28), pp. 36-38.

Altschul A (1984b) Does good practice need good principles?, part 2, *Nursing Times*, *80*, (29), pp. 49-51.

Ammon-Gaberson KB and Piantanida M (1988) Generating results from qualitative data, *Image: Journal of Nursing Scholarship*, *20*, (3), pp. 159-161.

Arens K (1989) *Structures of knowing: psychologies of the nineteenth century*, Kluwer Academic, Boston.

Argyle M Furnham D and Graham J (1981) *Social situations*, Cambridge University Press, London.

Askham J (1982) Telling stories, *Sociological review*, *30*, (4), pp. 555-573.

Asquith S (1977) Relevance and lay participation in juvenile justice, *British Journal of Law and Society*, *4*, (1), pp. 61-76.

Atkinson P (1977) The reproduction of medical knowledge, in Dingwall R (ed.) *Health care and health knowledge*, pp. 85-106, Croom Helm, London.

Bakhtin M (1984) *Problems of Dostoevsky's Poetics*, Manchester University Press, Manchester.

Bales R (1951) *Interaction process analysis*, Addison-Wesley Press, Inc, Cambridge, Massachusetts.

Banton R Clifford P Frosh S Lousada J and Rosenthall J (1985) *The politics of mental health*, MacMillan, Houndmills.

Barker P (1982) *Behaviour therapy nursing*, Croom Helm, London.

Barker P (1989) Reflections on the philosophy of caring in mental health, *International Journal of Nursing Studies*, *26*, (2), pp. 131-141.

Baruch G (1981) Moral tales: parents' stories of encounters with the health professions, *Sociology of Health and Illness*, *3*, (3), pp. 275-295.

Becker H (1958) Problems of inference and proof in participant observation, *American Sociological Review*, *23*, (6), pp. 652-660.

Becker H (1967) Whose side are we on?, in Douglas J (ed.) (1970) *The relevance of sociology*, pp 99-111, Appleton-Century-Croft, New York.

Becker HS and Geer B (1957) Participant observation and interviewing: a comparison, *Human Organization*, *16*, (3), pp. 28-32.

Belknap I (1956) *Human problems of a state mental hospital*, McGraw Hill, New York.

Benner P (1984) *From novice to expert: excellence and power in clinical nursing practice*, Addison-Wesley, Menlo Park.

Benner P (1985) Quality of life: a phenomenological perspective on explanation, prediction, and understanding in nursing science, *Advances in Nursing Science*, *8*, (1), pp. 1-14.

Benner P and Wrubel J (1989) *The primacy of caring*, Addison-Wesley, Menlo Park.

Bennett WL and Feldman MS (1981) *Reconstructing reality in the courtroom*, Tavistock, London.

Berger P and Luckmann T (1967) *The social construction of reality*, Pelican, Harmondsworth.

Bernstein RJ (1976) *The restructuring of social and political theory*, Methuen, London.

Billig M Condor C Edwards D Gane M Middleton D and Radley A (1988) *Ideological Dilemmas*, Sage, London.

Bloor M and Fonkert JD (1982) Reality construction, reality exploration and treatment in two therapeutic communities, *Sociology of Health and Illness*, *4*, (2), pp. 125-140.

Bloor M and McIntosh J (1987) Power, surveillance and client resistance: a comparison of the techniques of surveillance used in therapeutic communities and health visiting, paper presented at the B.S.A. Med. Soc. Group (Scotland) conference, Glasgow, 31-10-87.

Blumer H (1969) *Symbolic interactionism: perspective and method*, Prentice Hall, New Jersey.

Bott E (1976) Hospital and society, *British Journal of Medical Psychology*, *49*, pp 97-140.

Brown J and Sime J (1981) A methodology for accounts, in Brenner M (ed.) *Social methods and social life*, pp. 159-188, Academic Press, London.

Brown J and Canter D (1985) The use of explanation in the research interview, in Brenner M (ed.) *The research interview: uses and approaches*, Academic Press, London.

Bunch EH (1982) Balancing the mandates and conducting business as usual: the organization of work and communicating with schizophrenics on a psychiatric ward, unpublished DNS thesis, University of California, San Francisco.

Bunch EH (1985) Therapeutic communication: is it possible for psychiatric nurses to engage in this on an acute psychiatric ward?, in Altschul A (ed.) (1985), *Psychiatric Nursing*, pp. 43-62, Churchill Livingstone, Edinburgh.

Burgess R (1984) *In the field: introduction to field research*, George Allen and Unwin, London.

Burke K (1969a) *A grammar of motives*, University of California Press, Berkeley.

Burke K (1969b) *A rhetoric of rhetoric*, University of California Press, Berkeley.

Burton F (1978) *The politics of legitimacy: struggles in a Belfast community*, Routledge and Kegan Paul, London.

Campbell M (1984) Information systems and management of hospital nursing: a study in social organisation of knowledge, unpublished PhD thesis, University of Toronto.

Canter D Brown J and Groat L (1985) A multiple sorting procedure for studying conceptual systems, in Brenner M (ed.) *The research interview: uses and approaches*, pp. 79-114, Academic Press Ltd, London.

Carr P (1980) To describe the role of the nurse working in a district general hospital psychiatric unit, unpublished PhD thesis, University of Manchester.

Carter (1959) The critical incident technique in identification of the patient's perception of therapeutic patient-patient interaction on a psychiatric ward, *Nursing Research, 8,* (4), pp. 207-211.

Caudill WA Redlich F Gilmore HR Broom EB (1952) Social structure and interaction process in a psychiatric ward, *American Journal of Ortho Psychiatry, 22,* pp. 314-334.

Chapman G (1987) Text, talk and discourse: nurses' use of language in a therapeutic community, unpublished PhD thesis, University of London.

Chapman G (1988a) Reporting therapeutic discourse in a therapeutic community, *Journal of Advanced Nursing, 13,* (2), pp. 255-264.

Chapman G (1988b) Text, talk and discourse in a therapeutic community, *International Journal of Therapeutic Communities, 9,* (2), pp. 75-89.

Cicourel A (1964) *Method and Measurement in Sociology,* Free Press of Glencoe, London.

Cicourel A (1976) *The social organisation of juvenile justice,* Heinemann Educational, London.

Clark C with Asquith S (1985) *Social work and social philosophy: a guide for practice,* Routledge and Kegan Paul, London.

Clark E (1988) Nursing research in professional development, module 1 of *Research awareness,* Distance Learning Centre, South Bank Polytechnic, London.

Clarke M (1986) Action and reflection: practice and theory in nursing, *Journal of Advanced Nursing, 11,* (1), pp. 3-11.

Clinton M (1985) Training psychiatric nurses: why theory into practice won't go, in Altschul A (ed.) *Psychiatric Nursing,* pp. 132-149, Churchill Livingstone, Edinburgh.

The Committee on Psychiatric Nursing of the Group for the Advancement of Psychiatry (1955) Therapeutic use of the self: a concept for teaching patient care, in *Group for the Advancement of Psychiatry Reports vols. I and II,* report no 35, pp. 1-12.

Conant LH (1965) Use of Bales' interaction process analysis to study nurse-patient interaction, *Nursing Research, 14,* (4), pp. 304-309.

Cormack D (1976) *Psychiatric nursing observed,* Royal College of Nursing, London.

Cormack D (1983) *Psychiatric nursing described,* Churchill Livingstone, Edinburgh.

Darbyshire P (1990) High-flown theory, *Nursing Times, 86,* (2), pp. 54-56.

Davis BD (1984) What is the nurse's perception of the patient?, in Skevington S (ed.) *Understanding nurses,* pp. 67-80, John Wiley and sons, Chichester.

Denzin NK (1970) *The research act in sociology,* London, Butterworth.

Denzin NK (1978, 2nd edition) *The research act,* McGraw-Hill, London.

Denzin NK (1989) *Interpretive interactionism,* Sage, London.

Dickoff J James P and Wiedenbach E (1968) Theory in a practice discipline, *Nursing Research, 17,* (5), pp. 415-435.

Diers D (1979) *Research in nursing practice,* JB Lippincott, Philadelphia.

Diers D and Leonard RC (1966) Interaction analysis in nursing research, *Nursing Research, 15,* (3), pp. 225-228.

Dingwall, R (1977) *The social organisation of health visitor training,* Croom Helm, London.

Douglas JD (1971) *American social order,* The Free Press, New York.

Dreyfus H (1983) Why current studies of human capacities can never be scientific, *Berkeley Cognitive Science Report No. 11,* Cognitive Science Programme, Institute of Cognitive Studies, University of California and Berkeley.

Dreyfus HL and Dreyfus SE (1986) *Mind over machine,* The Free Press, New York.

Dreyfus H and Rabinow P (1986) *Michel Foucault: beyond structuralism and hermeneutics,* Harvester, Brighton.

Eco U (1979) *A theory of semiotics,* Midland, Milan.

Emerson RW (1982, originally published in 1841) Circles, in Emerson RW *Selected essays,* edited and with an introduction by Ziff L, pp. 225-238, Penguin, Harmondsworth.

Erikson KT (1968) Patient role and social uncertainty, in Rubington E and Weinberg MS (eds.) (1973) *Deviance: the interactionist perspective,* MacMillan and Co, New York.

Faugier J (1990) Revealing hidden fears, Nursing Times, *86,* (11), pp. 66-68.

Faulkner A (1979) Monitoring nurse-patient conversation in a ward, *Nursing Times, 75* , (35): occasional paper 23, pp. 95-96.

Fay B (1975) *Social theory and political practice,* George Allen and Unwin, London.

Fielding P (1982) An investigation of student nurses' attitudes toward old people in hospital, unpublished PhD thesis, University of Southampton.

Flanagan JC (1954) The critical incident technique, *Psychological Bulletin, 51,* (4), pp. 327-358.

Foucault M (1971) *Madness and civilization,* translated by Howard R, Tavistock, London.

Foucault M (1979) *Discipline and punish: the birth of the prison,* Peregrine, Harmondsworth.

Foucault M (1980) *Power/knowledge,* Harvester, Worcester.

Foucault M (1982) The subject and power, afterword in Dreyfus HL and Rabinow P *Michel Foucault: beyond structuralism and hermeneutics,* Harvester, Brighton.

Freidson E (1970) *Profession of medicine,* Harper and Row, New York.

Garfinkel H (1967) *Studies in ethnomethodology,* Prentice-Hall, Englewood Cliffs, New Jersey.

Garfinkel H (1968) The origins of the term "ethnomethodology", (excerpts) in Turner R (ed.) (1974) *Ethnomethodology,* pp. 15-18, Penguin, London.

Giddens A (1976) *New rules of sociological method,* Hutchinson and Co Ltd, London.

Giorgi A (1975) An application of phenomenological method in psychology, in Giorgi A Fischer C and Murray E (eds.) *Duquesne Studies in Phenomenological Psychology vol 2,* pp. 82-103, Duquesne University Press, Pittsburgh.

Glaser BG and Strauss A (1965) *Awareness of dying,* Aldine, Chicago.

Glaser B and Strauss A (1967) *The discovery of grounded theory,* Aldine, Chicago.

Goffman E (1962) *Asylums: essays on the social situation of mental patients and other inmates,* Aldine, Chicago.

Goffman E (1963) *Behaviour in public places: notes on the social organization of gatherings,* Free Press of Glencoe, New York.

Goffman E (1967) *Interaction ritual,* Penguin, Harmondsworth.

Goffman E (1969) *The presentation of self in everyday life,* Penguin, Harmondsworth.

Goffman E (1972) *Relations in public,* Penguin, London.

Goffman E (1974) *Frame analysis: an essay on the organization of experience,* Harper and Row, New York.

Gold RL (1958) Roles in sociological field observations, *Social Forces, 36,* (3), pp. 217-223.

Gray-Snelgrove RH (1982) The experience of giving care to a patient dying of cancer: meanings identified through the process of shared reflection, unpublished PhD thesis, University of Toronto.

Grypdonk M (1987) The introduction of the nursing process in a home health agency, paper presented at the International Nursing Research Congress, University of Edinburgh, July 29-30, 1987.

Habermas J (1963) Theory and practice in a scientific civilization, in Connerton P (ed.) (1976) *Critical sociology: selected readings*, Penguin, Harmondsworth.

Habermas J (1970) Systematically distorted communication, in Connerton P (ed.) (1976) *Critical sociology: selected readings*, Penguin, Harmondsworth.

Habermas J (1971a) Technology and science as 'ideology', in Habermas J (ed.) *Toward a rational society*, pp. 81-122, Heinemann Educational, London.

Habermas J (1971b) The scientization of politics and public opinion, in Habermas J (ed.) *Toward a rational society*, pp. 62-80, Heinemann Educational, London.

Habermas J (1976) *Legitimation Crisis*, Heinemann Educational, London.

Hagell EJ (1989) Nursing knowledge: women's knowledge. A sociological perspective, *Journal of Advanced Nursing, 14*, (3) pp. 226-233.

Hammersley M and Atkinson P (1983) *Ethnography: principles in practice*, Tavistock, London.

Hargreaves W and Runyon N (1969) Patterns of psychiatric nursing: role differences in nurse-patient interaction, *Nursing Research, 18*, (4), pp. 300-307.

Harper D (1987) *Working knowledge*, University of Chicago Press, Chicago.

Harré R (1970) *The principles of scientific thinking*, MacMillan, London.

Harré R (1978) Accounts, actions and meanings: the practice of participatory psychology, in Brenner N, Marsh P and Brenner M (eds.) *Social contexts of method*, Croom Helm, London.

Harré R (1979) *Social being*, Basil Blackwell, Oxford.

Harré R (1981) Expressive aspects of descriptions of others, in Antacki C (ed.) *The psychology of ordinary explanations of social behaviour*, pp. 139-156, London, Academic Press.

Harré R (1982) Ethogenic methods: an empirical psychology of action, in Breakwell GM Foot H and Gilmour R (eds.) (1985) *Social psychology: a practical manual,* The British Psychological Society and MacMillan Press Ltd, London.

Harré R (1983) *Personal Being,* Basil Blackwell, Oxford.

Harré R and Secord PF (1972) *The explanation of social behaviour,* Basil Blackwell, Oxford.

Harré R, Clark D and DeCarlo N (1985) *Motives and mechanisms,* Methuen, London.

Hays JS and Larson KH (1963) *Interacting with patients,* MacMillan, New York.

Henderson V (1966) *The nature of nursing: a definition and its implications for practice,* MacMillan, New York.

Heyman B and Shaw M (1984) Looking at relationships in nursing, in Skevington S (ed.) *Understanding Nurses,* pp 29-47, John Wiley and Sons Ltd, Chichester.

Hobson RF (1985) *Forms of feeling: the heart of psychotherapy,* Tavistock Publications, London.

Hochschild AR (1983) *The managed heart: commercialization of human feeling,* University of California Press, Berkeley.

Hughes D (1980) Lay assessment of clinical seriousness, unpublished PhD thesis, University of Swansea.

Hughes D (1988a) When nurse knows best: some aspects of nurse/doctor interaction in a casualty department, *Sociology of Health and Illness, 10,* (1), pp. 1-22.

Hughes D (1988b) Paper and people: the work of the casualty reception clerk, paper presented at the BSA Medical Sociology Group Conference, York, 16-18 September, 1988.

Hughes E (1951) Studying the nurse's work, in Hughes E (ed.) (1971) *The sociological eye,* Aldine, Chicago.

Hughes E (1962) Good people and dirty work, reprinted in Hughes E (ed.) (1971) *The sociological eye,* Aldine, Chicago.

Hunt JC (1989) *Psychoanalytic aspects of fieldwork,* Sage, London.

Inoue S (1980) Interaction and interpretation in everyday life, in Denzin NK *Studies in symbolic interactionism, vol 3,* pp. 1-24, JAI Press, Greenwich, Connecticut.

Jeffery R (1979) Normal rubbish: deviant patients in casualty departments, *Sociology of Health and Illness, 1,* (1), pp. 90-107.

John AC (1961) *A study of the psychiatric nurse,* Livingstone, Edinburgh.

Joint Committee of the Manchester Regional Hospital Board and the University of Manchester (1955) *The work of the mental nurse*, Manchester University Press, Manchester.

Kaplan A (1964) *The conduct of inquiry: a methodology for behavioural science*, Chandler Publishing, San Francisco.

Kappeli S (1987) A matter of definition, *Nursing Times*, *83*, (44), pp. 67-69.

Kasch CR (1986) Toward a theory of nursing action: skills and competency in nurse-patient interaction, *Nursing Research*, *35*, (4), pp. 226-230.

Kelly M and May D (1982) Good and bad patients: a review of the literature and a theoretical critique, *Journal of Advanced Nursing*, *7*, (2), pp. 147-156.

Kendell RE (1975) *The role of diagnosis in psychiatry*, Blackwell Scientific Publications, Oxford.

Kennison BJ (1983) Nurses and patients: the clinical reality of sickness vols. I and II, unpublished PhD thesis, University of Michigan.

Kreckel M (1982) Communicative acts and extralinguistic knowledge, in Von Cranach M and Harré R (eds.) *The analysis of action*, Cambridge University Press, Cambridge.

Kuhn TS (1970) *The structure of scientific revolutions*, University of Chicago Press, Chicago.

Kvale S (1983) The qualitative research interview: a phenomenological and a hermeneutical mode of understanding, *Journal of phenomenological psychology*, *4*, (2), pp. 171-196.

Labov W and Fanshel D (1977) *Therapeutic discourse: psychotherapy as conversation*, Academic Press, London.

Lemert E (1962) Paranoia and the politics of exclusion, in Rubington and Weinberg (1987) *Deviance: the interactionist perspective*, MacMillan, New York.

Llewelyn S (1985) The experience of patients and therapists in psychological therapy, unpublished PhD thesis, University of Sheffield.

Lofland J and Lofland LH (1984) *Analyzing social settings: a guide to qualitative observation and analysis*, Wadsworth, Belmont, California.

Lyman and Scott (1970) *A sociology of the absurd*, Appleton-Century-Croft, New York.

McCarthy T (1976) Translator's introduction, in Habermas J *Legitimation Crisis*, pp. vii-xxiv, Heinemann Educational, London.

McHugh P (1968) *Defining the situation*, Bobbs-Merrill, Indianapolis.
MacIlwaine H (1980) The nursing of female neurotic patients in psychiatric units of general hospitals, unpublished PhD thesis, University of Manchester.
MacIlwaine H (1981) How nurses and neurotic patients view each other in general hospital psychiatric units, *Nursing Times, 77*, (27), pp. 1158-1160.
MacIlwaine H (1983) The communication patterns of female neurotic patients with nursing staff in psychiatric units of general hospitals, in Wilson-Barnett J (ed.) (1983) *Nursing research: ten studies of patient care*, John Wiley and Sons, Chichester.
MacLeod MLP (1990) Experience in everyday nursing practice: a study of 'experienced' surgical ward sisters, unpublished PhD dissertation, University of Edinburgh.
MacLeod Clark J (1981) Communication in nursing, *Nursing Times, 77*, (1), pp. 12-18.
MacLeod Clark J (1982) Nurse-patient verbal interaction: an analysis of recorded conversations in selected surgical wards, unpublished PhD thesis, Chelsea College, University of London.
Mair M (1987) Kelly, Bannister and a story telling psychology, paper presented at the 7th International Congress on Personal Construct Psychology, Rhodes College, Memphis, Tennessee, U.S.A., August 1987.
Mair M (1989) *Between Psychology and Psychotherapy*, Routledge, London.
Manaser JC and Werner AM (1964) *Instruments for study of nurse-patient interaction*, MacMillan, New York.
Marks IM (1977) *Nursing in behavioural psychotherapy*, RCN, London.
Marks I (1981) *Cure and care of neuroses*, John Wiley and Sons, Chichester.
Marks IM (1985) *Psychiatric nurse therapists in primary care: the expansion of advanced clinical roles in nursing*, Royal College of Nursing, London.
Marsh P Rosser E and Harré R (1978) *The rules of disorder*, Routledge and Kegan Paul, London.
May D and Kelly MP (1982) Chancers, pests and poor wee souls: problems of legitimation in psychiatric nursing, *Sociology of Health and Illness*, 4, (3), pp. 279-301.
Mead GH (1934) *Mind, self and society*, edited and with an introduction by Morris CW, University of Chicago Press, Chicago.

Meichenbaum D (1977) *Cognitive behaviour modification: an integrative perspective*, Plenum, New York.
Melia K (1981) Student nurses' accounts of their work and training: a qualitative analysis, unpublished PhD thesis University of Edinburgh.
Melville H (1963, originally published 1851) *Moby Dick*, Dent, London
Menzies I (1970) *The functioning of social systems as a defense against anxiety*, Tavistock Pamphlet No 3, London.
Nightingale F (1924) *Notes on nursing*, Harrison and Sons, Ltd., London.
Nisbett RE and Wilson TD (1977) Telling more than we can know: verbal reports on mental processes, *Psychological Review*, *84*, (3), pp. 231-259.
Ogden CK and Richards IA (1949) *The meaning of meaning*, Harcourt and Brace, London.
Parsons T (1951) *The social system*, Routledge and Kegan Paul, London.
Paykel ES Mangen SP Griffith JH and Burns TP (1982) Community psychiatric nursing for neurotic patients: a controlled trial, *British Journal of Psychiatry*, *140*, pp. 573-581.
Paykel and Griffith (1983) *Community psychiatric nursing for neurotic patients*, Royal College of Nursing, London.
Peplau (1952) *Interpersonal relations in nursing*, GP Putnam's Sons, New York.
Peplau (1960) Talking with patients, *American Journal of Nursing*, *60*, pp. 964-966.
Peplau (1978) Psychiatric nursing: role of nurses and psychiatric nurses, *International Journal of Nursing Review*, *25*, (2), pp. 41-47.
Peplau H (1988) The art and science of nursing: similarities, differences and relations, *Nursing Science Quarterly*, *1*, (1), pp. 8-15.
Poe EA (1967, originally published 1841) Descent into the maelstrom, in Poe EA (ed. Graham K) *Selected Tales*, Oxford University Press, Oxford.
Polanyi (1967) *The tacit dimension*, Routledge and Kegan Paul, London.
Pollock L (1989) *Community psychiatric nursing: myth and reality*, Scutari, Harrow.
Pollock L and Tilley S (1988) Submitting for approval, *Senior Nurse*, *8*, (5), pp. 24-25.

Potter and Mulkay (1985) Scientists' interview talk: interviews as a technique for revealing participants' interpretative practices, in Brenner M Brown J and Canter D (eds.) *The research interview: uses and approaches*, Academic Press, New York.

Potter J and Wetherell M (1987) *Discourse and social psychology*, Sage, London.

Raffel S (1979) *Matters of fact*, Routledge and Kegan Paul, London.

Render HW (1947) *Nurse-patient relationships in psychiatry*, McGraw-Hill, New York.

Reynolds W and Cormack D (1982) Clinical teaching: an evaluation of a problem oriented approach to psychiatric nurse education, *Journal of Advanced Nursing*, *7*, (3), pp. 231-237.

Ricoeur, P (1971) The model of the text: meaningful action considered as a text, reprinted in Rabinow P and Sullivan M (1979) *Interpretive social science*, pp. 73-101, University of California Press, Berkeley.

Roberts H (1985) *The patient patients: women and their doctors*, Pandora Press, London.

Robinson K (1985) Knowledge and its relationship to health visiting, in Luker K and Orr J (eds.) *Health visiting*, Blackwell Scientific Publications, Oxford.

Rock (1979) *The making of symbolic interactionism*, MacMillan, London.

Rubington and Weinberg (1987) *Deviance: the interactionist perspective*, MacMillan, New York.

Ruffing-Rahal MA (1986) Personal documents and nursing theory development, *Advances in Nursing Science*, *8*, (3), pp. 50-57.

Sackmann S (1989) The role of metaphors in organization transformation, *Human Relations*, 42, (6), pp. 463-485.

Sacks H (1984) On doing 'being ordinary', in Atkinson JM and Heritage J (eds.) *Structures of social action*, Cambridge University Press, Cambridge.

Schatzman L and Strauss AL (1973) *Field research*, Prentice Allen, Englewood Cliffs, New Jersey.

Scheff T (1966) *Being mentally ill*, Aldine, Chicago.

Schuetz A (1943) The problem of rationality in the social world, *Economica*, *10*, pp. 130-149.

Schutz A (1944) The stranger: an essay in social psychology, *American Journal of Sociology*, *49*, (6), pp. 499-507.

Schutz (1968) On multiple realities, in Gordon C and Gergen K (eds.) *The self in social interaction*, pp. 61-70, John Wiley and Sons, New York.

Schutz A and Luckmann T (1974) *Structures of the life-world*, Heinemann, London.

Scottish Health Service Planning Council (1988) *Scottish Health Authorities review of priorities for the eighties and nineties*, HMSA, Edinburgh.

Scull A (1982) *Museums of madness: the social organization of insanity in nineteenth century England*, Penguin, Harmondsworth.

Secretaries of State (1989) *Caring for people: community care in the next decade and beyond*, HMSO, London.

Selden R (1985) *A reader's guide to contemporary literary theory*, The Harvester Press, Brighton.

Shanley E (1988) 'Inherently helpful' people wanted, *Nursing Times, 20*, (84), pp. 34-35.

Shotter J (1984) *Social accountability and selfhood*, Basil Blackwell, Oxford.

Silverman D (1985) *Qualitative methodology and sociology: describing the social world*, Gower, Aldershot.

Simm JA (1978) The social organisation of psychiatric nursing: theoretical comments upon sociological and hospital research and empirical observations on the behaviour of nursing staff, unpublished PhD thesis, University of Manchester, UMIST.

Sladden S (1979) *Psychiatric nursing in the community*, Churchill Livingstone, Edinburgh.

Smail D (1984) *Illusion and reality: the meaning of anxiety*, JM Dent and Sons, London.

Smail D (1987) *Taking care: an alternative to therapy*, JM Dent and Sons, London.

Smith DE (1978) 'K is mentally ill': the anatomy of a factual account, *Sociology, 12*, pp. 23-53.

Smith G (1980) *Social need: policy, practice and research*, Routledge and Kegan Paul, London.

Smith PA (1988) Quality of nursing and the ward as a learning environment for student nurses: a multimethod approach, unpublished PhD thesis, University of London.

Stacey M (1976) The health service consumer: a sociological misconception, in Stacey M (ed.)*The sociology of the National Health Service, Sociological Review, monograph* 22, pp. 194-200, Keele.

Stanislavski K (1980) *An actor prepares*, Methuen, London.

Stelling J and Bucher R (1973) Vocabularies of realism in professional socialization, *Social science and medicine, 7*, pp. 661-675.

Stockwell F (1972) *The unpopular patient*, RCN, London.

Strauss A (1987) *Qualitative analysis for social scientists*, Cambridge University Press, Cambridge.

Strauss A Schatzman L Bucher R Ehrlich D and Sabshin M (1964) *Psychiatric ideologies and institutions*, The Free Press of Glencoe, London

Sugden J (1980) Nursing activity and some variables in the psychiatric treatment process, unpublished MPhil thesis, University of Edinburgh.

Swaffield, L (1990) Quest for quality, *Nursing Times, 86*, (12), pp. 16-17.

Szasz T (1979) *The myth of psychotherapy: mental healing as religion, rhetoric and repression*, Oxford University Press, Oxford.

Teasdale K (1989) The concept of reassurance in nursing, *Journal of Advanced Nursing, 14*, pp. 444-450.

Thompson IE Melia KM and Boyd KM (1983) *Nursing Ethics*, Churchill Livingstone, Edinburgh.

Tilley S (1985) Multiple phobias and grief: a case study, *Behavioural Psychotherapy, 13*, pp. 59-68.

Tilley S (1990) Negotiating realities: making sense of interaction between patients diagnosed as neurotic and nurses in two psychiatric admission wards, unpublished dissertation, University of Edinburgh.

Tilley S and Weighill VE (1986) How nurse therapists assess and contribute to the management of alcohol and sedative drug use among anxious patients, *Journal of Advanced Nursing, 11*, (5), pp. 499-503.

Totman, R (1980) The incompleteness of ethogenics, *European Journal of Social Psychology, 10*, pp. 17-41.

Towell D (1975) *Understanding psychiatric nursing*, Royal College of Nursing, London.

Travelbee J (1969) *The process of psychiatric nursing*, FA Davis and Co, Philadephia.

Travelbee J (1979) *Intervention in psychiatric nursing*, FA Davis and Co, Philadelphia.

Turner BS (1987) *Medical power and social knowledge*, Sage, London.

United Kingdom Central Council for Nursing, Midwifery and Health Visiting (1984) *Code of professional conduct for the nurse, midwife and health visitor*, UKCC, London.

Vidoni C (1984) The relationship between the nursing staff's perception of the patient's behaviour and the patient's perception of his feeling state prior to the seclusion episode, unpublished DNS thesis, Catholic University of America.

Vygotsky LS (1978) *Mind in society: the development of higher psychological processes*, Harvard University Press, Cambridge, Massachusetts.

Webb C (1981) Classification and framing: a sociological analysis of task-centred nursing and the nursing process, *Journal of Advanced Nursing, 6*, (5), pp. 369-376.

Webb C (1989) Action research: philosophy, methods and personal experiences, *Journal of Advanced Nursing, 14*, (5), pp. 403-410.

Weighill VE, Tilley S and Keenan G (1986) Weight groups: reflections on working together in primary care, *Health Visitor, 59*, pp. 106-108.

Whyte WF (1960) Interviewing in field research, reprinted in Burgess RG (ed.) (1982) *Field research: a sourcebook and field manual*, pp. 111-122, George Allen and Unwin.

Wieder DL (1974) Telling the code, in Turner R *Ethnomethodology*, pp. 144-172, Penguin, Harmondsworth,.

Wilson T (1970) Conceptions of interaction and forms of sociological explanation, *American Sociological Review, 35*, (4), pp. 697-709.

Wilson-Barnett J (1988) Lend me you ear, *Nursing Times, 84*, (33), pp. 51-53.

Wooff K and Goldberg D (1988) Further observations on the practice of community care in Salford: differences between community psychiatric nurses and mental health social workers, *British Journal of Psychiatry, 153*, pp. 30-37.

Wooldridge PJ (1971) Meta-theories of nursing: a commentary on Dr. Walker's article, *Nursing Research, 20*, (6), pp. 494-495.

World Health Organisation (1978) *Mental disorders: glossary and guide to their classification in accordance with the ninth revision of the International Classification of Diseases*, World Health Organization, Geneva.

Appendix 1

Letter to patients

Dear

I am interested in finding out more about how psychiatric nurses and selected patients understand their interaction, especially their conversations with each other. To find out more about this I plan to spend time on this ward to try and become more aware of how patients and nurses interact with each other. I also plan to ask selected patients and nurses to tell me about their conversations.

I would like your help in this research. This would involve you agreeing to set time aside at your convenience to tell me about your conversations with nurses. What you tell me will be strictly confidential. That is, I will not report to any nurse what you have told me. However I would then like, with your permission, to ask the relevant nurse about the conversation. Again, what the nurse tells me will be confidential. That is, I will not report to you what the nurse tells me. My aim is to build up a picture of how both of you understand your conversation together, in the hope that the knowledge thus gained will be of help to future nurses and patients. I would like to tape record what you tell me and type your account of the conversation. After this the tapes will be erased. If you do not want a tape recorder to be used I would like to take notes on what you tell me. I would also like your permission to consult your case notes.

If this work results in material for publication. I will ensure that no participant can be identified from its content. If there were any material you specifically wanted omitted from publication I would respect this wish.

You are entirely free to agree or not to agree to take part in this research. Neither agreement nor declining will affect your treatment. If you agree to take part, please read and sign the accompanying consent form. Your agreement, if given, can be withdrawn at any time, without affecting your treatment.

Yours sincerely,

Stephen Tilley
Scottish Home and Health Department Research Training Fellow

Letter to Nurses

Dear

I am interested in finding out more about how psychiatric nurses and selected patients understand their interaction, especially their conversations with each other. To find out more about this I plan to spend time on this ward to try and become more aware of how patients and nurses interact with each other. I also plan to ask selected patients and nurses to tell me about their conversations.

I would like your help in this research. This would involve, firstly, your setting aside time at your convenience, to tell me about your conversations with selected patients. The patients will also have been asked or will be asked, about the conversations. Both what you tell me and what the patient tells me will be strictly confidential. That is, I will not repeat to the patient what you have told me, nor to you what the patient has told me. The aim of my asking both is to build up a picture of how both of you understand your conversations together. My hope is that this knowledge will be of use to future nurses in their practice. I will need to record what you have told me on tape for transcription (after which the tapes will be erased) but will ensure that no participant can be identified by name, grade, etc.

The second sort of help I would like is for you to set time aside as your work commitments permit, for interviews on aspects of your work and the ward's functioning relevant to this research. The aims of the interviews will be clarified, participation will be voluntary and confidentiality is again ensured.

The kind of research I want to do depends on your help and co-operation. If any questions arise about the research I will be happy to answer them.

If this work results in material for publication, I will ensure that no participant can be identified from its content. If there were any material you specifically wanted omitted from publication I would respect this wish.

You are entirely free to agree or not to agree to take part in this research. If you agree to take part, please read and sign the accompanying consent form. Your agreement, if given, can be withdrawn at any time.

Yours sincerely,

Stephen Tilley
Scottish Home and Health Department Research Training Fellow

Consent Form (Patients)

I understand the content of this letter outlining the aims and plan of this research and agree to participate by being interviewed about interaction, especially conversations, with nurses.

I understand that this information is confidential and that all reasonable measures will be taken by the researcher to ensure that individual participants cannot be identified.

I also agree that the researcher may read my case notes.

Signed...

Date...

Appendix 2

Example 1: Shifting the stone

Power was expressed in the metaphors in different nurses' accounts of interaction with P3. NC spoke of P3 getting worries 'out of the way'. SN said that he helped P3 'talk through' thoughts of his dead father. P3 'got it out of the way'. NA2 talked of 'getting things in the open', getting them 'aired'. Talking 'took a weight off P3's shoulders'. NA2 'latched onto' something P3 was saying and 'picked it up', 'got it out of the way'. NB said that P3 let him into his private world - it was like P3 had 'lifted a stone' and NB 'had to go in'. P3 'got it off his chest'.

The metaphors suggest that the power involved shifting a weight that lay oppressively on P3, blocking him. What was blocked was his voice, his ability to say what he felt. Talking it (the block) through with the nurses he talked through it (the block). My understanding of 'the block' and of the work involved in shifting the stone was informed by my interaction with P3. In order to tell me about the conversations with the nurses he had to tell me that he had thought of his father:

> P: I've been speaking to Julie too. She (?) been asking me how I was getting on, and I told her that I'd been all right and that, but I'd dreamt about my Dad again... And it makes you scared a wee bit...
>
> R: You've been talking with Linda about how you'd got on and the X-ray, and uh, the uh, her her plans for for Christmas.
>
> P: Aye.

R: And with Julie about the dream you'd had, and how you'd got on...

P: At home, how I'd handled it. I'd handled it quite good except for, eh, dreaming of my Dad.

R: Well thanks very much for telling me about those.

I heard and felt P3 offer an opening onto his fear and grief. My understanding of the power of the invitation and the power the nurses needed to enter P3's world were informed by my feelings in hearing P3, and my reluctance to enter the world opened by the metaphor.

Example 2: A deaf woman crying out

SNP5 told me that she saw P5 as a woman who sat alone, her hearing aid turned off, cut off, deliberately not hearing. One day when P5 wailed and shouted the nurses told her that she was disturbing the other patients. They put her in a sideroom (cut her off). SN was put in with her. SN was with P5 in the world P5 disclosed in that closed room. SN saw P5 as like a tightly coiled spring. She heard P5 say (something she said she had never been able to say before) 'My God. Please forgive me. I love my bairns.'. SN tried, without thinking - she had no time to think - to make P5 feel less guilty about breaking down. SN said that she thought back to admitting P5, to feelings she picked up from the family.

Comments

The feelings and 'vibes' the nurses picked up were potent. Picking up the vibes enabled them to act in the situation with P5 and P3. The vibes told them what to do. When they told what they picked up and did the nurses used metaphors in which they were involved and implicated with the patients: NB shifting his stone, SN cut off, feeling guilty, terribly distressed. Through use of metaphors nurses told how they saw and responded to something in which they were implicated with the patients. Their participation in the situation was a constitutive aspect of the stone shifting, the cutting off and the release.

The metaphors conveyed how nurses and patients reflexively constituted the reality of the situations of interaction and the reality of the sites. SN was shut off by the same act that shut off P5: together they defined the power of others to shut them out. NB shared a place and experience with P3, constituting the site as a place where such sharing could take place.

My understanding of the metaphors, their power, was informed by my feeling with the nurse in the room with the patient, with the nurse with the patient lifting the stone. The knowledge embedded and embodied in these metaphors was a form of power. Ricoueur (1971, p. 101) argues that:

> Understanding is entirely mediated by the whole of explanatory procedures which precede and accompany it. The counterpart of this personal appropriation is not something which can be felt, it is the dynamic meaning released by the explanation which we identified earlier with the reference of the text, that is, its power of disclosing a world.

The interpretation of metaphor is this monograph suggests that metaphors mediate understandings which convey feeling as well as having potential for 'disclosing worlds' (cf. Denzin's, 1989, 'cognitive-emotional' interpretive interactionism).

Appendix 3

Validity relates to the aims of the research and to the methods used to realise those aims. The main issue related to validity in qualitative interpretive research is whether the actor's interpretations and understandings have been presented in such a way that the reader can understand the phenomenon from the actor's point of view. Where two actors are concerned the aim is to do this in such a way that the perspective of each is recognised. The threats to validity lie in the process of data creation and in analysis. In creation of data, imposition of the researcher's perspective through leading questions, or lack of sensitivity leading to failure to enable the actor to present her understandings will limit the value of the data (Kvale, 1983). In analysis, the threats include failure to pick out themes that convey the actor's meanings, and picking out concepts that are meaningful to the researcher but do not reflect the actor's understandings.

Attempts were made to limit these threats to validity. It is accepted that my understandings were involved in the entire process of the research, and that what I brought to the research inevitably contributed to the products. However, I made efforts to ensure that avoidable biases were minimised. For example, in asking actors to tell about conversations rather than focusing on 'goals', I may have reduced the likelihood of 'set' replies. I definitely asked leading questions on occasion, but hearing the early transcripts heightened my awareness of doing so and may have kept this to a minimum. In addition, there are indications in the data that the actors were able to 'turn down' my leads, that is, to tell me when my questions or interpretations did not make sense. I was certainly also aware on listening to tapes of having not picked up what, with hindsight, seemed clear leads to further understandings. However, again, the fact that I was aware of this meant that in future interviews I worked harder to keep open to what the actor was saying. Patients and nurses knew that my aim was to understand from their point of view. In addition they knew that the other would be telling about the conversation. These two features may have reduced the likelihood both of their omitting features that were significant in conveying their interpretation and of deliberately misleading me. In analysing the data from field notes and accounts, there were threats to validity in mis-hearing and mis-transcription. I have addressed these issues in the main text. There were also threats related to selective interpretations, premature closure of analysis and obsessive over-interpretation (Ammon-Gaberson and Piantanida, 1988). Regarding the first point, it is clear that my understanding and interpretation was involved in all stages of analysis, and that, broadly, interpretation was guided by my interests in doing the study. I was aware of the possibility of premature closure at times, in particular when I followed theoretical leads (for example, when I realised the similarity of my core categories to the characteristics of interaction as outlined by Giddens, 1976). However, I responded by returning to the data and asking whether another story could be told, and to look for disconfirming evidence. The danger of 'shuffling' (Ammon-Gaberson and Piantanida, 1988) was real. I tried to remedy these tendencies with self-injunctions to 'return to the data'.

The strongest reply to the threats to validity was return to the sources of the data that formed the basis of the understanding. I have indicated that I tried as much as possible to feed back my understanding of what the actor was saying in the interview to clarify that I had 'got it'. That actors could and sometimes did contradict me meant that the 'lead' in understanding (at least sometimes) lay with them. If there were especially important points I checked out more directly that I had understood. For example, in Site One I had developed on the basis of several sorts of data an understanding that nurses in interaction with patients started from collective understandings reached in 'Kardex' meetings or handovers. In a second level account interview with a nurse I asked her directly if the way she had tackled a problem with a patient was based on the collective understanding. She claimed that part of it was, but that part of it was her own 'personal' understanding:

> R: Right, and uh, for her, and the kind of information and advice and (?) and all, perception of her that you had and so

on, did that come from a collective picture of her? You know, you..

N: Yes, that could (?). Eh, yeah.

R: You see what I mean? ..Th-, there's a, what I'm, what I'm, I'm, sort of, operating on the basis that there are, kind of collective picture of patients that people have here and share and..

N: That, that would be collective, but, eh, the way...that sort of, the suggestion that I planted was done on the spur of the moment, (?).. Right?..Eh, but, it was on the basis of collective information, although my individual, eh, plan of care sort of thing of P2 ..I decided on doing it that way, right?..Cos I, I was pretty sure she would take something from that..

This led me to look more closely at the relationship of shared and personal knowledge. The point here is a more general one. The validity of each type of data was enhanced by the fact that I was constantly relating data of various sorts and from various sources - fieldwork observations to accounts to interviews. This meant that I had the chance to 'check out' understandings at various points (cf. Denzin, 1970, on 'triangulation').

The validity of the interpretations was enhanced by feeding back to the nurses the sense I had made of the site and asking whether they could recognise themselves in the account I gave of them and their work. The response of nurses in Site Two, that they could recognise their practice, including the interpretation of 'responsibility' as a key to their work with these patients, warrants these understandings. It could be argued that they had little choice but to accept what was fed back to them, or that the interpretations were simply not relevant. However, that interpretation would be inconsistent with their readiness to 'correct' some key points, for example, regarding the relationship between gender and the kinds of work done in groups (see Chapters 5, 6. and 7). Feedback sessions in Site One with as many of the 'surviving' nurses as possible (two out of three), produced another round of interpretation, further understandings in response to the views I shared with them.

The issues of reliability are closely related to those of validity. The usual questions - whether another researcher would produce the same 'results' using the same methods and whether the study could be replicated later with the same results - are not relevant. The study was intended to interpret the actors' interpretations of the interaction they took part in producing. They were understandings of there and then. The understandings of actors changed from day to day: indeed the purpose of using the methods I used was to be sensitive to changes in interpretation and interaction based on interpretation. The actors and conditions had changed by the time I went to give feedback to Site Two. It is also likely that another researcher would have 'found' different things in the sites, interpreted them differently. There are few middle-aged American-but-trained-in-Scotland psychiatric nurses doing this sort of research (to select just a few characteristics that I was aware of as shaping my understandings). However, insofar as I was able to bring to my awareness (and actors sometimes noted) these features which shaped some of my background understandings, I used them in the research. For example, as a man asking mainly women patients about their interaction, I noted a patient's remark that her talk with nurses was 'women's talk', and tried to attend thereafter to how I read the site in terms of gender, and checked out my readings. The question of reliability of analysis of field notes and interviews is more problematic. I could have asked other researchers to analyse a portion of the data. However, since the thread that ran through all of the data was my developing understanding of the data, and since that understanding was informed by background understandings and what had 'percolated' through from various sources during the fieldwork (for example, as a result of learning all I knew about Site Two after I had been in Site One; or, as a result of sharing the sites through time with those I came to understand), it would have been impossible to ascertain the meaning of agreement or disagreement between my interpretation and that of someone who had not been involved in the same process of understanding.

One further point regarding validity and reliability should be made. I have said that I gave feedback to the Sites. However, the feedback was to an extent selective. In one Site, because most of the nursing staff had changed by the time I gave feedback, I discussed with nurses, some of whom were working in different wards, what form of feedback would be most helpful. We agreed that I would feed back to as many as possible of the nurses who had taken part in the study, rather than to the whole team currently working in the ward. This meant that some understandings which related to conditions and staff at the time of the study could not be confirmed by all staff.

Appendix 4

P: I think we (Note: the patients in a group meeting with the nurses) talked about when coming to hospital that we meet, need an awful lot more support than when we go out of hospital, and we can also help each other, one another when we're in hospital at the beginning because the people who are getting better going out they know what they've been through, with being so ill...And that's where the nurses are so understanding, so they do help you and they know how to help you, and they really do make you well. It might take a while because you've got to learn to crawl before you walk. I always say its like a swimming pool, because I mean you can't just jump into the deep end without jumping into the shallow end at first. So therefore the nurses when you come into hospital they do help you, they run round you and see what they can do and how they can help you and they show you where your bed is and, and tell you the o-, o-, occupational therapy activities you've to take in and your rota on the dishes, and when the meals are and the coffee breaks are, they're very helpful and they do give you a lot of help. But like I say, at the beginning it's most important because you don't know what you're coming into and at the same time you're not feeling well whatsoever, you're feeling really ill.

Appendix 5

P: And then, we spoke about, eh, he suggested that I should get a holiday. And I told him I can't afford it. And he was telling me that he had been away on holiday, to Skegness. But, that it was quite expensive. (Sighs 'Eh'). That was really all...(He made) good suggestions, which I had, I, I thought of myself, like, I need to, I need to get a job, and I could **do** with a holiday, but that means, eh, saving up money and I cannae do that till I get a job...But it was a good conversation...It just sort of seemed that he was i-, he seemed interested in me as a person, no just a, patient, if you see what I mean...He just seemed to be interested in, why I was there and, eh, he seemed to want to know, what kind of family I had...And, I don't know, it was just as if he wanted to understand maybe why I drank, or why I was anxious. I I, I quite like the conversations, cos, it lets you know, eh, what the nurses are like, **away** frae here...Knowing what he (?), his wife does, and knowing that he's got two girls. And that they go to Skegness. Just, things like that.

R: It may sound a stupid question, but why is that good?

P: I don't know (sighs). You can, sortae relate to them. Like, for me it would be different if, if he wasnae married, and, didnae have a family. I dinnae think I could relate to him so much, then...Where uh, I could relate, to him.

R: Because he wouldn't have..

P: The pressures o', like say, bills, or saving for a holiday, or,

R: Right, I've got you. Right...Some of the things that **you**, can understand.

P: Mnhmn.

Appendix 6

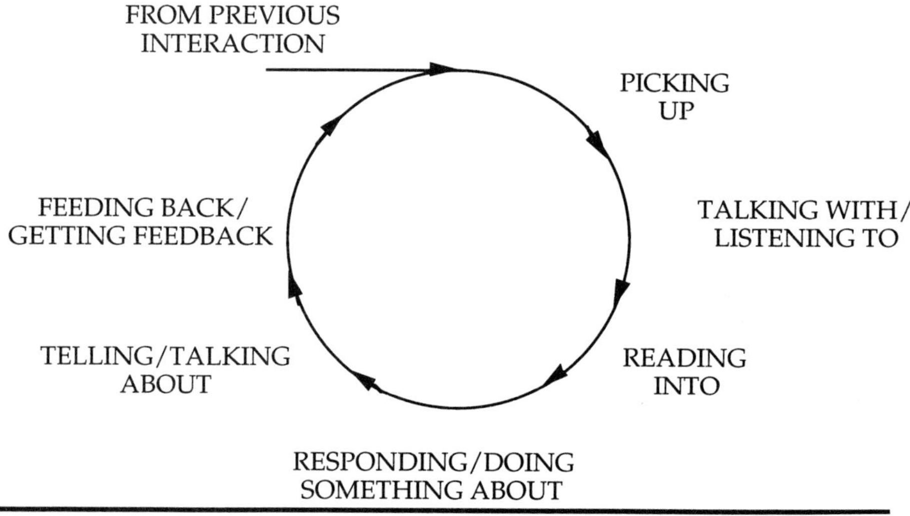
FROM PREVIOUS
INTERACTION
PICKING
UP
TALKING WITH/
LISTENING TO
READING
INTO
RESPONDING/DOING
SOMETHING ABOUT
TELLING/TALKING
ABOUT
FEEDING BACK/
GETTING FEEDBACK

Appendix 7

N: Yeah. She originally came to us **via** (...) after having, a, panic attack, uh which was in fact so, disturbing to everyone **around** her (...) which was the main reason that she came to us on an in-patient basis in the **first** place. (? As or ? Uh) she, was felt to be depressed, and having some problems coping, so, basically, drug therapy was seen as being a way of lifting her mood. It lifted, and as far as we could assess, um, the panic and problems of coping seemed to resolve, and she seemed to be much more able to **cope**.

R: Mn.

N: However (laughs), we found out that that wasn't quite correct. (...She was discharged..) However, within a day or two of going, the panic attacks seem to have become much worse. So, she again had to be, come on an in-patient basis. When she came in, the panic attacks had then dropped, so obviously, there was something out there that was a little bit **too** challenging for her.

R: Mn.

N: So we, tried to talk with her, to try and find out what this **was.** And, between ourselves and the medical staff came up with this idea that uh, **probably** it was something fairly long-standing..and, there was a lot of anxiety that she had which was put off, on these panic attacks so, so (? it was) thought to bring in the psychologist to try and handle it from there, and, basically we then saw it as being simply a management of, building up her confidence, and having, nurses available to, work with her, on her programme.

R: Mnhmn.

N: Uh as the programme ran through she, **initially** didn't seem to feel too confident about that. (? N laughs or R does) (? 'This seems) very much like black magic', you know, 'Do these things and you will feel better'. But uh, it did seem to start taking (? on) from there. And, from there on, really as I say, it's just been, a kind of supportive role we've had, since she does **not** seem to be willing to look at the, issues, which we suspect, of, a marital nature which is the **real** problem. (? Um), she's not willing to do anything exploring **that**, to any depth, therefore we're just looking to, ease her off her symptoms.

R: Those were the, the, **things** out there, that were, causing anxiety that you referred to,

N: Yeah.

R: on her first discharge, those are the, **marital**,

N: (?)

R: problems y-

N: **That**

R: you **suspect**.

N: seems to be the, the energy comes from that, and just, putting the anxiety off to things in the environment on a general not-coping basis.

R: Right, right. OK. So, in some senses, she came the first time, was helped, through medication with the depressive problems, em, was discharged, and, returned again very, **quickly** with **anxiety**, problems which, you thought were related to, underlying issues, probably,

N: Yes.

R: to do with the marriage, and, this was never, this was something that was not, s-, you know taken up by her or seen by her as, the **issues**. And um, a programme was, she was referred to the psychologist, for, what?, for help in assessing, what the i-, the issues were or, for

N: I- i-

R: (? a specific) (?)

N: initially, and then, a desensitisation programme thereafter.

R: That was based on the psychologist's assessment..

N: Yes,

R: Right.

N: working down the hierarchy.

R: Right. Um, and the nurses helped out in th-, in the carrying out of that programme, and then, as that, as she got more **comfortable** with that, played a largely supportive role.

N: (?)

R: OK. Now that's, that's uh, good information, now d-, if I ask, you know, how you think **she** sees her, **stay** or the issues are and so on, do you have, do you have a, a conception of that?

N: Um..broadly speaking I have to admit, uh, no, um, she tends not to relate to us,

R: (? Mn.)

N: except in a conversational,

R: Mnhmn.

N: thing, so I'd suspect that she sees the, doctor and now the psychologist as, the **curer** (Note: N's concept of 'curer' spoken as in inverted commas)

R: Mnhmn.

N: and ourselves very much as, **hotel services** and somebody to talk to.

R: Mnhmn, mnhmn.

N: Uh, our role in, a **lot** of people's views is is a fairly minimal one as they **perceive** it.

R: Mnhmn. Mnhmn.

N: Um, she may see us as being, **generally supportive**,

R: Mnhmn.

N: but um, probably not seeing it, from a, a planned or, calculated angle, just that we're **nice people.**

R: Right. Right. Um, so that the doctors would have helped out with the drugs in the, the first instance and the psychologist helped out with the agoraphobic symptoms,

N: Mnhmn.

R: with the nurses' assistance, in the second, admission, and that's, that's, so the nurses have been kind of **adjuncts**, to that.

N: Yes.

R: Um, OK. From, from, back again to, from **your**, point of view, the, what **has** been the nurses', **role**, throughout that then? Throughout her stay? You've described it, you know, as, as what the stay was **about**, in terms of depressive symptoms and, um, anxiety and, and agoraphobic, symptoms, what **overall** has been the nursing role, do you think, for her?

N: Uh, **i- initially** assessing.

R: Mnhmn.

N: And, then, as I say, reassurance and, generally trying to engage with her,

R: Mnhmn.

N: to, give her the opportunity to talk over these issues, which **have** been raised, but which she is **not** wanting to do any **work** on. Um, involvement also with the support group,

R: Mnhmn?

N: again, to give her opportunity to vent her feelings and think through the issues, which again, have not really been taken up.

R: Mnhmn, mnhmn.

N: Um, latterly, as I say, we've withdrawn a bit to a more broadly supportive role.

R: (? Right, OK), is that, is that a, **policy**, a **plan**, to withdraw, uh..?

N: Y-yes, uh, she's **signalled** to us she's not really wanting to engage in anything terribly **deep**, in the way of conversation, so, time for exploratory work you could say's, now no longer available, so (?that) it's just building her up, emotionally.

R: Right. OK, well that's, very helpful, good information, um, I think that covers the points that I was, that I was interested in. Um, what, what uh, that helps me do is,

Note: break in recording.

R: ..as well, you know, how how, the perception is. So, my understanding of what you were saying was, um, because of, use, you use the term 'resistance', because of the **reluctance**

N: Mn.

R: um, to, engage, with the real issues, um, on P4's part, then, tha-, the **conflicts** will still remain, there, whatever they are that, aren't being addressed. And, (? th-) that'll lead to, probably, further admissions or, you know, further **problems** which may require intervention at some point.

N: Yeah.

R: Yeah.

N: Cos, th-, there's a, (? in a), nature of, the way she seems to look at things she doesn't seem to be really challenging **much**, you know, letting **lots** of things go past,

R: Mn.

N: without really **looking** at them and saying an **opinion** on things.

R: Mn.

N: And she's obviously, **not** wanting to, too **deeply**, really at anything, even her **cure**,

R: Mn.

N: you know, if you could call it that, of being here, (?) we're, we're saying 'This will work', but, she seems to be willing just to take **that** pretty much at face value. Which I, I feel is, indicates that, indicates that she herself's not really going to be able to cope, and that these issues, that she's **not** tackling will probably cause anxiety, which will cause **other** issues,

R: Mnhmn.

N: to be **not** (sniggers) tackled.

R: Mnhmn. The, general, not

N: Yeah.

R: tackling,

N: Yeah, so

R: style..

N: she would) say, going to the **shops**, you know, 'What will I get?', you know, she'll not be able to tackle that, either.

R: Mnhmn. And that ties, seems to tie in with the, idea that you presented her, with opportunities, to confront these things,

N: Mnhmn.

R: and so on, and (? ch-), in fact, (? are you saying) in a sense, **challenged** her to do so, at, at times?

N: Yes.

R: Um, but that hasn't been taken up, there's been a, a..

N: 'E-, everything's

R: **resistance** (? to or ? and) that.

N: fine at home, it's just these, symptoms that is the problem.'

R: Right. Right. OK, so there's a, there's a, **divergence** of, views on, what's, what the real,

N: Mnhmn.

R: issues **are**, in a way, but,

N: Yes.

R: but even that divergence can't be, confronted directly, because, the uh..what is it? sidestepped? or or, the possibility that there might be another ex-, another, cause or, whatever, is just not recognised, or..?

N: For the purposes of the admission, no.

R: Right.

N: Th-, th-, those questions are not addressed.

R: Do they get **put** to her as, as possible explanations of things, or..

N: (Sighs, sounds uncomfortable) Um..

R: By, you know by the nursing staff, again, do you think or, or is it just more

N: O- o-

R: an opportunity..?

N: only on a fairly tentative basis.

R: Right.

N: Uh if, if you, put a question, over, and in the question you'd, in-built, you know, an **opener**, let u-, say (? you), 'Do you not feel that it could be, situation at **home** that might be..

R: Mn.

N: adding to, your anxiety?'

R: Mn.

N: If you get a straight 'No' from that, then obviously you can **not** move any further.

R: Right.

N: Whereas, if, 'Well, there are some things that are **problems**.',

R: Mnhmn.

N: and (chuckles) then you say 'Well, what **kind** of problems?',

R: Right.

N: then you can move in from there, but, as long as 'Everything, at home is **fine**, there is nothing wrong' (Note: these latter two in quotations too?),

R: Right.

N: then obviously, she's not willing to look **at** that.

R: Right, right. So, it's a matter of, offering, **openings**, which, if they're closed down, **can't** be followed up, um, and, nothing gets, nothing gets done..

N: Mnhmn.

R: Right.

N: (?We) may get rid of her symptoms, the things at home **may** continue on, but, she **might** not develop any psychiatric-type symptoms,

R: Mnhmn.

N: she might just (laughs) end up with a broken marriage, which, a lot of people, encounter

R: (? Mnhmn.)

N: without actually engaging in, contact with the psychiatric services.

Appendix 8

The right attitude was based on the problem as defined. An example of how attitude changed with response by the patient was found in Site Two. A nurse described how the view of P10 changed during her admission:

> N: Well. When she came in, initially the presentation seemed to be, that of an alcohol withdrawal, in a lady who, also suffered panic attacks. Uh, that was, the first, picture. Um, as her time with us enlarged a bit, it appeared that, uh, she did not feel the alcohol problem was such a a major thing, but the panic attacks, which was the main reason for her taking the medication...Um, she, had apparently, had, once her notes appeared on the ward, it became obvious that she'd tried medication, psychology, medical support, and (? it) didn't seem to work for her. So, we were tending to speak with her to try and explore things a bit to find the basis (? of) these panics. And what came up was the fact that, uh, she felt that they (? were), been with her that long that she couldn't really give them up. That is was very much part of her life style. And, that if she didn't have them, she would feel (laughs) insecure.
>
> R: If she didn't have a panic? So they were a part of her.
>
> N: ..She, didn't **seem** to wish to make the, contact between the fact that she had abused alcohol, and, previously she had a-, abused, minor tranquillisers that she'd been on (? to help her to) relax, and she'd, done that to, **control**, the panic attacks. So we (laughs) tried to tie that together, but she didn't really make the connection.

R: (?). How did, h-, how did it come out, um, that, that was part of her but she couldn't (? actually) pick it up, did that come from, did the nurses..?

N: Yeah. In speaking with her, she was quite definite (? in) that point, that uh, it **was** a problem. But, similarly, she couldn't see that she could give it up, because it **was** part of her life - (? the panic attacks). We were kind of pushing at, how you, how you could, help her handle (? them)...

R: Was that in one to one nurse, interaction with her, or, (?) involved with her, or..?

N: Uh, one to one. Uh, she had mentioned it to myself, (?) with one or two other of the nursing staff, so (?), thought was uh, well, (laughs) 'Are we going to **go** anywhere with her?' So, from there on we were, really just, offering support and reassurance, until, we could come up with a definite (? What are we doing?). And, that was, a referral to the AA, uh, sorry, the alcohol problems clinic, initially, and, they came up and saw her and she did not **see** herself as having an alcohol problem, which was how she was (?), so they therefore stepped back, since obviously, if there's no alcohol problem, she (?). However, her, her main problem was anxiety. However, in her interactions with, **our** medical staff, and nursing staff thereafter, the anxiety was not the problem, it was the drink. So, as such, we weren't really, being **pushed** to, offer her, treatment for, the panic attacks. She's had some generalised literature, uh, the psychologist had a chat with her, but apparently her problem was alcohol, **not**, anxiety. So, she'd effectively **stopped** us, from treating her. And, yesterday, absented herself from the ward. She does seem to be coping a lot better, because she actually managed to tell everyone, except the nurses, about her going...

R: She's now, I think you've included what I was, (?), how did, how, how do you think **she** saw her problem. It sounds as if you think she saw (? it), um, to do with, anxiety, and, alcohol and sedatives in the past (?) to (?) that's the major problem, (?). Is that right?

N: Yes..Um, she, does seem to have domestic problems. And the husband and the children, the relationship with them, do seem to get on top of her, (? at times). But, she didn't see them as being any particularly big thing, it was the other way round,

> the fact that she wasn't doing so well meant that she couldn't cope with them. So, in some ways, we were, we were offering her a holiday, so that she could get away from the pressures of home.

The nurse's account tells of a complex history of interaction interpretable as repeated attempts on the part of the staff to understand what the 'main thing' with the patient was, in order to respond with treatment; repeated attempts to work, when the patient wanted a holiday. (Note: This was the patient advised by a student nurse (See Chapter 5 and Appendix 5) that she needed a holiday.) The nurses were balked, from this point of view, by the patient's changes of story and the incompatibility of her view of her problems with theirs. The nurse's account legitimated 'just supporting', given that they were not being 'pushed' to offer other help. The account illustrates the context of interaction. The nurses worked in moral orders, in which different specialist services negotiated the terms of help with each other and with the patients. The nurse summarised the medical view, as seen by the nurses:

> N: The medical staff, saw her as being somebody that had problems coping and used and abused alcohol. And, because of her not linking in with the Alcohol Service and not really, suggesting (? psychology's) would be much good, medical staff tended not to get in that (? definitely), and to launch a plan in fact for her, it was very much 'Well, let's see if the Alcohol Service'll take her, let's see if the psychologist'll take her'. But uh there, there wasn't that much active, medical attention. The biggest bit was, after the, previous ward round where, decided that she would, **not** use the professional services, terrifically well, therefore, it would be a better idea to get her linked in with, a similar function but with a more social organisation, (? such as) voluntary. And the trick was to work out if it was an anxiety management group, or, the drinking problems to go for...

Appendix 9

N: Um, I've seen quite a lot of P5 during the shift, but she hasn't said much, at all.

R: Right, OK, so can you tell me the con-, whatever conversation you had with her, there, just before you (?) came in?

N: Yes, um, well she, first of all she broke down and she was sobbing uncontrollably so she was taken in the clinic, and, um, in between the c-, the sobs and the cries, she kept repeating, um, 'My bairns, I love my bairns' and, um, 'I've never been able to cry before'..and 'God, please forgive me'. And that was basically all that was said, but she kept repeating this again and again.. and these were obviously the thoughts that were in her head.

R: Mnhmn, mnhmn.Wh-, what were y-, what were you saying during this time, do you remember at all? You know, (?) what you were saying?

N: I was trying, I was saying, uh, 'Yes I realise that you love your children'..Um, and 'It's good that you do have a good old cry'..Um..maybe try and make her feel less guilty about being hysterical and about breaking down. And, I kept telling her that the doctor would be coming soon, to give her the medication she needed...to make it better for her. Um..

R: So you were actually trying to, um, make her feel less guilty about being out of control (?)

N: Yeah..

R: (?) crying (?)

N: Uhuh. I tried to reinforce the belief that it's good to cry, and that you should do it more often.

R: Mnhmn, mnhmn, right. OK. Was that, were those thoughts in your mind when you were doing it?

N: Yes, it was, it was purely instinctive. I didn't really have much time to think about what I should be saying. I just said, whatever, I thought was (?)

R: Right, OK. That's, that's interesting, (?), it's difficult to, to kind of look back and say 'Well, what was I thinking at the time', but.. were those thoughts like a a she's I mean, can you, can you recollect sort of what was going through your mind, when you (?)

N: Uh..Yes, since she's come into the ward she's been very, very silent..she's never really communicated with anybody... And of course, she has a hearing problem..so she purposely shuts herself off by taking out the hearing aid, so that she can't listen to other conversations and so she doesn't feel (?) to join in.

R: Uhuh.

N: And, it was this that was in my mind, that she's been keeping all this (?wound?) up inside of her..and then now, it's just all coming out, all at once, a, as a, some kind of a, release.

R: Mn. Mn. And that was actually in your mind..

N: That's what was going through my mind, yeah, that this is a very, tormented woman who's been bottling up all this emotion..for days, weeks, months, who knows? (Note: N very animated) And now, finally, it's all coming out, so I kept thinking that, it was, even though it was very distressing for her, it's probably, very good for her, very beneficial.

R: OK. Anything else you can recall about (?)

N: Um..I, I kept thinking about, when her daughter came in with her, and her daughter has a lot of anger towards her mother, because she's, I think she's lost patience with her and P5 is very aware of this, and feels guilty about the, anger that she's caused, her daughter. And it's just (? and clears throat), just a lot of inner torment that she's gone through.

(Note: portions of tape not transcribed)

N: While I was sitting there with her..all these things came back to my mind.

R: Right. Well that's very helpful information, to me. Anything else you'd like to add, (?)?

N: Mn, just that it was very distressing for me.

R: For you, (?).

N: Very, yeah.. At a time like that you don't, really have the opportunity to think back, Oh, what did they tell me in College, how to react to this kind of situation..You don't really have time, you just have to follow your instincts at a time like that and say whatever, feels right to say.

R: Right, right. Aye. That, distress, are you, do you take it away with you, I mean will you take it away with you? Is it (?)

N: I'll try not to, but it'll be something that I'll always remember, I think.

Appendix 10

1. Site One Sorts

A trained nurse

1. male and female
2. psychotic, neurotic and others
3. alcoholic, anorexic/personality disorders, organic, mood disturbances, schizophrenia
4. where from - which team will look after on discharge
5. over 65, would be housed elsewhere if there were another ward
6. not acute, should be housed elsewhere
7. religion
8. could be sent home if there were industrial action tomorrow
9. smokers
10. been here before or not, whether they know the ward culture, for example it's not on to smash windows here
11. where they will go on discharge

A trained nurse

1. ill or not ill and have problems (social)
2. name
3. who they talk to
4. isolate themselves
5. need reassurance, take up time
6. have family support
7. activities/sport

A trained nurse

1. psychotic v. organic v. dependent
2. problems with families
3. housing/social problems
4. need special observation or attention

A trained nurse

1. acute/still ill/for rehabilitation/very ill/ready to go out the door
2. diagnosis

A student nurse

1. dependency levels
2. learned behaviour
3. patients helped by ward environment or not
4. dependency on staff or on institution
5. dependency outside or only in
6. ones there's hope for or not

2. Site Two Sorts

A trained nurse

1. male/female for sleeping arrangements
2. disturbance of function
3. cope outside
4. will need us again
5. dependency needs here - 'hotel' function
6. safe on the street or would cause concern
7. need a secure eye on them/most nursing care/physical needs/able to talk and to work with
8. rewarding/give job satisfaction/cute but unrewarding/like a string with lots of knots

A trained nurse

1. know what I'm doing with them
2. depressive/affective
3. satisfaction nursing them or not

4. psychotic/not
5. age
6. dependence on system v. won't see again
7. family support
8. happy here or not
9. close observations or not
10. I get on well with relatives or not

A trained nurse

1. nursing input required
2. diagnosis
3. time I spent personally thinking about them
4. time spent talking to them
5. priority in medication (hangover from secure unit days)
6. medical input
7. knowledge the patient and their situation/time spent on them in report

A student/learner nurse

1. male and female
2. know them well
3. ones we've helped and ones who are the same
4. ones I like or don't
5. I understand their illness or not
6. how they relate to each other

A student/learner nurse

1. dementia/situational/acutely disturbed
2. acutely ill/quite ill/getting well/ not ill/ no improvement
3. share feelings with other patients or not
4. observation level

Appendix 11

N: Em, I was just wondering how P8 had got on when she went home for the weekend, em, because she seems fine in here, but, obviously she's in for a reason, and I thought it was loneliness was the main, thing..

R: Mnhmn.

N: And I said, 'It must be terrible, going to an empty house, em, after being used to the company', and she was saying Yes, she enjoyed the company here. Even though she didna speak all the time, it was just nice that there was somebody there that she could speak to if she felt like it. That going home and, having to go out and try and make contact with people just for conversation. So what I gather, she had only spoken to a neighbour. Cos her bread was blue mouldy. And she had to take **that** in....Uh, she was saying that she might get a bit, mixed up, and I said 'Oh but we all do' because P8 and I went to the, Safeways once, and we didna ken that we had to unload, the messages onto the conveyor belt, and the, the lassie was a wee bit annoyed with us. And I says, '**I** get mixed up at times, too'. But you've just to **accept** that (Note: last sentence maybe 'spoken' to P8)

...

R: Yeah! Eh, and when she came back, did you talk about anything, in particular?

N: I don't think we were speaking on anything, about anything in particular. It was mainly about her weekend, that I was, anxious to see how she'd got on herself.

...

R: Right. So, you know, sh- she seems fine in here, but you thought that You know, there's got to be a reason for her **being** in here, and, you thought it was loneliness.

N: Mnhmn.

R: Is that a, um, a kind of, collective view that that's one of the problems she faces, is that something that you've discussed with her before, or that the nurses have, you know, noted as being a problem for her, do you think?

N: Yes,

R: Is it something that came out of that conversation?

N: I- it's been discussed.

R: Aye.

N: Em, I think it come out of her conversation, because, she's in here they say it's bereavement, em, but her husband died (...), and when I tried to speak to her about it, she says that all the friends had rallied round initially, and she had loads of company, and then, as is always the case, they sort of trail off, think that she's doing well.

R: Mn. Mn.

N: And, maybe it's just hit her now.

R: Right. And uh, so you were, asking about the weekend and how she'd gone home **to** an empty house, she said, she'd thought of coming back almost, and, all her experiences there. Um, and then about, what happens **after**,.. um, and the possibility of voluntary, work. So looking ahead toward things that might help, her,

N: When she goes out.

R: with the loneliness, when she goes out.

N: Because observing her in here, she's keen to do things, she'll, **very** anxious to come along and make the toast, make the tea, she's anxious to fill her time, creatively, purposefully, that's the word. Eh, that I, that's why I thought the (voluntary organisation).

R: Right. Right. So that was you, sort of, em, based

N: Looking at what she was,

R: on your, observations,

N: aye,

R: and, and knowledge of her.

N: what she was doing in here. And eh, she said how much she had enjoyed the Coffee Club, so I thought Well, this is a way of showing her that she can be a **help** to the community. (? If) she's experienced, volunteers helping her, she might be able to help somebody else.

R: Right.

N: And she's a sensible woman.

R: Right.

N: And this is her first, time in a psychiatric hospital.

Appendix 12

N:..morning I think. Em, yeah. She'd come back from pass that day and I was just telling her about what had been decided at the case conference on the Monday...Like, Ruth Boal (social worker) was going to go in and see her with Dr. X. Em, the home, the health visitor was going to visit her. Sean, her son would go to the nursery on the Tuesday, and they would get a home help on the Monday and Wednesday and she would go to the Centre on three days a week and that she was to start at the Centre the following day, that was the, that would be the Tuesday it would have been the Wednesday she was to start and I was just telling her how to get there, get there eh...Just information, really, and eh well she also felt that she told me how her weekend had gone and she felt that the drugs had a lot to do with it and I let her know that the drugs really didn't have much to do with how she had been at home, eh, it was mainly up to her, a lot of it was up to her. And she says well you know, 'Do you think that's, you know, do you not think it is the drugs?', I said 'No, I think I think a lot's something to do with you and you've got to try maybe to get on with Phil', cos I think they were having some difficulties with their relationship...Em..(now ?) she agreed with that, that they had a bit difficulty because he, he would tell her what to do at home, he'd been used to being at home hisself, you see, for so long, eh, that he had different ways of doing it and P2 was a bit sort of huffed at him telling, telling her what to do...and, felt that they didn't really have enough time at home together, so I was just sort of reinforcing that you know she she had to sort of, do a bit of work with her relationship with Phil and try and got on a bit better. And that when she did go out she would have a lot of support...

Appendix 13

N: I've **tried** to bring up about her husband twice or thrice, because we think this is what it is. And eh, she just said 'Oh, well, that was a long time ago, and I had a lot of friends after he died', but she says 'Some of them havenae come near me since'. And I says 'Well, this is the time that you **need** them'. That you get a lot of folk initially, when you're bereaved, but I says 'Later on you still need them, and they don't seem to realise it'. I said 'Maybe you should go out more'.

N: And I said to her that I knew how **I** felt, if somebody was coming it was a lot of extra work. That you did clean the hoose and you baked and, you prepared for them, where it was better if somebody came unexpectedly, eh, and then they had just to take you as they found you. You know, with all this, work. And I says 'And it would be nice for **you** to go to somebody else for a change, instead of **you** having, all the work'. So she had actually went out at the weekend as well.

..

R: Right. It sounds like, you were, uh, tying in, her worries about, you know, catering for other people, you know, having them in and all, with her anxiety, with her, her, getting uptight about having to do that and all. Suggesting a way around that. Is that right? Is that the the (?)..?

N: Yes, I think so, because I think this is half her problem, for years she's had nine people for lunch on a Saturday. And **she** wants, the staff to say 'Don't have them'. She wants the easy way out, for somebody to say to her, 'Don't have them', so that she can go to her son and say, 'I've not to have you'.

R: Mn. Mnhmn?

N: Em, but we cannae turn around and say that to her, it's her decision whether she has them or not. I said it might be better if it wasnae, as organised, or if she went to them instead.

R: Right. Is that something, that, the staff, together, work out, or is that something that you're, you know, that that that's something you're just **aware** of, as a, as..?

N: That's just me, I think (laughs).

R: Right, right.

N: Whether it's right or no. I'm only putting myself in her **place**, because (Note: mentions own circumstances that meant she could identify with P8's problems). And I **know**, it can be a strain, though you love your family, if they're coming **every** week, and you've to prepare a meal every week, I I, I **appreciate** it must be a strain.

...

N: Well I just hope that I'm saying and doing the right things, because I don't seem to have any guidance, eh, **from** the staff.

R: Mnhmn?

N: There don't seem to be meetings and they say 'Right, we'll have to, to tell P6 to do this, and we'll have to tell P8 to do that', but I'm just really using my own experience. And maybe that's why I relate better to...(Note: mentions characteristics of self and situation she shares with some patients).

R: Ah, right, right. OK. That's, that's interesting, um, that, you know, there aren't, sort of, places where, you know, people work out a strategy, you know, the staff work out a strategy and say 'This is what we'll do'.

N: No.

R: So you're left to, each person, as far as you know, if left to their own,

N: That's what **I** feel,

R: devices.

N: we're left to our own devi-, devices, and I've spoke to the staff about it and they said that we're just really here to **listen**. But I feel just listening to people's problems, you've got to **suggest** something. You cannae tell her what to do, but if you can empathise a wee bit, and s- say, 'Oh, I know how you feel, but, it's much easier if you you make the effort to go out to them, and then you don't have all this work'.... Cos I really feel it's just, I've just drawn from my own experience...

R: Right. So your experience actually matches, in some ways, a lot of the people's, in here, a lot of the patients in **some** respects.

N: Uhuh...I don't say I'm in the same situation, but I feel that, I can put myself in **their** situation, because, (? of) similar problems, or, similar things cropping up.

Appendix 14

N: Eh, it was just, today, I was talking to P8 and and P6, actually, and eh, they were talking about you and,

R: (Laughs)

N: wondering what they would say to you today.

...

N: Well, I said to P8, I says, 'Tell (Note: researcher) that I've been pestering you about five times to go for tomatoes for me'. 'Oh no, I'll no do **that**.'

R: (Laughs). Right.

N: Eh, I says, 'But I **have** been pestering you', I says, 'I cannae get oot, the day', I says, 'and I need tomatoes to go hame, so I've asked (laughs) you about three times', eh, 'No, I'll no tell him that'. Where I was trying to get her to tell you, the things, **tae**, that, maybe I was doing wrong (laughs).

R: Yes. No. That's right, I understand what you're saying. Yeah, yeah.

N: Eh, eh, 'No, no, you might get into bother for asking a patient to go for messages for you.'

R: Right. Right. That's, that's good information, I'm glad you mentioned that, cos that fits in..

N: But I asked P8 especially, because she likes something to do. And I felt, she'll no go out to the shops **herself**. But if she thinks she's doing me a favour, she might go oot and, (? not be so bored).

R: yes. Yes, uhuh. Aye. OK.

N: So if she says onything, you could say, uh, that I..

Appendix 15

R: OK well, this is to have a chance for me to ask you again about any conversations you've had with the nurses today, or or yesterday evening..

P: None at all.

R: None at all..

P: Very little.

R: Very little.

P: Very little.

R: Aye.

P: Just taking the medicine.

R: Just at the medicine time.

P: Mnhmn.

R: Aye.

P: They give out the green medicine.

R: Uhuh, aye.

P: That's all.

R: Aye. Any other times at all, even short conversations with them, or is it just..?

P: No.

R: No.

P: (?) I'm old of course.

R: You're old.

P: Aye.

R: Do, do you think that's connected with..?

P: Awww, seventy-seven year old.

R: Ah, uhuh. What, how do you think that's connected with not speaking to the nurses?

P: Well, they don't speak to me...They don't eh...Oh there was one this morning, n-, nursing officer.

R: Uhuh.

P: I'm sure, I think that's what he was, very nice too, very nice. He was speaking, talking about my own condition of course....

(Note: there follows an extensive account of this conversation.)